ELECTROPHYSICAL AGENTS IN PHYSIOTHERAPY

ELECTROPHYSICAL AGENTS IN PHYSIOTHERAPY

THERAPEUTIC & DIAGNOSTIC USE

SECOND EDITION

Hilary Wadsworth

A.P.P. Chanmugam

Science Press

Preface

Views on the treatment of disease and disability by physical agents such as electricity, light, heat and sound energy have changed a great deal in recent years. Although change is inevitable and desirable, it becomes necessary to review the situation to ensure that change was not due to fashion, but to scientific evidence. Vast strides have been made in the last twenty years in pathophysiology, photometry, biomedical engineering and computer sciences for clinical application and surgery. In comparison to these strides physical therapy using physical agents has not developed sufficiently. Why? We have been given a wealth of knowledge on the physics and physiological effects of these agents. We have been presented with streamlined machinery by manufacturers. Yet development is minimal.

Perhaps the answer lies in following suggestions — antibiotics, analgesics, vitamins and corticosteroids have replaced some use of physical agents. There is also a lack of sufficient evidence concerning the therapeutic effects of the physical agents, nor have extensive scientific trials been undertaken in this sphere. With the advent of the electron microscope and other scientific instruments new knowledge has been gained in relation to the biophysical and biochemical changes in the body. This knowledge has not been related to the use of physical agents in physiotherapy. Another factor contributing to the lack of development is that physical agent prescriptions have been too empirical. Insufficient inquiry has been made into the rationale for prescription. Should it be microwave, short wave or other modalities? Or perhaps a combination of modalities? What definite rationale governs the choice of agents? Yet another reason is that treatment by physical agents is a time-consuming, frequent, protracted method using skilled personnel who are often in short supply.

The book is designed to be used, in conjunction with *Electricity, Fields and Waves in Therapy* by Alex Ward, Science Press, to help all personnel prescribing and administering physiotherapy treatment. This book will assist therapists to judicially select, within the limits of available scientific evidence, the modalities of physical agents available, bearing in mind that the all-important goal is the speedy rehabilitation of the patient, minimising disability and pain. In our experience there is insufficient literature describing suitable techniques of application of modalities, with scientific assessment of effectiveness. We have collected as much data as possible from trials and research in the last five years, and have collated it into suggestions for rational treatments. We have stressed the detailed technique of application of each modality, as well as suggested rational selection of modalities for patient treatment.

It is to be hoped that therapists will conduct further trials of their techniques in the future so that some of the assumptions we have made can be confirmed, or disproved. Until then, we hope that this book will help to make physiotherapy treatment using electrophysical and other agents as logical as possible within the limitations of our current understanding.

Hilary Wadsworth
A.P.P. Chanmugam

Acknowledgements

The authors wish to thank the many people who have given their assistance, support and encouragement during the preparation of this book. In particular, the assistance of Mrs Esme Stephens and other members of the staff of the School of Physiotherapy, Cumberland College of Health Sciences, has been invaluable, as has the secretarial and editorial assistance provided by Mrs Mary Conning.

In addition, the assistance of Mr Giovanni De Domenico in the preparation of the second edition has been inestimable. The comments and criticisms received concerning the first edition have also been most useful, and it is to be hoped that we have been successful in overcoming some of the inadequacies which existed.

Illustrations, taken from 'Basic Guidelines for Interferential Therapy', G. De Domenico (1981), have been included with permission of the author and of the publisher, Theramed Books. Sincere thanks are also extended to Mr Jim Reid of Theramed Australia for his generous assistance in the preparation of additional illustrations for this edition.

Contents

1 Heat and the Skin

Some Key Points in this Unit

Heat is a form of energy. Heat is transferred from a body of higher temperature to a body or environment at a lower temperature.

The quantity of heat needed to raise the temperature of 1 gram of water by 1° C, say 14.5° to 15.5° C, is 4.2 joules (1 calorie).

The heat capacity (C) of a body is the ratio of the quantity of heat (Q) supplied to a body to its corresponding temperature rise (T).

$$C = \frac{Q}{T}$$

The heat capacity of a body is numerically equal to the quantity of heat needed to raise its temperature by one degree Celsius.

Specific heat capacity of a material is the quantity of heat in joules that must be supplied to one gram of material to raise its temperature by one degree Celsius. The units are J/g/°C.

Temperature is measured on the Celsius temperature scale, formerly called centigrade.

Electromagnetic waves are forms of energy. They consist of a transverse electric field together with a transverse magnetic field, and were first described by James Maxwell in 1861. Light waves, radio waves, microwaves and X-rays are all electromagnetic waves with different frequencies but the same velocity. The velocity of electromagnetic waves is denoted by c and its value is 3×10^8 m.s.$^{-1}$.

Photon and Quanta. According to Planck in 1900, energy is emitted in discrete packets of quanta. The quantum of electromagnetic radiation is the photon. The energy of a photon is calculated from the frequency of the wave.

$$E = hv$$

where E = energy of photon; v = frequency; h is Planck's constant, which has the value of 6.63×10^{-34} J.Hz^{-1}.

Hyperaemia is an increased content of blood in a part with distention of blood vessels. It may be *active* from the active dilatation of blood vessels, or it may be *passive* hyperaemia from hindered drainage when veins and lympatics are occluded, or in congestive heart failure.

Vasodilatation is the increase of the lumen of blood vessels, that is, the blood vessels are dilated.

Denaturation is the alteration of the characteristics of an organic substance, especially a protein, by chemical or physical action.

1.1   Some Ideas on Heat and the Electromagnetic Spectrum

Every living organism produces heat. The heat is either lost to the environment or stored in the body. In man's natural environment the predominant form of radiation is thermal, and it is with this radiation that we are most familiar. The reason is partly that our senses are adapted to receive this form of radiant energy, thereby giving us the sensations of sight, warmth, cold, and pain, and partly that the atmosphere around us is suited to transmit thermal radiation.

Heat is continually produced in the body as a by-product of metabolism. It is lost from the body by radiation, conduction and evaporation. In respect to heat transfer between man and his environment, the sun is by far the most important source of radiant heat, and radiation from our skin to the environment is an important source of cooling. As much as 70% of body heat production may be lost by radiation exchange with the cold surfaces in our environment.

An understanding of the kinds of electromagnetic radiation that produce heat, the physics of heat, and a knowledge of the structure of the skin are essential to enable the physician and the therapist to produce maximum benefit from the use of therapeutic heat. Knowledge of the physiological responses of the body to heat and the effects of thermal radiations on any pathophysiological states of the body help in the use of heat in the treatment of patients.

Heat is a form of energy. Thermal energy can be thought of as vibrations of the molecules of the substance. This motion of the molecules and their electrons causes the emission of electromagnetic waves. Waves are emitted in discrete packets called photons. Both the average energy of the photons and their rate of emission increase as the temperature of the source is increased. Photons of a particular energy have a characteristic wavelength or frequency. Absorption of photons by a body leads to an increase in its heat energy.

Some derived SI units

QUANTITY	UNIT	SYMBOL	DEFINITION
frequency	hertz	Hz	One cycle per second
force	newton	N	The force which when applied to a mass of 1 kg causes an acceleration of 1 metre per second per second in the direction of the force
pressure	pascal	Pa	The pressure which arises when a force of 1 N is applied uniformly over an area of 1 m^2
work, energy	joule	J	The work done, or energy expended, when a force of 1 newton moves through a distance of 1 metre
temperature	degree Celsius	°C	$t(°C) = T(K) - 273.15$
electric potential	volt	V	The potential difference between two points on a conductor carrying a current of 1 ampere when the power dissipated between the points is 1 watt

THE ELECTROMAGNETIC SPECTRUM

Vibrations at a nuclear and electronic level give rise to photons of a wide range of frequencies. The electromagnetic spectrum is an array of the various electromagnetic waves in order of length or frequency.

One wavelength is the horizontal distance between the crests of any two adjacent waves. Electromagnetic wavelengths are measured in nanometres (nm). One nanometre equals one thousand millionth of a metre, 10^{-9} m. One *cycle* is the complete sequence of events that takes place during the passage of one wave. *Frequency* is the number of cycles which pass a point in unit time.

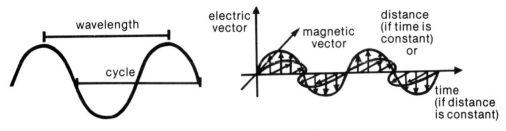

an electromagnetic wave

Electromagnetic waves travel in straight lines at the velocity of about 300 000 000 metres per second. The velocity is the same for all electromagnetic waves, so the frequency varies inversely with the wavelength.

$$c = \lambda v$$

where c = velocity of light (metres per second)
λ = wavelength (nanometres)
v = frequency (cycles per second, Hz)

Medical applications of electromagnetic waves

REGION	DATE, DISCOVERER, AND SOURCE	WAVELENGTH	FREQUENCY	MEDICAL USE
X-ray (including gamma)	1895 Roentgen bombardment of metals with electrons 1898 M. and Mme. Curie radioactive nuclei	10^{-15} m to 10^{-9} m	10^{23} Hz to 10^{17} Hz	diagnosis (TB, cancer) and therapy
ultraviolet	1801 Ritter electron transitions in atoms	10^{-9} m to 4×10^{-7} m	10^{17} Hz to 10^{15} Hz	sterilisation of equipment; surface lesions (180 to 390 nm)
visible	1702 Newton as for UV	390 nm to 700 nm	10^{15} Hz to 10^{14} Hz	diagnosis
infrared	1839 Herschel vibrations of atoms and molecules	700 nm to 15 000 nm	10^{14} Hz to 10^{12} Hz	superficial heating of tissues
microwaves	1885 Hertz motion of electrons in an oscillating circuit	1 mm to about 10 m	10^{11} Hz to 10^{7} Hz	deep heating of tissues (2450 MHz)

Wavelength in Metres

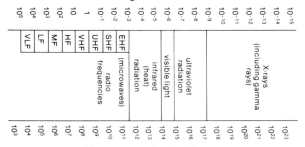

Frequency in Hertz

The electromagnetic spectrum

1.2   Structure of the Skin

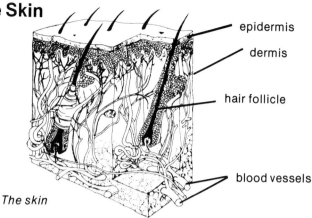

epidermis

dermis

hair follicle

blood vessels

The skin

The skin is one of the largest organs of the body. It comprises about 16% of our body mass. The skin covers the body and protects the deep tissues. Its free surface is not smooth, but is marked by delicate grooves, or flexure lines, which create patterns that vary from region to region. They are deeper on non-hairy regions such as the elbows, knees, palms, and soles. The complicated surface patterns on the fingers have such marked variations that they are a dependable way to identify an individual.

The skin is composed of two main layers, the surface epithelium, the *epidermis*, and the subjacent connective tissue layer, the corium or *dermis*. Beneath the dermis is a looser connective tissue, the superficial fascia or *hypodermis* which in many places is largely transformed into subcutaneous adipose tissue. The hypodermis is loosely connected to underlying deep fascia, aponeurosis, or periosteum. The skin is continuous, with several mucous membranes at mucocutaneous junctions. Such junctions are found at the lips, nares, eyelids, vulva, prepuce, and anus.

THE EPIDERMIS

The epidermis is non-vascular and consists of stratified squamous epithelium composed of cells of two distinct lineages. The epidermis varies from 0.07 to 0.12 mm in thickness over most of the body, except on the palms and the soles where it reaches a thickness of from 0.8 to 1.4 mm. This is present from birth.

There are two systems of cells in the epidermis:

(*a*)   the malpighian or keratinising system which comprises the bulk of the epidermis, and is a derivative of the ectoderm covering the embryo;

(*b*)   the pigmentary system of the skin, which consists of the deeper layers of the epidermis that do not keratinise, but are capable of forming melanin. These arise from the embryonic neural crest.

The *superficial keratinised portion* of the skin consists of (*a*) stratum corneum; (*b*) stratum lucidum; and (*c*) stratum granulosum. The *stratum corneum*, or horny layer, consists of several layers of flat horny cells, lacking a nucleus, and with protoplasm replaced by keratin. Keratin is the most insoluble protein of the body, and it gives the upper layers of skin a horny appearance. These lifeless cells are closely packed with no attachment and are constantly being shed.

The *stratum lucidum*, or clear layer, is formed of layers of flattened, closely compacted, eosinophylic cells, in which traces of flattened nuclei and refractile droplets of eleidin in the cytoplasm may be seen. Lucidum is seldom seen in the thinner epidermis of the general body surface.

The *stratum granulosum*, or granular layer, consists of three to five layers of flattened cells containing numerous granules that stain readily. These are kerato-hyalin granules. The origin and chemical nature of these granules are yet to be determined, but they are associated with the formation of keratin.

The superficial keratinised cells of the skin are continuously being exfoliated from the surface and being replaced by cells that arise from mitotic activity in the basal layer of the epidermis. The cells produced there are displaced to higher levels by the birth of new cells below. As they move up, they produce keratin, which gradually replaces the metabolically active cytoplasm. The cell dies, the nuclei and other organelles disappear, and it is shed as a lifeless residue of a cell. The whole process of cytomorphosis takes 15 to 30 days, depending on the site on the body, and a number of other factors.

The germinative system. The deep part of the superficial epidermis consists of the *stratum malpighi* which is subdivided again into (*a*) stratum basale, the germinative layer; and (*b*) stratum spinosum, the prickly cell layer.

The *stratum basale*, or germinative layer, consists of a layer of columnar cells with oblong nuclei. The cells are placed perpendiculary on a basement membrane. These cells are adjacent to the dermis. The cells of the malpighian layer are rich in free polyribosomes and have granular endoplasmic reticulum. The mitochondria are sparse and the Golgi apparatus negligible. In the basal layers are also present bundles of tonofibrils (cytoplasmic fibrils).

In between the tonofibrils are dense materials corresponding to kerato-hyalin granules. Also found in the basal layer or in the underlying connective tissue of the dermis are specialised cells with many branching plasmic dendrites called melanoblasts. Although melanin granules are found in the malpighian cells, they are formed only in the melanoblasts, for these cells alone possess the enzyme tyrosinase which is necessary for the synthesis of the pigment.

The *stratum spinosum* is composed of several layers of polyhedral cells, which are joined to one another by well-developed plaques called desmosomes. From these desmosomes the tonofibrils radiate into the cytoplasm of the cell. The processes give the cells their prickly appearance. In the upper layers of the stratum spinosum are numerous spherical granules. The exact nature of these granules is not known, but they may secrete a substance which makes the cell membrane thicker.

Pigmentation of the skin. The color of the skin is due to three factors:
(*a*) Tissue has an inherent yellowish color due to carotene (in the stratum corneum, fat of the corium, and the subcutaneous tissue).
(*b*) The oxyhaemoglobin imparts a reddish hue.
(*c*) Shades from brown to black are due to the pigments melanin and melanoid present in varying quantities.

Throughout the malpighian layers, particularly in the deep layers, elaborately branched cells, called dendrite cells or the Langerhorn cells, are present, which, following irradiation of the epidermis with ultraviolet rays, exhibit an uptake of active tyrosinase and further activation results in the production of melanin. They are also capable of DNA synthesis.

Melanin is formed as a product of specialised cells called melanocytes, which are found mainly in the dermo-epidermal junction. The melanocytes, with their pigment-containing processes, extend upwards for long distances among the interstices of the malpighian cells. They are not attached to the other cells by desmosomes. The melanocytes in the cheek and forehead and in the genital, nasal, and oral epithelium are about twice as numerous as in the rest of the body. The number of melanocytes is the same in all races. Differences in color are due to the amount of pigment produced.

Melanin is formed on a specific particle, the melanosome. It is an elongated body with rounded ends, about 0.6 μm long, with a fibrillar internal structure. The size and shape vary with the species. In man they are elongated, except in redheads when they are spherical. Lack of melanin in the epidermis is due to absence of melanocytes; or in albinism, due to the inability of the melanocytes to form melanosomes. The activity of the melanosomes is influenced by hormones and by the physical environment.

Biochemical changes in pigmentation. A colorless precursor, thought to be the amino acid tyrosine, is brought by the blood to the dendrite cells which produce melanin. Here under the influence of an enzyme dopoxidase, which is now believed to be identical with the mammalian tyrosinase, the tyrosine is converted into melanin. During the oxidation process the tyrosine goes through several intermediate stages until it is polymerised, and finally oxidised into melanin. Ultraviolet reactions in the skin accelerate chemical changes and produce more melanin.

If secretions of skin are treated with dihydroxyphenylaline, those cells which contain dopoxidase convert it into melanin. This is the *dopa reaction*, and it demonstrates that dendrite cells are capable of manufacturing melanin.

THE DERMIS

The corium (or dermis) is a tough, flexible and highly elastic structure. It is thicker in the palms of the hand and in the soles of the feet, thicker on the posterior than on the anterior aspect of the body, and on the lateral than on the medial sides of the limbs. It is thin and delicate in the eyelids, scrotum, and penis.

The thickness of the dermis cannot be measured exactly, since it passes into the subcutaneous layer without a sharp boundary. The average thickness is 1 to 2 mm and about 3 mm in the palms and soles.

The outer surface of the dermis in contact with the epidermis is uneven and thrown into papillae. The deep main portion of the dermis is called the reticular layer, and the outer surface is called the papillary layer. The two cannot be clearly separated.

The *reticular layer* consists of dense connective tissue. The collagen fibres form bundles running in various directions, but most are more or less parallel to the surface. Elastic fibres form thick networks between the collagen fibres, and are more numerous in the region of the hair follicles, sebaceous, and sweat glands.

The directions taken by the parallel collagen fibre bundles are termed the *cleavage lines*, and surgical incisions along the cleavage lines heal with minimal scar tissue. If the skin becomes stretched by fat deposition, pregnancy, or growing tumors, the fibres in the reticular area partially rupture, resulting in scar formation and the appearance of white streaks.

In the *papillary layer*, the collagen and elastic fibres are fewer and form a continuous fine network in the papillae beneath the epidermis. The cells of the dermis are more abundant in the papillary layer. The papillae are highly sensitive vascular eminences. The papillae are few in number and minute in parts endowed with slight sensibility, but more numerous in sensitive areas, such as the palms of the hands. Within the papillae tissue is a capillary loop.

Hair follicles. Hairs are slender keratinous filaments that develop from the matrix cells of the follicular invaginations of the epidermal epithelium. The hair does not grow continuously. Phases of growth alternate with periods of rest. The structure of the hair follicle varies markedly at different parts of the cycle. In the resting hair the follicle is relatively short, its epithelium is similar to the surface epidermis and the hair shaft is anchored firmly to the follicle by fine keratin filaments. During the phase of growth, the follicle elongates and the epithelial cells surround the dermal papilla and differentiate into several types. The cells of the outermost layer are the most heavily keratinised. The pigmentation of the hair is due to the epidermal melanocytes located over the tip of the dermal papilla.

The human hair exhibits regional differences in the competence of the hair follicles to respond to male sex hormones. The characteristic regression of scalp hair varies with the genotype. Baldness is a hereditary trait that requires a physiological level of androgen for its development, but no amount of androgen can induce baldness in an individual not carrying that trait. Body hair is increased by androgens and scalp hair is decreased. The psychogenic overlay on patchy baldness of the scalp and its interrelation with hormones has yet to be defined.

Sweat glands are found in almost every part of the skin and are classified as two types: (*a*) eccrine; (*b*) apocrine.

Eccrine glands are the most numerous and are found all over the body. They consist of a tube coiled up in the form of a little ball. The secreting part of the gland lies deep in the true skin. The size of the sweat glands varies. They are especially large in regions which sweat profusely, such as in the axilla and groin. Their numbers vary according to the region. They are plentiful on the palms of the hand and the soles of the feet. They are least numerous on the neck and the back.

The *apocrine glands* occur in the axilla, eyelids, areola, and nipple of the breast and the external genitalia. They are larger than eccrine glands and produce a thicker secretion. Unlike the eccrine glands, they are connected to the hair follicles.

Sweating under physical stress begins on the forehead and face and spreads to the rest of the body. Under nervous strain, the palms and soles start sweating first.

The *composition of sweat* is 99% water, with sodium chloride and other compounds such as urea and lactic acid, and potassium ions. The density is 1.004 $g.ml^{-1}$. The pH is sometimes acidic, sometimes alkaline. In abnormal states the sweat may contain compounds not usually present, such as bile pigments, albumin, sugar and blood. The amount of water lost through the glands is 0.5 to 2.5 litres per day. Insensible water loss amounts to 50 ml per hour in man, and muscular exertion increases it to about 1200 ml per hour. Water is lost from the skin by the sweat glands and by osmosis.

Sweating is controlled by the sympathetic nervous system. The eccrine glands are innervated by cholinergic nerves, and the apocrine glands are innervated by adrenergic nerves. No sweating occurs in denervated areas. The sweat centre in the brain is believed to be in the preoptic area immediately anterior to the hypothalamus. The sweat centre is influenced by emotional state, nausea, and asphyxiation.

It is thought that the sweat glands in the palms and soles have both cholinergic and adrenergic fibres, since many emotional states that excite the adrenergic fibres of the sympathetic system are known to cause local sweating of hands and feet during emotional stress. It is believed that moisture from the sweat helps the surface of the hands and feet to gain traction against smooth surfaces, and prevents drying of the thick cornified layers of skin. The eccrine glands do not function simultaneously or under the same conditions on all parts of the body.

Sebaceous glands. One or more sebaceous glands are associated with each hair follicle. The sebaceous glands are small, sacculated, glandular organs lodged in the substance of the corium. They are found in most parts of the body, but are especially abundant in the scalp and the face. They are not present in the palms and the soles of the feet.

Each gland consists of a single capacious duct, which comes out of a cluster of 2 to 5 oval alveoli, or sometimes as many as 20. The ducts open into hair follicles.

The sebaceous glands produce a secretion by complete fatty degeneration of their cells. It is known as *sebum*. Sebum acts as a natural lubricant to hair and skin and protects the skin from moisture and exfoliation. It is also bactericidal. It is stimulated by the activity of the hormone androgen, particularly during adolescence when the sebaceous glands are highly active. If secretions cannot be discharged due to a blocked duct, little white pinheads are seen at the skin exit of the duct. Acute inflammation of the hair follicle and sebaceous gland by staphylococci gives rise to a boil.

Hypodermis. The subcutaneous layer consists of loose connective tissue and is a deeper continuation of the dermis. It has numerous collagen and elastic fibres which run parallel to the surface of the skin. They are few where the skin is freely movable, as on the flexor aspects of the body. Depending on the part of the body and its function, the hypodermis contains fat cells which can reach a thickness of 30 mm in the abdomen. The subcutaneous layer has many blood vessels and nerve endings.

1.3   Circulatory System of the Skin

The circulation of the skin serves two functions:
(*a*)   nutrition of the skin tissues;
(*b*)   conduction of heat.
To perform these two functions the circulatory system in the skin is characterised
by two major types of structures.

NUTRITIVE SYSTEM

The arteries that supply the skin are in the subcutaneous layer. Their branches
form a network parallel to the surface between the dermis and the hypodermis.
From here branches are given off to nourish the subcutaneous stratum with its fat
cells, sweat glands, and deeper portion of the hair follicle. At the boundary
between the papillary layer and reticular layers of the dermis they form a dense
subpapillary network or the *rete subpapillare*. This gives off thin branches to the
papilla.

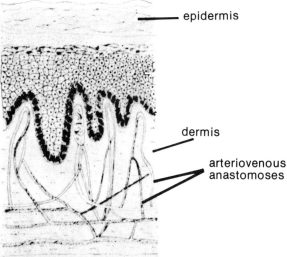

The circulation of the skin

Each papilla has a single loop of capillary vessels with an ascending arterial and
descending venous limb. The veins that collect the blood from the capillaries in
the papilla form the first network of veins, then follows a network of veins at the
junction between the dermis and the subcutaneous tissue. This is at the same level
as the arterial rete cutaneum. Into the network the veins from the sweat glands
and sebaceous glands enter. From the deeper network pass the large subcutaneous independent veins accompanying the arteries.

HEAT CONDUCTION SYSTEM

Vascular structures concerned with heating the skin consist principally of
(*a*)   an extensive subcutaneous venous plexus which holds large quantities of
        blood that can heat the surface of the skin when the blood is warm;
(*b*)   in some areas of skin, arteriovenous anastomoses, which are mainly large
        vascular communications directly between the arteries and venous plexuses.

Arteriovenous anastomoses are most commonly found in the skin of the hands and feet, the skin of the nose, lips and external ear, the mucous membrane of the nose and alimentary canal, the coccygeal body, the erectile tissue of the sex organs, the tongue, the thyroid gland, and the sympathetic ganglia. They may occur in other locations. The structure of the arteriovenous anastomosis consists of a coiled or straight connecting vessel where the former has a thick muscular coat and a fine lumen. It is innervated by fine unmyelinated sympathetic fibres which can cause complete closure so that the circulation goes through the capillary bed. When patent, blood passes directly from artery to vein excluding the capillary bed from the circulation for the time being.

The digital anastomoses have a special arrangement by forming a large number of small units called the *glomera*. They are found in the deep layer of the dermis and have one or more afferent arteries. The afferent artery comes off at right angles from the main cutaneous artery, and after a short distance gives off a number of fine periglomeral branches that become enlarged, and makes an S-curved shape. It narrows down to become continuous with a short vein, and goes back to the receiving deeper cutaneous vein, receiving as it goes the venules from the papillary layer of the skin. In the child at birth they are relatively few. They develop in the early years, and then in old age they undergo atrophy and sclerosis and are fewer in number.

Structurally the vessels in the digital anastomoses are unusual in that they have small endothelial muscular elevations where the vessel enlarges, and other variations in the veins. The muscular wall is thick and looks epitheloid. The anastomosis is innervated by the vasoconstrictor sympathetic fibres that secrete norepinephrin. On constriction, blood in the veins can be almost nil, and on complete dilation, they allow rapid flow of warm blood into the plexuses. Environmental adjustment lies in the glomera of hands and feet. The finger glomera make minute-by-minute adjustment. The glomera are important in regulating heat loss.

The arteriovenous anastomosis in the alimentary canal serves a different function to the heat-regulating function of the digital anastomosis. During absorption from the villus, the anastomosis is closed. In between, it becomes patent and regulates the pressure in the portal vein. Arteriovenous anastomoses in the body are important in regulating local and general body temperature. Other functions are regulation of blood pressure, pressor reception, and epitheloid secretions.

Blood flow. In the resting skin the blood volume is 0.25 litres per square metre of body surface area. This amount of blood is 20 times as much as is needed to supply nutrition to the tissues. On maximum heating the blood volume is increased to 7.5 times the resting level. A large portion of this high volume flows through arteriovenous channels by-passing the usual capillary routes and thus blood, as it perfuses all the veins, conducts heat to the outside. The plexuses also act as a storage depot for blood.

Lymphatic system. The skin is rich in lymphatic vessels. In the papillary layer they form a dense network of vessels beginning in the papilla as blind outgrowths — which are deeper than the blood vessels. There are three layers of lymphatic plexuses in the dermis, communicating with the plexus in the deep fascia by trunks running through the subcutaneous fascia. They are not connected with the hair or glands of the skin.

1.4 Sensory Receptors of the Skin

The stimulation of our sense organs informs the nervous system of environmental changes to which adaptive changes must be made in response to the stimulus. Each different type of sensation that we experience is called a modality of sensation. The characteristic of a sensation by which we distinguish it clearly from all other sensations is known as its *modality*.

Clinicians describe sensations as detailed in the following table. This is influenced by anatomy and histology. We shall deal chiefly with cutaneous sensations.

FIBRE TYPE	SENSATION	NERVE	SIGNS AND SYMPTOMS	
A(δ) A C	CUTANEOUS SENSATIONS pain	exteroceptors all sensory nerves	decreased sensation	HYPOAESTHESIA
			complete loss of sensation	ANAESTHESIA
			diminished ⎞ pain	HYPOALGESIA
			increased ⎬ sensi-bility	HYPERALGESIA
			loss ⎠	ANALGESIA
A(δ) C	temperature	all sensory nerves	complete loss diminished increased	ATHERMAESTHESIA HYPOTHERMAESTHESIA HYPERTHERMAESTHESIA
A(∝) (β) (γ)	DEEP SENSATIONS proprioceptors	motor branches of spinal nerves	loss of muscle joint tendon sensibility or position sense	⎧BATHAESTHESIA ⎨ ⎩BATHYHYPOAESTHESIA
B	VISCERAL SENSES organic sensation	visceroceptors autonomic nerves	hunger, nausea	
C	visceral pain	autonomic nerves	referred pain	

A sensation has several parameters: *quality* (subjective distinguishing between hot, cold, warm); *intensity* (a fundamental parameter pertaining to the finite threshold strength of stimulus); *locus* (the brain knows the location of the stimulation, as coming from some part of the body or the outside world); *discrimination* (the ability to discriminate the spatial aspects of a stimulus, its location, size, shape); and *affect* (the subjective responses to afferent impulses).

Each sensory nerve fibre transmits only one modality of sensation. This is called the *law of specific nerve energies*. The sensor transducer action of the peripheral terminals of the sensory neuron consists of conduction along nerve tracts, to central tracts, to transformation of signals at synaptic junctions, to appreciation of the parameters of the stimulus, to interrelation with emotion, past experiences and other sensations, and then response-coded or patterned from two levels of psychological neural levels.

Mechanoreceptors

TYPES	SITE
TOUCH AND PRESSURE RECEPTORS free nerve endings	all tissues of the body, chiefly in the corium, but also found in the epidermis, epithelium of certain mucous membranes, cornea, tympanic membrane, root of hair, tendons, periosteum, the walls of blood vessels, and around the sweat glands they have both myelinated and finely myelinated nerve fibres
MEISSNER'S CORPUSCLES tactile corpuscles	found in the papillae of the skin of hand, foot, front of forearm, lips, palpebral conjunctiva and tip of tongue
PACINIAN CORPUSCLES lamellated corpuscles	found in the subcutaneous tissues of the palm of hand, plantar aspect of foot, genital organs, arm, neck, nipple, periosteum, interosseous membrane of arm and forearm, near joints, mesentery, pancreas
HAIR END ORGANS	each hair follicle is innervated by deep cutaneous plexus of nerves, both myelinated and non-myelinated
PROPRIOCEPTORS neurotendinous organs of golgi neuromuscular spindles the vestibular apparatus	 tendons of muscles muscles ear
PRESSORECEPTORS AND STRETCH RECEPTORS	lung and heart, detecting changes in pressure stretch of lung and stretch due to blood in heart

The main types of sensory receptors are: mechanoreceptors, chemoreceptors, thermoreceptors, and receptors for electromagnetic radiation and pain.

Mechanoreceptors respond to physical stimuli that cause mechanical displacement of tissues and are further classified according to their function.

There are two types of *thermoreceptors*, one for detecting cold and one for warmth. The skin has discrete cold-sensitive and warm-sensitive spots. On the forearm there are 13 to 15 cold spots per square centimetre, and 1 to 2 warm spots per square centimetre. Temperature is carried by Group III A fibres and small unmyelinated C fibres. The specialised endings of Krause's end bulbs for warmth and Ruffin's end organ for cold have been disproved. Many authorities have regarded them as regenerated or degenerated changes in nerve bundles. Temperature receptors are thought to be the highly branching group of fibres. Warmth receptors discharge at a temperature of 20° to 45°C. Maximal discharge rate is at 37° to 40°C. Cold receptors discharge at 15° to 29°C and maximally at 15° to 20°C. Above 45°C the warmth receptors stop discharging, and pain receptors are stimulated. Temperature sensations are believed to be due to the combination of cold and pain receptors.

The accompanying table contains the main features of the two types of *chemoreceptor*.

Chemoreceptors

TYPES	SITE
ovoid structures composed of elongated receptor cells	taste buds of the mouth, olfactory cells of the nose, which detect chemical substances in the air
tiny nodules (5 mm long) composed of epitheloid cells in a network of connecting cells	the carotid and aortic cell bodies that detect changes in O_2 concentration in blood

Electromagnetic receptors are neuroepithelial cells, for example the rods and cones of the retina which respond to light.

Pain receptors (nocioceptors). Three kinds of pain are sensed: deep pain from muscles, tendons, joints and fascia (bathyaesthesia); superficial or cutaneous pain; and visceral pain.

Many kinds of stimuli may elicit pain — electrical, mechanical, extremes of heat and cold, and a variety of chemicals. One explanation of the wide range of pain stimuli possible is that the various noxious agents all release a chemical substance in the skin and this substance stimulates the pain end-organs.

1.5   Biophysical Properties of the Skin

Electrical properties of skin. The skin of a healthy person contains a certain amount of water with salts dissolved in it. The quantity of water is governed by the number of sweat glands present, which varies from a high concentration in the palms and soles to a much lower level in the trunk and extremities. Moist skin conducts electricity and dry skin resists it. Chemically pure water does not conduct electricity, but if it contains even small amounts of salts, water becomes a conductor.

Surface electrical resistance of skin is a function of its water and electrolyte content. The electrical resistance of the skin is quite variable. When it is dry, skin resistance is 1000 000 ohms (1 megaohm, M Ω) and when artificially heated it may go down to 200 000 ohms. When the skin is moist, the resistance is about 20 000 ohms. Skin resistance can be measured by a sensitive dermohmeter, which in its simplest form is a milliammeter connected to a battery and a resistance to limit maximum current flow.

Skin resistance is inversely proportional to temperature. It is increased in the presence of oedema, whether localised or generalised. Exercise lowers skin resistance due to the increase of vasodilatation.

Ischaemia raises skin resistance and decreases muscle excitability. In elderly atherosclerotic patients the skin resistance is measured in millions of ohms.

Innervation alterations cause a change in skin resistance. The changes occur in logarithmic progression from the normally innervated cutaneous areas to the partially denervated and then the completely denervated areas.

Thus when applying a low frequency current to the skin, the skin should be warmed and moistened to reduce the skin resistance. Lower intensities of current will then be needed to overcome the skin resistance and produce the desired reaction.

Thermoregulatory sweating. The surface electric resistance of the skin is an index of its sweating. The control of sweating is a function of the autonomic nervous system. Thermoregulatory sweating may be used to demonstrate lesions of the sympathetic nervous system. A post-ganglionic lesion will show interference of a sweat pattern corresponding to the sensory distribution of a nerve. A more central lesion will show a sweat pattern disturbance corresponding to a dermatome.

Electrolyte conductivity in skin. The body is composed largely of water, and the skin is therefore impervious to water in order to prevent it from entering or leaving through its epithelium.

Skin epithelium consists of proteins and lipids in a state of electrical neutrality. The pores have a negative charge above a pH of 4 and a positive charge for a pH below 3. The epithelial layers of the skin act as a porous membrane and the extracellular fluid in the dermis is an electrolyte solution. Although the skin will not absorb an electrolyte if soaked in it, it will allow its passage if the dissolved ions are pushed through by an electric current, as most solutions used in ion transfer have a pH of 4 or more. Thus in electro-osmosis there is passage into the skin of the solvent with its dissolved substances.

Inside the dermis the negative ions move to the positive pole by the principle of ion transfer. By osmotic and ionic interchange between intercellular fluid and the capillary wall, there is further migration of ions. The converse also occurs and charged particles emerge out of the capillaries into the intercellular fluid.

These principles are applied when using direct current iontophoresis in the treatment of patients.

Skin temperature changes occur when thermal radiation is applied to the body, and this is influenced by the thermal conductivity of skin, the density, the specific heat of living skin, and the circulation architecture. The product of these factors in the skin or any other tissue will influence temperature evaluation. Fatty tissue will be more quickly heated as it has a lower specific heat, and once heated will not readily lose heat.

As water has a higher thermal conductivity than fat, moist skin will conduct heat faster via its circulation. Biological tissues with a greater density of connective tissue or fat will have a lower thermal conductivity than areas where there is a predominance of muscle tissue under the skin. It is the water content of tissue that influences skin temperature elevation on heating by the physical modalities.

Thermal conductivity can be conditioned by consecutive exposures to the physical modality, and a greater heat tolerance can be obtained. This varies with different people. The amount of melanin in the skin also influences thermal conductivity. Dark skin is heated about twice as rapidly as white skin.

Skin reflectance. Reflection from the skin follows Lambert's cosine law, which states that the intensity of radiation is proportional to the cosine of the angle between the ray and the perpendicular to the plane being irradiated. Skin reflectance also depends on the spectral ranges, such as visible and near infrared, microwave, and also the color of the skin. With infrared in the region of 3 to 100 μm, reflecting power of the skin is small and reflectance is low for black and white skins. With infrared and visible light in the region of 0.4 to 2.8 μm, there is a greater reflectance, which is greater for white skins than for dark skins.

With microwave at 2450 MHz the distribution of heat depends critically on the skin and subcutaneous fat thickness. A large part of the total energy which passes through subcutaneous fat to muscle is reflected, especially at the boundary separating skin from subcutaneous fat.

Skin transmittance depends on skin color, skin thickness, and the thermal radiation or electrical energy used. In high frequency currents and ultrasonics, the dielectric constant and specific resistance of skin and subcutaneous tissue in the region play a decisive part in determining transmittance.

1.6   Biochemistry of the Skin

The functioning of the connective tissue in the skin is dependent on the properties of its extracellular substances. The fibres are responsible for its tensile strength and resilience, while the ground substance is an essential medium between cells and blood. Its consistency and hydration can have an important influence on this vital exchange.

Collagen fibres are composed of the protein collagen, which has a high glycine content. Proline and hydroxyproline are also present. The fundamental molecule or unit of collagen is tropocollagen, which is made up of three polypeptide chains. Collagen as a substance is capable of inducing hydroxyapatite crystal growth when exposed to metastable solutions of calcium and phosphate. These conditions are not present in normal connective tissues, so tendons and ligaments do not calcify. This has been explained by there being some component in tendon and ligament which prevents calcification. This property of collagen to induce crystal formation is important in calcification and can occur at any site.

The principal component of *elastic fibres* is the protein elastin, with some glycine and proline, but there is a high content of valine and a new amino-acid, desmocine. Like collagen it has an effect on hydroxyapatite crystal fibre formation, and it is possible that it is involved in the pathological calcification of skin, aorta, and other sites.

Reticular fibres are believed to be identical in chemical composition to collagen fibres, but vary in their physical nature, being immature fine collagen fibrils.

The *ground substance*, or *matrix*, is an amorphous, viscid, semi-fluid substance, containing hyaluronate, which is responsible for its consistency. This property is thought to stop the spread of bacteria in tissues. Some bacteria produce the enzyme hyaluronidase and depolymerise the hyaluronate. Ground substance also contains tropocollagen.

1.7   Body Temperature

No single temperature can be considered as normal. Although man is homeothermic and the mechanisms involved in homeothermy tend to stabilise internal body temperature, they cannot completely prevent temperature variation in response to internal and environmental thermal stresses. Normal body temperature implies specific conditions under which the measurement is taken.

Core temperature. The term *body temperature* means the temperature of the interior, called the *core temperature*, and not the skin temperature or that of the tissues immediately underlying the skin. The core temperature is regulated accurately, and does not normally vary from the mean by more than $0.1°C$. Surface temperature rises and falls with the temperature of the surroundings. The rectal temperature is representative of the core temperature and varies least with environmental changes in temperature. Oral temperature is at least $0.6°C$ lower than rectal temperature, but this is affected by many factors such as ingestion of hot or cold fluids, environment, humidity, sex, sweating, stress, drugs, tobacco, alcohol, changes in posture, and rate of rise of temperature.

Surface temperature. Various parts of the body are at different temperatures, and the magnitude varies with the environmental temperature. The extremities are generally cooler than the trunk.

Subjective classification of external temperature

FEELING	CELSIUS
very cold	0° – 13°
cold	13° – 18°
cool	18° – 27°
neutral	27° – 33°
warm	33° – 37°
hot	37° – 40°
very hot	40° – 43°

THERAPEUTIC RANGE: 5° – 44°

The temperature of the skin is a function of a maximum which occurs at about 1 mm beneath its surface and a minimum at about 1.8 mm. Each is related to the arteriolar and the deep venous plexuses respectively. The environmental temperature and humidity greatly influence the skin temperature. As the environmental temperature rises, there is an increase in perspiration. Each major portion of the body shows a critical temperature for the beginning of perspiration.

Since the layer of subcutaneous fat is about 4 mm thicker in women than in men, the skin temperature of women is 1°C lower in the cold zone and 1.7°C higher in the hot environmental zone. Women do not show active sweating until the air temperature is 32°C, whereas men begin to perspire when the temperature reaches 29°C. Evaporation of perspired water removes increasing proportions of the total heat produced until the air and skin temperatures are the same, at which time all of the heat is lost by evaporation. Evaporation will lower the skin temperature by about 3°C and will also change the thermal characteristics of skin.

Each anatomical area of the body has its own temperature characteristics related to histological structure, texture, blood and nerve supply, hair covering, sweat glands and local reflex actions.

(a)   The posterior trunk has a stable skin temperature.
(b)   The forehead is unresponsive to heat and cold, especially cold.
(c)   The finger tips, palms, soles, lobes of the ears, and parts of the face react rapidly to a cold environment. If the body is warm, these areas show vasodilatation and a rise in skin temperature when first exposed to cold, a reflex which protects the areas from frostbite.

Isotherms. Visualise the body as a central core at uniform temperature surrounded by an insulating shell, composed of the thickness of the epidermis. The shell thickness is increased when heat has to be conserved. Core isotherm patterns are controlled particularly for heat conservation. Isotherms are surfaces connecting points of equal temperature.

Schematic isotherms in body cooling — warm body on right, cooler on left. Insert shows circulatory system in the leg, illustrating the arrangement for heat exchange

(Aschoff and Wever, 1958)

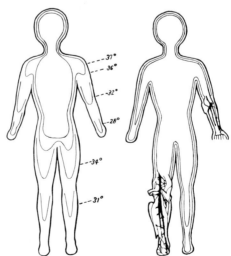

Temperature gradient. Body temperature, although generally kept constant, always shows more or less regular variations due to rhythmic diurnal changes, variations in the menstrual cycle in females, and other causes. In the core no completely uniform temperature exists, since the temperature of each organ in the core depends on the relative level of metabolism of the specific organ and the blood supplying it. The shell, having a lower mean temperature than the core, produces a *temperature gradient* from core down to skin. The main factor in the temperature regulation of mammals is their capacity to alter the temperature gradient in the shell, and to change the ratio of shell volume to core volume. The main factor contributing to the existence of the temperature gradient is that, under ordinary conditions, environmental temperature is below body temperature, so the body loses heat (by conduction, evaporation and radiation).

Regulation of body temperature. The rate of heat production usually balances the rate of heat loss.

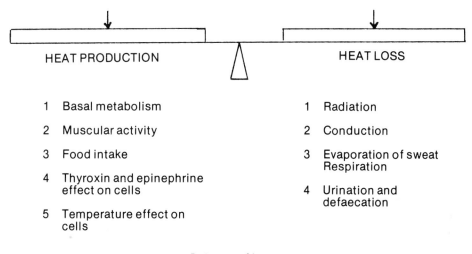

HEAT PRODUCTION	HEAT LOSS
1 Basal metabolism	1 Radiation
2 Muscular activity	2 Conduction
3 Food intake	3 Evaporation of sweat Respiration
4 Thyroxin and epinephrine effect on cells	4 Urination and defaecation
5 Temperature effect on cells	

Balance of heat

Thermostatic control of temperature occurs in neural centres in the spinal cord and in the hypothalamic region. The reflex and semi-reflex thermoregulatory centres include autonomic, somatic, endocrine and behavioral patterns. Reflex responses activated by the cold are controlled from the posterior hypothalamus; those activated by warmth, from the anterior hypothalamus. Increase of catecholamine from the adrenals is an important endocrine response to cold. In heating large areas of vascular field, the thermoregulating centres of the hypothalamus would increase reflexly the blood supply to the impoverished areas, and thus increase local skin temperature. This is the physiological basis of reflex heating.

New research has shown that other regions in the vicinity of the hypothalamus may contain important integrating mechanisms involved in defence against both cooling and heating, and must be included with the regions essential for thermoregulation.

1.8   Temperature Measurement

Mercury-in-glass thermometers include the familiar clinical thermometer. It is designed to cover a range from 34°C to 42°C, reading to 0.2 degrees.

Thermoelectric thermometers are widely used in temperature measurement. A thermocouple consists of a pair of wires of dissimilar materials welded together at one end. If the weld or measuring junction is at a temperature different from the free ends, a potential difference will be established. If the ends are connected, an electrical current will flow in the circuit as long as the difference in temperature is maintained. The current generated can be measured and calibrated in units of temperature.

Thermography. All bodies constantly lose energy by radiation. This radiation may be in the visible range (400 to 700 nm) as in the case of the sun, or in the far infrared (maximum at 9600 nm) in the case of a body at 37°C. Skin surface temperature measurements can be made with speed and accuracy by means of a sophisticated clinical radiation camera.

The detector converts the radiation to electrical signals, which are used to operate a cathode ray tube in the same way that a television tube displays a rapid series of pictures. For a permanent record, a Polaroid camera is used to photograph the screen.

Clinical applications. *Carcinoma* of the breast is associated with an elevated temperature of the skin over the tumor. Thermography is widely used in detecting such carcinomas.

Acute disc lesions can be detected by the formation of a 'hot spot' in the spinal region.

Male infertility due to the formation of a varicocele on part of the testes can be diagnosed by thermography of the scrotum.

Vascular disease. As a preventive measure for cardiovascular accidents, thermography is being tried out for early evaluation of the degree of stenosis of an arterial occlusive lesion.

Thermography is used to measure the infrared radiation emitted from the supraorbital regions of the forehead. Forehead temperature depends upon the degree of irrigation of the region by the opthalmic artery, and is therefore related to the patency of the internal carotid artery. Blood flow to any portion of the body depends on many factors, such as blood viscosity, blood pressure, calibre of blood vessels, and environmental temperature. Thermography offers an atraumatic technique for accurate peripheral evaluation of cerebral blood flow.

1.9   Physiological Effects of Heat and Cold

The application of external heat to restricted body areas produces many changes in the tissues by local, general or remote effects. The parameters which determine the extent of physiological response to heat include:

    size of area exposed
    intensity of radiation
    relative depths of absorption of specific radiation

integrity of the cardiovascular and nervous systems
structure of the skin and subcutaneous tissues
age of the patient
functioning of neural, hormonal and chemical control of vasculature
functioning of thermoregulatory centre
thermal conductivity, density, and specific heat of living skin and tissue
absorption coefficient in a specific tissue for each modality
electrical and acoustic properties of tissues
pathophysiology of the area to be treated
amount of temperature variation
rate of rise or fall of temperature
duration of tissue temperature elevation or reduction.

In the total analysis of the effects of heat on the tissues there is often interplay between local and general actions.

There are, in the main, three direct specific physiological actions of heat on the tissues, and many other indirect effects. The main effects are:

(*a*)   local and remote increased blood flow due to temperature rise or fall;
(*b*)   stimulation of the neural receptors in the skin or tissues;
(*c*)   increase or decrease of metabolic activity.

There are no reliable methods of measuring physiological heat conduction in the body.

VASCULAR CONTROL IN SKIN

The skin is an effective radiator system. The flow of blood to and from the skin is through the controlled mechanisms of heat transfer to and from the core and shell (skin). Heat transfer is by combined conductor and circulatory convection. Heat tends to flow along a temperature gradient by transfer of thermal energy between adjacent atoms. The tissues of the body are not good conductors. Values reported for various tissues vary a great deal. Vascular tissue is said to be the best conductor, due to the profuse distribution of the capillaries.

Blood vessels penetrate the subcutaneous tissues and are distributed in the sub-papillary portion of the skin. Immediately beneath the skin is a continuous venous plexus which supplies the most exposed areas of skin by direct arteriovenous shunts which by-pass the cutaneous capillaries. The function of heat exchange in the skin does not involve large or varying requirements for energy conversion or oxygen consumption. *The flow of blood through cutaneous vessels is not adjusted primarily to the requirement of skin for oxygen, but rather to the functional requirements of the body for dissipation or conservation of heat.* The plexuses also function on occasion as a reservoir of blood, a function which is also independent of the nutritive requirements of the skin.

Reactive hyperaemia is an increase in the amount of blood in a region when its circulation is re-established after a period of occlusion. Blood flowing into the dilated vessels makes the skin become fiery red. The arteriolar dilatation is due to hypoxia and is effected by the release of chemical substances. Cutaneous reactive hyperaemia occurs after temporary arterial occlusion.

Various mechanisms which produce vasodilatation or vasoconstriction in the vascular bed in skin. (Rueh and Patton)

TYPE OF MECHANISM	VASOCONSTRICTION	VASODILATATION
neural	sympathetic nerve	axon reflex
hormonal	L-epinephrin norepinephrin	bradykinin (glands) acetylcholine
local chemical		unidentified metabolites CO O_2 histamine
radiations		X-rays ultraviolet infrared

VASCULAR CONTROL IN MUSCLES

Blood flow through muscle is regulated in relation to muscle oxygen requirements which vary widely between rest and vigorous exercise. Blood flow through resting muscle is in the region of 0.1 to 0.3 ml per gram per minute. In exercise it is increased 20 to 30 times. The blood flow to skeletal muscle is by thoroughfare channels and capillary networks, since arteriovenous shunts are rarely found in muscle tissue. This is in contrast to increased blood flow in skin which is by arteriovenous shunts. Regulation of muscle blood flow is through a combination of neural and local mechanisms.

Mechanisms affecting blood flow in skeletal muscles

TYPE OF MECHANISM	VASOCONSTRICTION	VASODILATATION
neural	sympathetic constrictor nerve	sympathetic vasodilator nerve
hormonal	norepinephrin	L-epinephrin acetylcholine
local chemical		unidentified metabolites ATP ADP

Substantial evidence indicates that increased blood flow through skeletal muscle can be initiated at higher levels of the central nervous system through the medulla, with or without synapses to the spinal cord. Following a temporary arrest of circulation in skeletal muscle, the circulation can be increased in proportion to blood flow debt, and is greater when the limb is warmed. Blood flow through a relaxed extremity is somewhat higher after vigorous exercise than during exercise.

The axon reflex is the simplest of all the reflexes controlling the circulation, and has been ascribed a role in the production of hyperaemia of the skin subjected to irritants. The concept is based on indirect evidence and has not been established fully. It is, however, widely accepted and difficult to disprove.

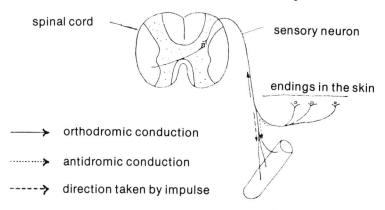

The axon reflex

Local Effects of Temperature Changes on the Tissues

Skin and superficial fascia — Circulatory effects. The local effects of heat lead to vasodilatation of the blood vessels at temperatures up to 42°C, with blood flow increasing by 4 to 5 times that of resting level. If the heating is prolonged for more than 30 minutes, then the blood flow reaches a plateau and declines. At temperatures of 45°C, with prolonged heating, the vasodilatation continues to operate, but there is a danger of a burn occurring. Vasodilatation with heating is due to the release of histamine-like substances that dilate the capillaries, and is also due to the axon reflex, as there is reflex dilatation of the arterioles. The increased capillary dilatation leads to increased capillary hydrostatic pressure and increased active capillary surface area. At a temperature of 45°C there is a doubling of capillary filtration.

At temperatures below 18°C there is vasoconstriction, and then there are cyclic phases of vasodilatation and vasoconstriction depending on other factors (see Unit 4).

Muscle — Circulatory effects. The various physical modalities, when absorbed by muscle, produce heat. There has been ample evidence showing that *muscle blood flow is not increased by heat*. Heat and exercise will increase blood flow more than exercise alone. In some pathological states there is increased blood flow present, and the effect of heat on such pathology must be studied carefully. Examples are in osteoarthrosis or disuse muscle atrophy.

Metabolic effects. The rate of metabolism of skin or muscle depends in part on temperature. It is increased by an average of 13% for a rise of 1°C. The initial rise in metabolism correlates with Van't Hoff's Law that the velocity of any simple chemical reaction increases 2 to 3 times for each rise of 10°C. Conversely metabolism falls with a drop in temperature. Heating beyond 45°C causes irreversible damage of tissue proteins and death of the tissues. Metabolic activity is also influenced by the velocity of temperature changes, and whether it is a rise or drop in temperature. A quick rise in temperature stimulates metabolism.

The effect of heat on biochemical activities of the body needs to be studied further in terms of clinical effects. At present there exists a wide gap of knowledge in this field. The speed of cellular oxidation increases with temperature (Van't Hoff's Law).

Collagen tissue. At normal tissue temperatures, collagen primarily exhibits elastic properties and only minimal viscous flow, but when heated to 39° to 44°C, the viscous flow becomes more dominant and tension relaxes markedly. This leads to a residual elongation of these tissues. For adhesions, it is more effective to use heat with a low tension stretch (Lehmann and others).

Joint stiffness is often associated with changes in the visco-elastic properties of joints. Heat can relieve joint stiffness, while cold increases joint stiffness.

Sensory nerve endings. Within the electromagnetic spectrum the band of wavelengths between 700 and 100 000 nm comprises the radiation which, when incident on the skin, arouses thermal sensations, and is thus considered as 'heat'. Apart from stimulating the sensations of hot and cold, heat produces definite *sedative effects*.

Physiological explanation of pain relief by strong heating is based on evidence that any sensory stimuli that reach the brain simultaneously with that of the pain stimuli can more or less attenuate the pain factor. If two pains occur at the same time in different parts of the body, the stronger pain diminishes the lesser. Historically, this leads to the theory of *counter-irritation*. Intensity of pain is diminished in proportion to increased or decreased heat gradient in skin rather than to temperature sensation.

Skin temperature also influences normal sensation of the skin. Two-point discrimination diminishes with cooling of the skin. There is some doubt about the direct effect of increase in temperature on the fusimotor system and, though heat alleviates pain, its effect on nerve conduction has still to be proved. Cold definitely reduces nerve conduction and thus relieves pain.

Temperature-evoked pain. It has been found that a skin temperature around 45°C is critical for evoking pain and reflex responses. It is also critical for producing cutaneous burns. Pain is related to skin temperatures only, whereas tissue damage is related to both skin temperature and the duration of the hyperthermic episode, which then starts the chemical reactions towards the production of burns. The skin can be conditioned by previous exposures altering the thermal conductivity and pain threshold for thermal radiations. Cutaneous pain threshold is independent of race and culture, sex and age, as seen in experiments done on Eskimos, Alaskans, Indians and whites in America, and Japanese. But different people do react differently to pain.

Magnitude of heat transfer and oxygen transfer. Local heating promptly opens the skin's arteriovenous shunts, or anastomoses. The opening of these shunts has a different effect on oxygen extraction from blood by the tissue and upon heat transfer between tissue and blood. Oxygen can transfer to the tissues only through the walls of the capillaries. Therefore when heat opens up the arteriovenous shunts, only a relatively small fraction of blood passes through the capillaries, most of the oxygenated blood being shunted into the numerous venules.

The magnitude of heat transfer between the blood and tissues depends on the time a unit volume of blood stays in the small vessels of the skin. Although blood passes more slowly through capillaries than through arteries and venules, the longer length of the venules permits a higher degree of temperature equalisation.

DEPTH OF HEATING

The different physical modalities available have heating patterns of varying depth. Surface heating is directed mainly to the superficial regions of the body, and is obtained by the use of such techniques as infrared, heating pads, wax, and warm baths. Deep heating is directed to all tissues under the subcutaneous region of fat.

Technically there are two methods available to produce deep heating:

(a) *Conduction* — Heat is transmitted by conduction from a high temperature induced in the superficial region. It creates the problem that, in order to obtain a sufficient temperature in the deep tissues, there will be an intolerable temperature at the surface.

(b) *Conversive* — Heat is developed in the deep structures directly by conversion of energy within a specific area, and this is *volume heating*. It is obtained by physical modalities such as ultrasound, short wave, and microwave diathermy.

High-water-content tissues such as muscle, liver, kidney, blood, and heart absorb heat quickly and maximally. Low-water-content tissues such as bone, fat and fascia impede heat transfer.

Subcutaneous fat tends to establish a temperature barrier. Fatty tissue, because of its low specific heat, is heated more than most skin or bone. Fat also has low thermal conductivity, and this causes a rise of temperature in the subcutaneous regions in comparison with the muscular region. At fat-muscle interfaces there is considerable reflection of microwaves and consequent heating of fatty tissues. Ultrasound is easily transmitted through fat, with little absorption. Short wave heats fat considerably because it has a poor blood supply and cannot dissipate the heat. The bone-muscle interface causes reflection of ultrasound and heating of areas adjacent to bone. Microwave is able to penetrate bone and heat structures around the bone. In the case of bones of small cross-section, microwaves will scatter rather than penetrate. Bone acts as an impediment to short wave diathermy.

Local heating over 45°C. Increased capillary permeability and increased capillary dilatation cause redness and oedema. A further flare of redness spreads out, due to the release of histamine-like substances, and vasoactive polypeptides, producing an effect on capillary and arteriolar dilatation. Blister formation is due to activity of proteolytic enzymes in the skin. Further rise in temperature will lead to denaturation and death of cells and tissues.

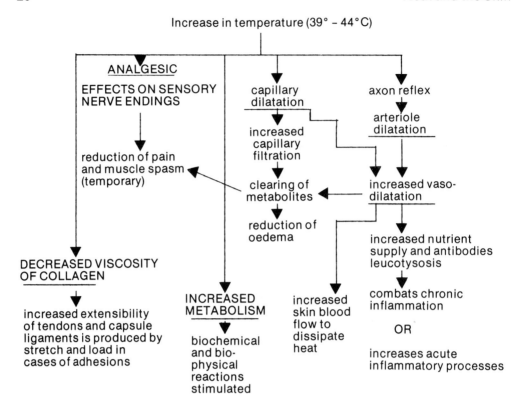

Increase in temperature (39° – 44°C)

ANALGESIC

EFFECTS ON SENSORY
NERVE ENDINGS

capillary
dilatation

axon reflex

arteriole
dilatation

reduction of pain
and muscle spasm
(temporary)

increased
capillary
filtration

clearing of
metabolites

increased vaso-
dilatation

reduction of
oedema

increased nutrient
supply and antibodies
leucotysosis

DECREASED VISCOSITY
OF COLLAGEN

increased extensibility
of tendons and capsule
ligaments is produced by
stretch and load in
cases of adhesions

INCREASED
METABOLISM

biochemical
and bio-
physical
reactions
stimulated

increased
skin blood
flow to
dissipate
heat

combats chronic
inflammation

OR

increases acute
inflammatory processes

Summary of the local physiological effects of heating

GENERALISED EFFECTS OF HEATING

When an area of the body is exposed to more than a minimal amount of heat and cold, the effects do not remain localised. Vasodilatation from heat spreads to adjacent areas. Heat applied to one leg affects the other leg or the arms. The remote effects of heat stem from the body's heat-regulating centre in the hypothalamus. Heating of the knee joint raises the temperature of the joint and increases the blood flow to the joint. How much of this is due to conduction of heat, and how much due to remote control is not fully understood.

Sweating is also governed by remote control. If sweating starts at a heated area, then remote periodic sweating starts at variable areas.

Heat applied to the abdomen has irregular effects on the blood supply. Applying external heating to the abdominal wall has the opposite effect on bowel blood flow to that on exposed skin areas. Heat to the abdominal wall diminishes intestinal mobility, and decreases acid secretions in the stomach. Cold has the opposite effect, thought to be due to indirect reflex heating, as oral administration of ice water decreases gastric mobility and acid production. Heat applied to the abdomen has variable effects on the blood flow of the liver, but always increases its excretory functions (Demling and Gromotka).

In experiments done on isolated gut by Valtonen in Finland, direct application of short wave diathermy on the smooth muscles of the trachea and intestines were found to produce relaxation.

The biological effects of heating by physical modalities may be contra-indicatory depending on whether they act at (a) cellular level, (b) organ level, (c) on the level of the heat and self-regulating mechanisms.

For example, the motor activity of the isolated part is increased when warmed, and decreased when cooled. When the whole or part of a mammalian body is warmed or cooled, the indirect effects of heat or cold are the opposite to that observed in the isolated gut. This is due to the regulating mechanisms of the body as a whole with the hormonal influence of epinephrin and thyroid, in which the function of one part of the body influences the functions of the other parts of the body.

Such factors must be taken into consideration when determining the selection of physical modalities for the treatment of superficial or deep structures in the abdomen and pelvis, for example salpingitis, parametritis of the pelvic organs, slow healing wounds, or haematomas of surgery in the abdomen. The application of heat or cold for gastro-intestinal or pelvic organ disorders, and the application of heat to the abdominal wall to obtain increased peripheral circulation in cases of Beurger's disease require careful consideration.

Summary of the general physiological effects of heating. Increased heat elimination by radiation, conduction, and convection.

Increased sweating with cutaneous heating, or when the body becomes over-heated. Large quantities of sweat are secreted owing to the stimulation of the anterior hypothalamus.

Increased circulation is due to direct effects, the release of histamine-like and other vasoactive substances which activate capillary dilatation, and the axon reflex acting on the arteriolar dilatation mechanisms.

Increase of pulse rate by 10 beats for each 6°C rise in temperature.

Lowering of blood pressure due to decrease in sodium concentration, loss of urea, and other nitrogenous substances.

Increased rate of breathing, due perhaps to alteration in hydrogen ion concentration (pH) or secondary alterations in O_2, and CO_2 concentration. During panting, only small quantities of air pass in and out of the lungs on each breath, so that mainly dead-space air enters the alveoli. Tremendous amounts of air pass over the tongue, trachea and mouth without great hyperventilation. This promotes cooling by evaporation, especially from the saliva of the tongue, as is seen in those animals which do not possess sweat glands.

Increased elimination through the kidneys, due to changes in the concentration of urea, NaCI, lactic acid, potassium, and other substances.

Increase of pH of blood.

Increase of lymphatic drainage due to increased capillary hydrostatic pressure.

This is mainly in the heated area but also indirectly affects the general lymphatic drainage.

Phagocytosis increases in the presence of inflammation, due to increased blood flow and other chemical reactions to heat.

1.10 Dosimetry

Dosage can be defined as the product of applied energy and duration of action. Heat dosage depends on three factors: intensity, duration and frequency of application. Heat intensity cannot be measured by any therapeutic apparatus, since the meters on the machine generally register the intensity of current supplied to the patient's circuit, or the power output from the transducer to the patient.

Dosage must be governed by biological factors, and most important is the actual tissue temperature evaluation, which cannot be assessed by modern commercial machines. The following dose concepts can be differentiated: *Power output* (dose rate) is the energy applied per unit of time, and is expressed in watts. 1 watt is the energy transformed into heat in 1 second when a potential of 1 volt is applied to a resistor of 1 ohm, causing a current of 1 ampere to flow in the apparatus.

Energy flux is defined as the dose rate per unit body surface area and is given in watts per square centimetre ($W.cm^{-2}$).

Total energy output is the product of the energy flux, the time of treatment, and the area of body surface under treatment. The total heat developed in the body by diathermy is a function of the total energy uptake. Safe threshold values of dosage can be exceeded by too sudden or too local development of heat. Approximate times of treatment are from 3 minutes to 30 minutes.

The turnover of heat in the human body is 8.4 mJ per day. This is an energy flux of 0.005 $W.cm^{-2}$. Therefore diathermy energy to increase temperature must be at least 0.05 $W.cm^{-2}$. Apart from looking at the energy flux of biological activities during the administration of diathermy, other factors such as depth of penetration, configuration of tissues, dilatation of blood vessels, and the existing temperature of the tissue to be treated must be considered.

Heat intensity. Two laws must be taken into consideration. *Van't Hoff's Law* indicates that the velocity of any chemical reaction increases 2 to 3 times for each 10°C rise in temperature. However, with increasing temperature there is a denaturing of the proteins involved in the chemical reactions (enzymes, protoplasm, and specific cellular proteins). This denaturing process is largely irreversible. *Kirchoff's Law* indicates that the greatest amount of heat is developed in the region of greatest current density.

$$H = I^2.RT$$

$$\text{where } H = \text{heat developed;}$$
$$R = \text{resistance;}$$
$$I = \text{intensity of current;}$$
$$T = \text{time.}$$

In short wave diathermy, the lines of force may cross or run parallel to the tissues, but in most areas it is a mixture of the two. In ultrasound and microwave, different types of tissues are in the area of wave propagation. Heat dissipation will be greater at the subcutaneous muscle level, as conversive volume heating is produced and there is less skin heating.

The current distribution will depend on the histology and size of the tissues, the prevailing pathophysiology, the conductivity (specific resistance) and dielectric constant of the tissues.

The relative amount of energy converted into heat at any given point is called the pattern of relative heating. The tissue temperature and temperature distribution will depend on the pattern of relative heating and the electrical properties of the tissues.

$$H = \triangle T \times \text{specific heat} \times \text{mass}$$

where H = the amount of energy converted into heat

$\triangle T$ = rise in temperature per second

This is further modified by the thermal conductivity of the tissues, the temperature of the part before treatment, and the pathophysiology of existing blood flow and metabolism.

Heat sensation. Dosage can only be guided by the feeling of warmth on the part of the patient. Degrees of heat sensation can be categorised broadly as

(*a*)   threshold value, gentle comforting warmth — *minimal*

(*b*)   distinct feeling of agreeable warmth — *medium*

(*c*)   intense feeling of heat, maximum heat tolerance is exercised — *maximum*

(*d*)   intolerable heat, burning sensation — *danger level.*

These guidelines are not reliable as they must depend on two factors:

(*a*)   intact sensation;

(*b*)   alertness on the part of the patient.

In acute stages, heat should be minimal and the patient should feel only a gentle glow.

In chronic stages, moderate heat could be given, depending on the desired effects. Patients must be warned not to try and take it as hot as possible, thinking that it will do them good. They should be warned, but not frightened, of the danger of burns.

It is important to ascertain what the meter reading signifies for each apparatus.

Duration of treatment is empirical. The average length of time used by physiotherapists is 15 to 30 minutes in routine treatments. *Bierman has shown that the maximum effect takes place at the 20th minute.* There is no evidence that hyperaemia is prolonged by increasing the duration. Further research is required to discover the amount of temperature increase needed to influence the metabolic activities of various tissues to produce reversal of pathological changes.

Frequency. There is no established rule regarding frequency. The aim of every physiotherapist is to shorten the period of rehabilitation and gain maximal benefit from a modality, so it is advisable to give daily treatment for the first course of 6 to 10 treatments. The next course could be on alternate days, but this is governed by the patient's response to treatment. Some acute cases are treated twice a day.

2 Conductive and Convective Heating

Some Key Points in this Unit

Conductive heating is the transfer of heat between two objects in contact, and at different temperatures, heat being transferred by conduction from the warmer object to the cooler one.

Convective heating is the transfer of heat energy by means of convection currents, which arise due to temperature and density differences in various parts of a fluid.

Specific heat of a substance is the heat required per unit of mass to change the temperature one degree Celsius. It is expressed as a ratio of the amounts of heat required to raise the temperature of equal masses of the substance and water by the same amount. The value for water is taken as one.

Thermal conductivity is the ability of a tissue to absorb heat and conduct it across the tissue.

Hydrocollator. An automatic heating unit which holds a supply of steam packs heated in water at a constant temperature ready for use.

Moist heat. The production of heat by a moist source.

Paraffin wax bath. An automatic heating unit which holds low melting point wax at a steady temperature, ready for use.

2.1 Heat Exchange by Conduction

As heat is a form of energy of motion, the transfer of heat on a molecular scale can be effected by the transfer of kinetic energy during the collision of molecules. Conduction is the diffusion of this energy from one body to another.

When an object is heated by a source in contact with it, the speed at which the heat will flow and cause a rise in temperature will depend upon the thermal conductivity of the source and the substance. The thermal conductivity of water is greater than that of fat. Tissues with high water content will conduct faster than tissues with low water content. The specific heat of the tissue will also govern the amount of heat needed to raise temperature by any particular amount. Fat has a specific heat of only 0.6, and can therefore be heated with less expenditure of energy than for water (specific heat = 1.0).

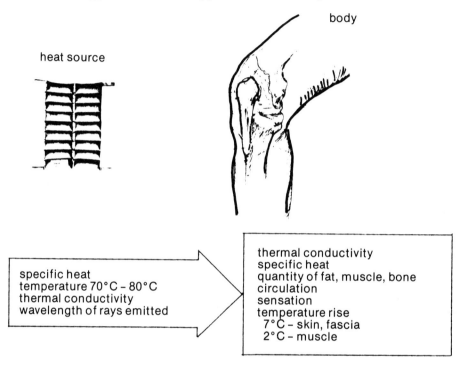

Transfer of heat by conduction

Sources of conductive heating include: solids — mud and peat packs, and electric heating pads; liquids — thermal water baths, and contrast baths, hot packs, and paraffin wax; and gases — hot air, and hot vapor baths. Heat is transmitted by conduction and some convection.

Commonly used modalities for therapeutic purposes are hydrocollator packs and paraffin wax baths.

2.2 Hydrocollator Packs

The use of moist heat as a therapeutic agent is one of the oldest forms of medicine. Today we have efficient automatic units producing a uniform and constant temperature to heat steam packs. They provide physiotherapists with a constant supply of ready-to-use heated packs. The heating unit is called a hydrocollator unit.

The hydrocollator unit is a stainless steel tank in which silica gel packs are heated. The capacities of the machines vary, and all units have insulated bases, the larger machines being insulated with fibreglass. The units contain a wire rack which acts as a divider for the packs and prevents contact of packs with the bottom of the tank. The heater is thermostatically controlled and maintains water in the unit at a temperature between 76°C and 80°C. It can be left on continuously as long as there is sufficient water in the tank.

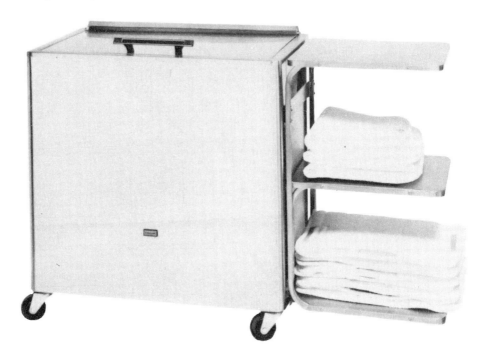

Hydrocollator unit

A hydrocollator pack is a fabric envelope containing *silica gel*. The main property of the gel is its capability to absorb many times its own volume of water and, when heated, to give off moist heat for 30 to 40 minutes. The packs are heated in a hydrocollator unit.

Packs come in varying sizes and shapes. They are designed to fit nearly any body contour and are used repeatedly, being returned to hot water after each use.

A special collar pattern pack for the neck is usually available. Packs are wrapped in
(*a*)   turkish towels
(*b*)   special terry cloth (absorbent)
(*c*)   large packs may be wrapped in bath blankets.

The packs generally last about six months. When they begin to wear out, the filler leaks out and makes the water cloudy — they should then be replaced.

Hydrocollator packs are used to give gentle moist heat to superficial regions of the body, mainly for the relaxation of pain and muscle spasm in superficial areas.

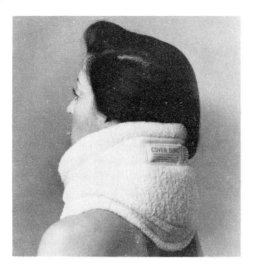

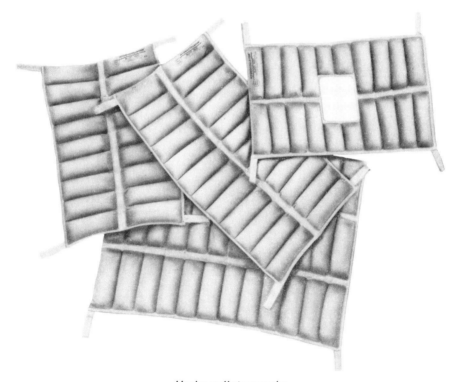

Hydrocollator packs

The part selected to be treated must be able to tolerate the pressure of the pack (approximately 500 to 800 gram), and to tolerate a 7° to 10°C rise in temperature. It is also necessary to ensure that the circulation can dissipate heat, and that skin sensation responses to thermal differences are normal, as it is easy to produce a burn.

The pack retains its heat for 30 minutes, but after 10 minutes the patient may regard the pack as cool and comfortable. Nevertheless the rise in temperature of the region under the pack averages 5°C.

The pack is applied to the body after being wrapped adequately in towelling or blankets. Care must be taken to have a layer of towelling, and to avoid excessive pressure by body weight being placed on bony points.

BIOLOGICAL EFFECTS OF HYDROCOLLATOR PACKS

Heat production. The effect of hydrocollator packs on the tissues is due mainly to the heat generated, and is subject to the quantity and depth of penetration of the long infrared rays emitted from the pack. When infrared is absorbed by tissues it produces heat. The penetration of the rays is no more than 0.5 to 1 mm deep. The conduction depth is governed by the properties of the underlying fat, muscle, connective tissue and bone.

Temperature elevation will depend upon the patency of the circulation and sensation, and the ability of the tissues to dissipate heat. Bone and fat will impede heat distribution — fatty tissue having a low specific heat will heat rapidly, and will cause heat conduction away from the site. Temperature rise takes place if the heat generated exceeds the rate at which the tissues can dissipate the heat.

Skin tolerance to heat is 44°C. Lower temperatures, such as 42°C, for over two hours can cause a burn. A temperature of 44°C over 30 minutes can cause a burn. Temperatures of over 45°C over 5 to 10 minutes will cause a burn. Therefore a safe but effective application of heat is 44°C for 20 to 30 minutes.

Thermal gradient in the tissues. Accurate assessments of temperature rises in skin, subcutaneous tissue, and muscle are not possible, but a rough gauge has shown that hydrocollator packs have the following characteristics:

Skin temperature. Within 7 minutes there is a maximum 7° to 8°C rise in temperature and then a drop of about 2°C over the remainder of the 20 to 30 minute application period. Within 60 minutes after treatment, the temperature returns to normal, a rapid drop occurring during the first 15 minutes after treatment.

Subcutaneous tissue and muscle temperature. In areas of tissue where there is no obstruction by fat or bone, the subcutaneous tissues show a rise of about 3°C maximally in about 20 minutes, which then disappears in about one hour, the maximum drop being after 15 minutes. In muscle there is an increase of about 1° to 2°C maximally after 30 minutes, and then follows the same drop in temperature pattern as skin and subcutaneous tissue. These findings have been corroborated by Abramson and his group and, recently, by Greenberg.

Hyperaemia. There is increased vasodilatation of the main venous channels in the skin through the opening of the arteriovenous anastomosis, by-passing the capillaries, since the main function of skin circulation is heat regulation. There is some increase in the flow of nutrients, antibodies, leucocytes, and oxygen to the tissues.

Skin blood flow increases more than twofold, and remains at a constant level for about 15 minutes. This is due to the release of histamine-like substances and *bradykinin* producing vasodilatation of the capillaries. The local reddening occurs after a 20-minute application of the packs. Blood flow to the joints is increased *reflexly*, and blood flow in distal muscles may be increased more than in proximal muscles.

Increased vasodilatation of superficial fascia and muscles is by heat conduction from the skin. Heat acts directly on muscle capillaries, and indirectly on arterioles by reflex vasodilatation. The quantity of heat generated is minimal compared with that produced by heat and exercise. Muscle circulation can be increased effectively only by exercise. Recent experiments have shown that, following hot pack and exercise, there is a total increase of blood flow, both in skin and muscle circulation, to about twice the amount that appears in exercise only, and the harder and longer the exercise, the longer-lasting is the muscle hyperaemia achieved. The amount of muscle blood flow increase is greater than that achieved by heat alone. So for a moderate increase of blood flow to muscle, heat is not necessary.

Sedative effects. Moist heat is a safe *analgesic* and a *muscle relaxant*. There are two mechanisms by which moist heat is thought to produce these effects.
(*a*)   Muscle spindle

The mechanism governing relief of muscle spasm is poorly understood. It is thought to be due to a decrease of *gamma fibre activity*, thereby decreasing muscle spindle activity via the direct effect of heat on the skin receptors. A quick warming of the spindles causes a temporary, complete inhibition of the firing of the spindles. *The central proprioceptive* mechanisms may also be affected by the reflex action of heat, since raising the body temperature causes decreased gamma activity.
(*b*)   Small myelinated 'c' nerve fibres

Heat reduces the conduction velocity of the 'c' nerve fibres. Again there are different theories of the mechanism underlying relief of pain by heat. There is thought to be some alteration in the thermal threshold of pain. Disease or injury is said to alter the thermal threshold of pain. Heat alters the temperature of the painful part, thus the pain threshold alters to new thermal limits. On the other hand metabolic, circulatory, tissue tension alterations, and the counter-irritant effect of heat, also play important parts in relieving pain.

Metabolic effects will be governed by the rate of rise, the amount of rise and subsequent fall in temperature. There is some increase in tissue metabolism, and change in rate of enzymatic activity. Hot packs over two or three areas may cause a temporary increase in sweating, dehydration and a decrease in blood pressure.

INDICATIONS FOR HYDROCOLLATOR PACKS

Pain and muscle spasm. The moist heat of the hydrocollator pack can relieve pain and muscle spasm in superficial regions. The mechanism causing relief is poorly understood. It is thought that the quick rise in temperature and alteration of the temperature of the painful area by 2° to 5°C causes reduction of nerve conduction velocity of the pain nerve fibres and raises the threshold of pain. The rise in temperature also causes increased circulation which then removes pain metabolites and thus breaks down the vicious cycle of pain and muscle spasm. The sudden rise in temperature can also create a counter-irritant effect, and thus cause a temporary relief of pain.

It must be understood clearly that the rise in temperature lasts only for about 20 to 30 minutes. If the effect of heat on pain and muscle spasm is to be utilised, the techniques of physiotherapy needed to restore range of joint movement and muscle strength must be applied immediately after the heat has been administered.

Inflammation. In cases of mild inflammation, temperature elevation of 2° to 5°C will cause an increase in phagocytosis and aid absorption of exudate. It has been used post-operatively for the healing of wounds following abdominal surgery, when there has been delayed healing with no infection, caused by mild haematomas or inflammation.

Oedema. Oedematous areas over a large section of an extremity, in chronic stages, can be treated with a hot pack in elevation to help absorption of the exudate. If the exudate is tenacious and excessive, other physical agents are more profitably utilised. The physiological mechanisms that occur are due to the increased permeability of cell membranes which cause the flow of fluid from the tissue spaces to the venous and lymphatic vessels. In oedematous areas the reverse vascular responses occur, as there is alteration of osmotic and hydrostatic pressures of the circulatory vessels.

Adhesions. Hot packs in conjunction with other physical measures such as mobilisation techniques, exercises and other measures will help to stretch adhesions and contractures of tissues. The raised temperature of the collagen will make it easier to stretch the adhesions. Again this is true only if the adhesions are placed superficially and are not tenacious.

CONTRA-INDICATIONS FOR HYDROCOLLATOR PACKS

Impaired skin sensation. This will be determined by a hot/cold skin test.

Some **dermatological conditions** are exacerbated by moist heat, such as eczema in the lower leg, athlete's foot in between the toes, and severe acne on the back. Any dermatological condition which appears after treatment must be reported.

Circulatory dysfunction. Patients with severe varicose veins, deep vein thrombosis and arterial disease must not have any heat applied directly over the part affected by circulatory disease, particularly in the limbs.

Analgesic drugs. If patients are under strong narcotics for pain, the time and dosage of the drugs must be ascertained. Heat is not administered immediately after intake of drugs, since pain tolerance to heat is impaired.

Infections and open wounds. Heat will increase the infective activity.

Cancer or tuberculosis in the area to be treated. Heat, by increasing the metabolic rate, may increase the rate of growth and spread of the disease.

Gross oedema with a very thin and delicate skin covering the area. The skin may be damaged by the pressure of the pack and the heat may tend to increase the oedema.

Lack of comprehension. Patients who cannot understand the nature of the treatment and comprehend the potential dangers, for example, children, very old patients, other nationalities.

Deep X-ray therapy within three months prior to treatment decreases blood flow in the area and may cause impaired skin sensation.

Liniments may cause hypersensitivity to heat, if applied recently. The patient should be asked to apply the liniment after a heat treatment.

ADVANTAGES

A hydrocollator pack is easy to apply, it saves time for personnel, and is efficient in heat conduction depending on area treated.

The packs are of various sizes which fit most clinical needs.

Moist heat has a more sedative effect than dry heat.

Maximal temperatures are more uniform than in electrically-heated pads.

The patient does not need much handling. The pads can be laid out ready for the patient to place on the affected part.

DISADVANTAGES

A hydrocollator pack is not easily applied around shoulders and hips.

It is somewhat heavy and should not be used on extremely sensitive patients, since it can increase discomfort.

Sometimes moist packs have a tendency to cause a skin rash.

TECHNIQUE OF APPLICATION OF HYDROCOLLATOR PACKS

Remove the pads and fill the tank three-quarters full of water. The water level should be kept slightly over the top of the pads at all times. This avoids the burning out of the heating element or scorching the packs.

Hold each pack by its loops so that its rectangular sections are horizontal and shake slightly to distribute the dry gel evenly. Place the packs in the water for 2 hours to soak. When placing them in the water, the packs must have the rectangular section facing vertically to permit the loops to stick out of the water.

Check that the thermostat is at 76° to 80°C. Switch on the machine. It takes approximately 2 hours to heat. The unit can be left plugged in for any length of time, provided the water level is maintained.

Check that the room temperature is 21° to 23°C.

Position the patient with the part to be treated relaxed and supported fully in a position which is comfortable, pain-free and accessible for pack application and maintenance.

Inspect the area to be treated for abrasions, cuts, wounds, scars, oedema and any circulatory dysfunction.

Test for hot and cold sensations.

Do not expose the patient unnecessarily. Wrap the rest of the body in order to maintain normal uniform temperature, since a change in body temperature will alter the physiological effects of the hot packs.

Explain to the patient the degree of warmth to be expected, the duration of the treatment, and the purpose of the treatment.

Ask the patient to inform you if any pain, discomfort, or burning sensation is felt during the treatment.

Remove the selected pack, holding it by the loops, and place it on a bath towel. Fold another towel into 4 to 6 layers and place it over the pack. Wrap the whole pack up with the bottom towel. The temperature of the wrapped pack should not exceed the 44°C skin tolerance. The hydrocollator pack when withdrawn from the machine should be 70° to 80°C. Higher temperatures cause discomfort.

Place the pack gently, with the folded towel side on the affected part. Maintain it in position with another towel, if necessary. Ensure that it does not exacerbate pain, produce discomfort, or occlude circulation.

Check that body weight is not occluding circulation, particularly over bony areas.

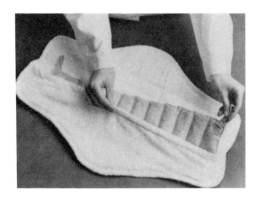

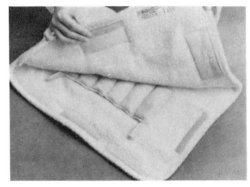

(a) Wrap pack in towels.   (b) Ensure that there are
                                                          4-6 layers.

Hydrocollator technique

Duration of treatment is usually 20 to 30 minutes. In cases of severe pain and muscle spasm as in polyneuritis the duration could be 30 to 45 minutes, but the pack must be renewed after 20 minutes.

Treatment must be given daily, particularly for the first course of treatment. The duration and frequency will be based on the acute, subacute, or chronic clinical features of the case. Subsequent courses of treatment will be based on the progress of the patient in relation to the pathology of the condition, and the assessed results of the therapy.

Remove the pack leaving the bottom towel in place. Return the pack to the machine. Dry the treated area and inspect for any signs of a burn or exacerbation of symptoms.

Proceed with other treatments as indicated.

CARE OF APPARATUS

The unit should be cleaned periodically (every month or so) with a good metal cleaner after removing the packs. If left out for an extended period of time, especially in the summer, the packs are likely to become mildewed. Cloudiness of the water in the tank is due to a slight leakage of the filler substance from the packs. This is not harmful and does not affect the packs or units in any way. The water level should be kept up to, or slightly over, the top of the packs at all times.

DANGERS AND PRECAUTIONS

Burn

A bright red patch may indicate the possibility of a burn, with blistering to follow. Burns could be caused by any of the following factors:

(*a*)   Insufficient towelling between the pack and the skin surface — part of the pack could have escaped out of the wrapping. Ensure that there is a minimum of six layers of towels well wrapped around the pack.

(*b*)   The temperature of the pack could be too high — check the thermostat of the machine.

(*c*)   Impaired skin sensation — particularly in elderly patients, who have fewer glomera to regulate heat dissipation; or in patients who have a peripheral neuropathy; or if the skin sensation test was performed inaccurately.

(*d*)   Impaired circulation due to circulatory disease, which was not detected from the case history or interview.

(*e*)   Hypersensitive skin from recent use of liniments or deep X-ray therapy.

Dehydration

If two or more areas or a large area have been heated, excessive sweating may produce some dehydration. A drink of water may help.

2.3   Hot Compresses

Hot local compresses are primarily for home use and are not practical for clinical use. The main principles of heating by the application of hydrocollator packs apply — heat by conduction, moist heat, minimal penetration. There is greater heat loss than with hydrocollator packs, and therefore the compresses have to be changed constantly.

TECHNIQUE OF APPLICATION OF HOT COMPRESSES

Equipment required

turkish towels, strips of woollen blanket or of any absorbent material
hot water at a temperature of 40° to 42°C or hot towel machine (electric)
plastic or rubber sheet
timer

Position the patient comfortably with the part to be treated fully supported.

Check the skin area to be treated.

Place a large towel in a basin with the free ends hanging out. Place a smaller towel inside the large towel. Pour hot water on to the towels, and wring them out. Make sure the towels are thoroughly wet.

Apply the towels to the desired area.

To maintain constant heat, cover the compress with a hot water bottle, or use an infrared lamp, or wrap in a blanket.

Apply the compress for 20 minutes, changing every 5 minutes.

Check the skin after the removal of the hot compress.

INDICATIONS

If hydrocollator packs are not available, hot compresses can be used as an alternative.

PRECAUTIONS IN APPLYING COMPRESSES

Make sure that the towels are wrung out properly.

Apply a compress which is only as hot as the patient can bear. If the compress is too hot, remove quickly, wipe any excess moisture from the skin and reapply.

In treating children, tolerance should be built up gradually during the first application to prevent a fear reaction by the child.

Fit the compress to the contour of the part to prevent air from entering and cooling the compress.

Avoid chilling the patient.

Have fluids ready to minimise dehydration.

2.4   Paraffin Wax

Paraffin wax for therapy is one of the most convenient, reasonably efficient methods of applying conducted heat to the extremities. Low melting point (55°C) paraffin wax is used. In order to keep the wax liquid at lower temperatures, and to prevent burns, liquid paraffin mineral oil is added to the melted wax. The paraffin wax then remains melted at a temperature of 40° to 44°C.

PHYSICAL CHARACTERISTICS OF WAX

Wax has a low thermal conductivity, and therefore it gives off heat slowly. When a part is dipped in wax and the wax allowed to set, there will be no rapid loss of heat from the treated part. The low thermal conductivity of the wax prevents the patient feeling as hot as in water of the same temperature.

The wax is self-insulating. The first layer creates a thin layer of air next to the skin (no absolute contact), which acts as an insulator.

Sweat does not evaporate and it also insulates.

After the removal of the wax, the part cools quickly.

EQUIPMENT

The wax is placed in a bath. Small baths are portable for home or ward use; larger baths are also available. Metal baths have an electric heating element with a large water jacket around the tank. A modern design from Leeds Polytechnic in collaboration with the Rheumatism Research Unit at Harrogate, England, is a bath 400 mm × 550 mm × 200 mm with a wall thickness of 25 mm, using an Isopad electric element with glass-wool thermal insulation.

The inherent advantage of the electric heating pad is that the thermal inertia of the water heating the wax is eliminated, and the initial warm-up is reduced from one hour to 30 minutes. The machine is lighter, since the heating element is placed between the outer fibreglass shell and the inner stainless steel container. The bath can be moved up and down by a load-screw driven by a handle at the top of the column. Patients can use the handle without bending. This enables patients to adjust to the right height for sitting and immersing hands or feet.

It is essential to have the bath heat unit thermostatically controlled, but one should not depend on this to determine the temperature of the melted paraffin. Thermometer readings should also be taken.

The baths vary in size and shape according to the manufacturer. However most are lined with monel metal which resists the corrosive action of perspiration. The bottom of the bath is covered with bakelite slats to prevent the patient from coming into contact with it.

OPERATION OF APPARATUS

The refined paraffin wax used has a melting point of 52° to 54°C. The paraffin wax bath has a capacity of 25 kg. To this you add 5 litres of light petrolatum oil which gives a 7:1 mixture. It lowers the melting point of the wax and thus helps to prevent a burn.

To melt the paraffin, turn the time switch one full turn. This causes the heat coils to operate continuously for one hour, which will make the paraffin melt quickly, but will raise the temperature too high for treatment purposes. If the thermostat is set properly, the temperature of the paraffin will then drop and be maintained at 40° to 44°C in 3 or 4 hours. It is important to check the temperature of the bath just before giving the treatment.

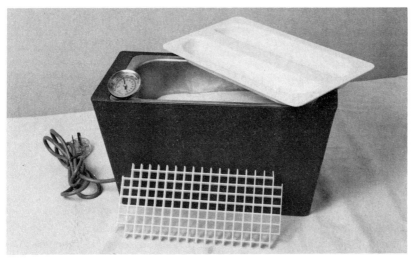

Paraffin wax bath

The paraffin bath can be plugged in day and night so that it will be ready for use at all times. The cost of continuous operation of the bath is about the same as that of a 40 watt lamp.

CARE OF APPARATUS

The part to be treated must be cleaned before putting it in the bath. Even though the bath is self-sterilising, it must be cleaned regularly, because of sediment that accumulates. In order to clean the bath, the paraffin must be liquid. Disconnect the unit from the electricity outlet. Dip the paraffin out of the bath with a small pan and pour it into another container. Remove the slats and clean them thoroughly. Now the remainder of the paraffin can be removed. The last of the paraffin and sediment may be removed with paper towels or some absorbent rags. Replace the slats, add the paraffin and plug the unit in. If the paraffin appears to cloud after it is heated, add a few ounces of oil until it clears. The complete paraffin and oil mixture should be changed every six months.

One method to keep the sediment under control has been reported by Margolin in New York. Eight thicknesses of cheese cloth are placed under the tank slats, with tapes to lower the slats into the bath. As sediment collects in large quantities, the slats and cheese cloth are removed and the slats washed.

PHYSIOLOGICAL RESPONSES TO PARAFFIN WAX THERAPY

Heat Production. There is a marked increase in *skin temperature* in the first two minutes, up to 12° to 13°C. This drops, while in the wax wrapping, to an increase of about 8°C at the end of 30 minutes. In the *subcutaneous fascia*, there is an increase of 5°C at the end of the treatment, in the *superficial muscles* there is only about 2° to 3°C rise in temperature at the end of treatment.

Circulatory effects. Stimulation of superficial capillaries and arterioles causes local hyperaemia and reflex vasodilatation. This is marked only in the region of the skin. The hyperaemia is due to the response of the skin to its function of heat regulation. The effects of vasodilatation in the muscle are negligible, but there may be some reflex heating in the joints. Skin and subcutaneous tissue temperature drops rapidly after 15 to 20 minutes, reducing vasodilatation. Exercise after wax is essential to increase muscle circulation, and to use the sedative effect of heat to obtain more range of movement and muscle strength.

Analgesic effects. The most important effect of wax is its marked sedative effect on the tissues. The moist heat is remarkably soothing to the patient. It is this effect that is utilised prior to exercise, in the treatment of superficially placed joints. It is very comfortable for the patient.

Stretching effects. Wax leaves the skin moist, soft, and pliable. This is useful for stretching scars and adhesions before applying mobilisation techniques.

INDICATIONS

Pain and muscle spasm. Wax reduces the pain and muscle spasm seen in hands and feet, as the moist heat encircles each finger and toe and relieves pain.

Oedema and inflammation. The gentle heat reduces post-traumatic swelling of the hands and feet, and also swelling in hands affected by rheumatoid arthritis or degenerative joint disease, particularly in the sub-acute and early chronic stages of inflammation.

Adhesions and scars. Wax softens the adhesions and scars in the skin and thus facilitates the mobilisation and stretching procedures.

CONTRA-INDICATIONS

Impaired skin sensation. This will be determined by a hot/cold skin test.

Some dermatological conditions are exacerbated by moist heat, such as eczema, athlete's foot, and dermatitis. Any dermatological condition which appears after treatment must be reported.

Circulatory dysfunction. Patients with varicose veins, deep vein thrombosis and arterial disease must not have any heat applied directly over the affected part.

Analgesic drugs. If patients are taking strong narcotics for pain, the time and dosage of the drugs must be ascertained. Heat is not administered immediately after intake of drugs, since pain tolerance to heat is impaired.

Infections and open wounds. Heat will increase the infective activity.

Cancer or tuberculosis in the area to be treated. Heat, by increasing the metabolic rate, may increase the rate of growth and spread of the disease.

Gross oedema with a very thin and delicate skin covering the area. The skin may be damaged and the heat may tend to increase the oedema.

Lack of comprehension. Patients who cannot understand the nature of the treatment and comprehend the potential dangers, for example, children, very old patients, other nationalities.

Deep X-ray therapy within three months prior to treatment decreases blood flow in the area and may cause impaired skin sensation.

Liniments may cause hypersensitivity to heat, if applied recently. The patient should be asked to apply the liniment after a heat treatment.

ADVANTAGES OF WAX THERAPY

Two or three patients can be treated at a time. Wax therapy is useful for patients with poor heat tolerance, and is useful for dry scaly skins, especially after removal of plaster of Paris following fractures. It can be combined with exercises which can be performed without supervision.

It is a useful modality that can be carried out at home for the chronic sufferer as in rheumatoid arthritis.

Wax can be moulded around the bony contours of hands and feet to apply heat evenly by conduction.

DISADVANTAGES OF WAX THERAPY

Sedimentation occurs at the bottom of the bath. The bath must be cleaned regularly and emptied at least twice a year. Contamination of the oil by atmospheric dust may occur unless it is covered by the lid when not in use.

Water tends to collect at the bottom of the bath.

TECHNIQUES OF APPLICATION OF PARAFFIN WAX

Technique I
Read the diagnosis and prescribed treatment carefully.

Explain the procedure to the patient and tell him what he may expect — warmth, tingling, and a drawing sensation in the fingers.

Check the contraindications and assess the patient's major signs and symptoms prior to treatment.

Skin test over the entire area to be treated, using hot and cold test tubes.

Check the temperature of the paraffin. It should be between 40° and 44°C on the thermometer, but as this may be inaccurate, test the wax by dipping a finger. Show this to the patient as a demonstration of the wax.

Inspect the part to be treated for cuts, scratches, rash, or infection.

Instruct the patient to wash and *thoroughly dry* the part to be treated. Remove any jewellery.

Position the patient and instruct him to dip the part in and out of the paraffin so that a thick coat of paraffin congeals on the skin. Repeat this 10 times. If treating a hand, instruct the patient to keep the fingers separated and caution him not to move them, thus avoiding breaking the paraffin glove. Remind the patient to dip the part to the same level each time, thus preventing fresh paraffin from entering the glove. Under this coating the skin sweats, and the resultant vapor, plus the enclosed air, acts as an insulator and prevents burning of the skin.

Warn the patient of the dangers of wax.

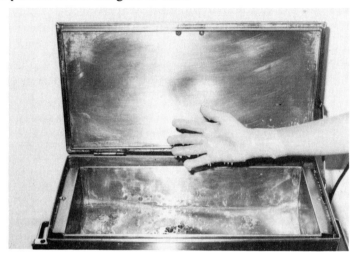

Immersion of hand in wax

Wrap the part in a layer of greaseproof paper and towels to help retain the heat.

Set a timer. Treatments are usually from 15 to 30 minutes.

When the treatment is completed, remove the towels carefully so that paraffin will not fall to the floor.

Remove the paraffin glove by loosening the top, then rolling the paraffin down towards the distal end of the extremity.

Inspect and dry the part treated. The skin should appear pink, soft, and pliable.

There should not be any excessive erythema, indicative of a burn. Assess for relief of symptoms.

Continue with other forms of treatment, a home program and record the treatment given and its effect.

Tidy the area and prepare for the next patient.

The paraffin glove, after removal, is deposited in a special container. At the end of the day, the paraffin in the container is melted, strained, and placed back in the paraffin bath.

Technique II

Dip and form a thin glove, and then keep the part immersed in the wax bath for a further period of 15 to 20 minutes. This will produce more heat in the tissues as a temperature gradient from the paraffin to the tissue is maintained at about 44°C.

Excessive heating is prevented by the solid layer of paraffin which has a low heat conductivity and retards the rate of heat flow.

Technique III

After dipping and immersion as in Technique II, place the part in a heat cabinet at 70°C, or place under an infrared lamp at a distance of 0.5 m.

Technique IV

Dip and form a coat twice and then immerse for 15 minutes. Remove the hand and place in a tray containing semi-liquid paraffin, and give the patient exercises for 20 minutes making shapes out of the solidifying wax.

Technique V

If oedema is present, after using Technique I place the hand in elevation under a hot air cabinet. Alternatively the hand may be kept in elevation wrapped in a blanket or towel for 20 minutes.

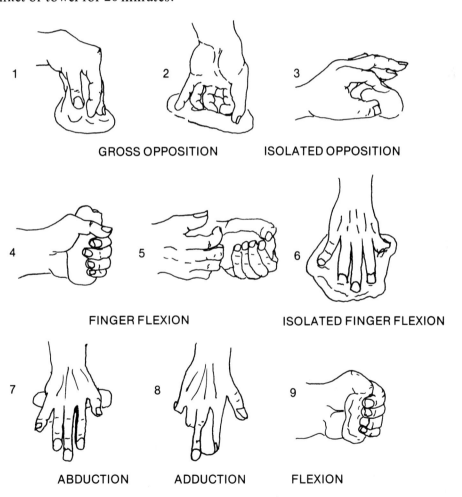

Paraffin wax technique IV

Paraffin wax technique

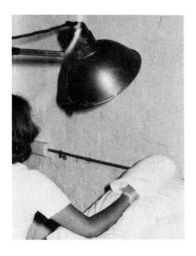

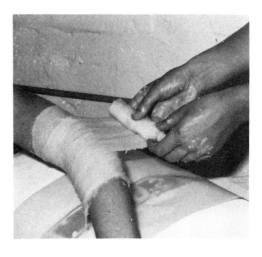

(*a*) technique III   (*b*) technique VI

Technique VI
Wax therapy to the knees and elbows may be given by applying around the joints elasto-crepe bandages which have been immersed in wax, and then further brushing more wax on the bandages using a paint brush. This technique is useful if the patient cannot tolerate dry heat and hydrocollator packs are not available.

Analysis of techniques
In Technique I there is a marked drop in temperature even before the covering is removed, and it is debatable whether wrapping is worthwhile. Technique V is useful for oedematous hands, with dry scaly skin. Technique VI has limited use, as there is insufficient rise in temperature, and it is useful only as a home technique. Techniques II, III, and IV are more useful. In II and III the temperature rise is maintained for a longer period.

2.5   Peloids — Mud Packs and Peat Packs

Peloids are mud and peat packs grouped together. They may be used as local packs or as immersion baths. Mud packs come from natural sources containing sulfur, iron, and silicates. Mineral sea mud contains the remains of sea life. Organic moor-peat contains decaying vegetable matter. The specific properties of mud and peat packs are attributed not to their chemical properties, but to their use as a source of conductive heat. The pressure of the peloid can help to stretch adhesions around joints, but there is a danger of impeding the venous circulation and of causing irritation of the skin due to its chemical composition.

METHOD OF APPLICATION OF PELOIDS

Peloids are heated to a temperature of 45° to 48°C and, enclosed in a cotton bag, are placed on the affected part. Since the peloids are poor conductors of heat, so application using a higher temperature is possible. If water is used in a mixture with mud or peat, the mixture is spread evenly on a cloth, and tested for the desired temperature. It is then placed on the body, moulded around the part, covered with plastic and a blanket and left for 20 minutes.

Remove the pack and sponge or spray with water. Rewrap the part until the patient has cooled down. The first treatment is at a temperature of 42°C, with successive treatments at 48°C.

The physiological effects are the same as with hydrocollator packs, plus the mechanical pressure responses causing stretching of adhesions and reabsorption of exudate.

INDICATIONS

Peloids have no advantage over hydrocollator packs or paraffin wax, but are often used for chronic osteoarthritis and rheumatoid arthritis, and any chronic post-traumatic joint stiffness.

CONTRA-INDICATIONS

Heart and kidney disease.
High blood pressure.
Vascular insufficiency.
Tuberculosis.
Acute inflammation.

2.6   Hot Air Baths

Hot air baths are small tunnels fitted with a hot air fan heater. The air temperature is kept at 70° to 80°C. They are mainly useful for traumatic injuries of the hands.

METHOD OF APPLICATION

The hand is kept in the hot air cabinet in elevation, and the patient can be given specific exercises to be done in the tunnel. It is a useful form of heat for the crushed hand with open injuries, joint stiffness and contractures. It is sedative in action, with some hyperaemia of the skin.

2.7   Contrast Baths

Contrast baths are an alternative method of applying heat with a certain amount of control to aid the normal body temperature-regulating mechanism. There is alternate immersion of the part in hot and cold water.

METHOD OF APPLICATION

Fill two baths of a suitable size, depending on the limb to be treated, one with hot water at 40° to 45°C, and the other with cold water at 15°C. The treatment should begin and end with hot water. Some therapists prefer to end with cold

water. Place the limb in hot water for 3 minutes. Immediately afterwards place
the limb in cold water for 1 minute. Repeat the cycle up to three times. Maintain
the hot and cold water at a constant temperature. The whole procedure should
not take more than 15 minutes.

PHYSIOLOGICAL EFFECTS

Marked vasodilatation occurs immediately. The skin temperature increases
rapidly. An increase of deeper circulation occurs reflexly. There is also a marked
sedative effect.

INDICATIONS

Post-traumatic swelling.
Pain due to swelling.
Chronic inflammation.

CONTRA-INDICATIONS

Advanced peripheral vascular disease.
Arterial insufficiency.
Diabetes.

2.8   Electric Heating Pad

Electric pads of various sizes are produced commercially. They are constructed
with a series of resistors to control the temperature produced by a heating
element wire surrounded by asbestos, cotton, or plastic covering.

2.9   Summary of Conductive and Convective Heating

The use of conductive heating by means of steam packs, paraffin wax baths and
contrast baths is a cheap, quick, and effective way of providing moist heat to
alleviate pain, muscle spasm and inflammation in restricted areas. Most forms of
conductive heating are similar in their action.

It is important to judge the biological effects of conductive heating by considering the several variables that govern the quantity of heat exchanged as well
as the rate of heat exchange, the temperature of the heat and source and body, the
specific heat of the tissues dissipating or absorbing the heat, the thermal conductivity of the tissues in the heat pathway, the time radiated, the existing
pathophysiology of the tissues, and the ability of the tissues to dissipate heat.

Thus some forms of conductive heating are more efficient, easier to use, or
more comfortable for the patient. The maximum safe exposure is at a temperature of 44°C, provided the mechanisms for heat dissipation are intact. Total
maximum depth of penetration is only to dermis level. Superficial tissues and
muscles only are heated to a maximum of 5°C rise for a varying period of 10 to
30 minutes following removal of the heat source.

Most fluids decrease in density with increased temperature. The density of
water at 10°C is 0.9997 and at 50°C is 0.9881 grams per millilitre. In a fluid of
non-uniform temperature where the colder portion is above the hotter portion, an
unstable situation occurs, and the colder fluid sinks, displacing the warmer fluid

which moves upwards. The fluid motion is called a *convection current*, and is seen in most hot water heating systems.

Heat is transmitted by movement in mass in a liquid or a gas. Convection involves the transfer of heat between a surface and a flow of hot fluid moving past the surface. The transfer of heat is by conduction from the molecular layer of fluid immediately on the surface, and the subsequent layers of molecules moving rapidly in respect to the surface.

Therapeutic devices include whirlpool baths, moist air baths, and hot air baths.

The physiological effects are similar to conductive heating, but are stronger.

References

Downey, J, Darling, R and Miller, J, 1968, The effects of heat, cold and exercise on the peripheral circulation, *Arch Phys Med*.

Halswell, M, 1969, Moist heat for relief of post-operative pain, *American J of Nursing, 67*, 4.

Harris, E D and McCroskery, P A, 1974, The influence of temperature on degradation of collagen by rheumatoidal synovial collagenase, *The New England J of Med*.

Krusen, Kottke and Ellwood, Handbook of physical medicine, Chapter 10.

Licht, Sidney (Ed), 1965, Therapeutic heat and cold, *Maryland: Waverley Press*.

Tuck, S, Chu, L S, and Augustin, C, 1964, Effects of paraffin bath and hot fomentations on local tissue temperatures, *Arch Phys Med, 45*, 87.

Whyte, H M and Reader, S R, 1951, Effectiveness of different forms of heating, *Ann Rheum Diseases, 10*, 449.

3 Conversive Heating

Some Key Points in this Unit

Conversive heating is relatively uniform heating produced by the conversion into heat of electrostatic or electromagnetic fields within the tissues.

An **electrostatic field** is set up between two electrodes by the application of a current to the electrodes.

An **electromagnetic field** is set up around the loops of a coil through which a current is passing.

A **condenser**, or capacitor, consists of two metal plates separated by an insulator. It has the ability to store a charge, and therefore store electrical energy.

A **dielectric** is the insulating or non-conducting material between the two plates of a condenser.

The **condenser-field method** of short wave diathermy uses the patient in the circuit as part of a condenser, so that an electrostatic field is set up in the tissues.

Short wave diathermy is a means of producing therapeutic heat in the tissues by the use of radio waves of high frequency.

Inductothermy is a method of applying short wave diathermy where the patient's tissues are placed in the electromagnetic and electrostatic fields created when a high frequency alternating current is passed through a coil.

Microwave diathermy is a means of producing therapeutic heat in the tissues by the absorption and conversion of electromagnetic radiations in the microwave band of frequencies.

A **magnetron** is a diode valve with a cathode and multisplit anode which produces the high frequency current required for the production of microwaves.

A **transducer** (director) consists of an antenna from which the microwaves are produced, and a reflector which focuses the microwaves and directs them towards the tissues.

Radiation is the process of propagating energy through matter or vacuum.

A ray is a beam of radiant energy.

Infrared radiation consists of electromagnetic waves with wavelengths from 770 nm to 15 000 nm.

Short infrared radiations extend from 770 nm to 4000 nm. They are also known as 'near infrared'.

Long infrared radiations extend from 4000 nm to 15 000 nm. They are also known as 'far infrared'.

3.1   Short Wave Diathermy

PHYSICS OF SHORT WAVE DIATHERMY

Production of short wave diathermy. Radio waves in the short wave band have frequencies in the range 10 MHz to 100 MHz. The short wave diathermy machines used by physiotherapists utilise the frequency of 27.12 MHz, with a wavelength greater than 11 m. Two main circuits are used:

(*a*)   the machine circuit, which produces the high frequency current, and amplifies its intensity;

(*b*)   the patient circuit, which is coupled to the machine circuit by inductors, and transfers the electrical energy to the patient in the form of an electrostatic or electromagnetic field.

The electrostatic field. In the condenser-field method, the electrostatic field is created by including the patient's tissues in the patient circuit as part of a condenser. Two electrodes are applied to the part, with spacing between the electrode and the skin, so that the electrodes are the condenser plates, and the patient's tissues together with the spacing are the dielectric of the condenser.

The high frequency alternating current is applied to the electrodes. The electric field, which exists around any charged object, is then concentrated between the two electrodes. As the patient's tissues lie between the two electrodes, the field will be concentrated in the tissues.

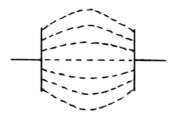

Electrostatic field

The electromagnetic field. In the inductothermy method, the electrode used is a thick insulated cable which completes the circuit from the machine. The cable is coiled in close relationship to the tissues, but separated from them by spacing.

As the high frequency current alternates in the cable, an electromagnetic field is set up around the centre of the cable, while an electrostatic field is set up between its ends. Because of the proximity of the patient's tissues, the two fields will be concentrated in the tissues.

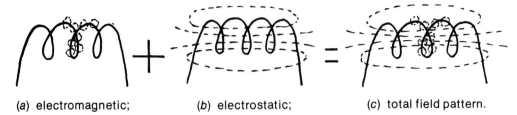

(a) electromagnetic;   (b) electrostatic;   (c) total field pattern.

Fields produced by an inductothermy cable

BIOPHYSICAL AND BIOCHEMICAL EFFECTS OF SHORT WAVE DIATHERMY

The basic events which take place when short wave diathermy is applied to the tissues occur as a result of the effects of the electric field on the tissue particles.

Effects of an electrostatic field. The *free ions* in the tissue fluid move backwards and forwards along the lines of force of the field as the charge alternates on the condenser plates. Because the charge alternates at a high frequency, the movement is minimal and may be termed a vibration of the ions. As a result of the vibration, friction occurs between ions, and the result of the friction is the production of heat in the tissue.

The *dipolar molecules* in the tissue, such as water molecules, will orient themselves towards the opposite charge on the condenser plates. As the charge is changing rapidly, a rotation of the dipoles will occur. As the molecules are coupled loosely with each other, a friction between molecules will occur, resulting in the production of heat in the tissue.

The *non-polar molecules* in the tissue, such as fat, undergo distortion of their electron cloud. As the field is alternating rapidly, the electron clouds oscillate back and forth. Minimal friction and molecular movement occur, so little heat is produced.

Effects of an electromagnetic field. The electromagnetic field produces eddy currents, which are circular currents at right angles to the lines of force. They tend to be more concentrated near the surface of the conductor, that is, in the superficial tissues. The friction of the tissue particles produced by these currents, and by the associated electrostatic field, results in the production of heat.

Heat production. The only proven physical effect of short wave diathermy is the production of heat as a result of the effects of the electrostatic and/or electromagnetic field set up in the tissues. Heat will be produced in all tissues affected by the field, but will be concentrated in the tissues of low resistance, such as those of high fluid content (blood and muscle). Very little heat will be produced in tissues of high resistance, such as fat and bone. Some heat will also be conducted to adjacent areas of lower temperature.

Physiological responses to the application of short wave diathermy depend upon the reactions of the tissues to temperature rise. Temperature regulation is a function of cardiovascular, hormonal and nervous control.

Heat applied to the skin (in a restricted area) results in an increased blood flow in the skin, which helps to distribute the heat to other areas. This increase in circulation is accompanied by vasodilatation. The mechanism of these changes applies also to short wave diathermy.

Mild heat produces reflex reduction of muscle tone. It is suggested that increased muscle blood flow plays some part in this mechanism, along with removal of the trigger irritation. Muscle spasm is probably an increased proprioceptor reflex mechanism, and the muscle spindles are the receptor end-organs for this reflex. As it has been shown that temperature increase at the muscle spindle decreases, and in some cases inhibits, the firing of the spindles, this may also contribute to the decrease in muscle spasm produced.

When the temperature at a nerve, or in subcutaneous tissues with a high proportion of cutaneous nerve fibres is elevated to above 45°C, then neural stimulation resulting in various reactions, and blood pressure and vascular responses, are seen.

Mild heating causes an analgesic effect in the underlying tissues, though the mechanism of the effect is not understood.

THERAPEUTIC EFFECTS OF SHORT WAVE DIATHERMY

The therapeutic effects of short wave diathermy may be used for the treatment of deep as well as superficial structures. The size of the lesion need not negate the selection of short wave diathermy as the method of treatment.

Pain. The relief of pain by short wave diathermy is useful in the treatment of traumatic and rheumatic conditions affecting muscles, ligaments, and joints. Relief of pain may also be helped by the relief of associated muscle spasm.

Muscle spasm may be reduced directly by short wave diathermy, or may be reduced by relieving the pain which contributes to it.

Inflammation. Resolution of chronic inflammation may be accelerated by treatment with short wave diathermy as a result of the increase in blood supply. This increases venous return from the area and aids the resorption of the oedema exudate.

Delayed healing. To promote the healing of open skin areas, an increase in the cutaneous circulation may be of assistance, provided the vascular responses to heat are normal. If the arteriolar and capillary dilatation do not allow sufficient increase in blood flow, heat should not be applied directly but may be applied proximally to an area with a good blood supply. This is done in an attempt to achieve reflex vasodilatation in the required area.

Infection. Treatment with short wave diathermy may assist in the control of chronic infection by increasing the circulation. This will increase the number of white blood cells and antibodies brought to the area to fight the infective organism, reinforcing the body's normal defence mechanism.

Fibrosis. Heat has been found to increase the extensibility of fibrous tissues, such as tendons, joint capsules, and scars, by from 5 to 10 times. The effect is produced by temperature increase within the therapeutic range.

DOSAGE

Duration of treatment. It is accepted that 20 minutes is the optimum treatment time as the tissue temperature will usually reach a 'steady state' in this time, and the increase in circulation will have reached its maximum. Shorter durations will not achieve maximum physiological effects, though they may be useful as a test dose to ascertain whether there are any untoward effects of short wave diathermy.

Intensity of short wave diathermy. The only safe measure of the intensity of treatment is the sensation of warmth described by the patient. The patient should feel no more than 'a mild, comfortable warmth' — anything hotter than this could result in the development of a burn.

Although most machines have a power output control, the power reading does not give any indication of the level of temperature increase in the tissues, as it cannot adjust for variations in the tissues included within the short wave diathermy field.

Care must be taken when increasing the intensity of short wave diathermy, as heat is not produced instantaneously. Two to three minutes on each intensity setting should be allowed for the heat to build up to the maximum for that setting. Only then, if the heat felt by the patient is not at the therapeutic level, should the intensity be increased to the next setting.

Frequency of treatment. Treatments may be given daily or on alternate days as indicated. The factors which determine the frequency of treatment include the response to treatment and the availability of the patient for treatment. Ideally treatment would be most beneficial if given once or twice each day.

INDICATIONS

Short wave diathermy may be indicated for the treatment of both deep and superficial structures.

In summary, short wave diathermy could be indicated for the treatment of:

disorders of the musculo-skeletal system
sprains
strains
muscle and tendon tears
capsule lesions
degenerative joint disease
chronic rheumatoid arthritis
joint stiffness
haematoma

chronic inflammatory or infective conditions
tenosynovitis
bursitis
synovitis
infected surgical incisions
carbuncles
abscesses
sinusitis
dysmenorrhoea

CONTRA-INDICATIONS

The contra-indications, as distinct from precautions, for short wave diathermy are specified as follows:

Over malignant tissues. The increase in metabolism resulting from the increase in temperature would accelerate the rate of growth and metastasis of the malignancy.

Over ischaemic tissues. The inability of the circulation to disperse the heat could result in temperature elevation to a level which would produce tissue destruction (burn). Also the inability of the circulation to provide the increased oxygen required by the resultant increase in metabolism could result in the development of gangrene.

Moderate and excessive oedema. Non-inflammatory oedema is particularly likely to be aggravated by the administration of any form of heat.

Over wet dressings and adhesive tape. Short wave diathermy will be more readily absorbed and a burn or scald could result.

Metallic implants. Any metal within the field of the short wave diathermy application will concentrate the field and result in the production of temperatures in the destructive range in adjacent tissues.

Pacemakers. The high frequency of short wave diathermy has been shown to interfere with or even inhibit the function of some pacemakers. Therefore it is advisable not to use short wave diathermy in the presence of any pacemaker, as the type is not always known.

Haemorrhagic areas. The increase in circulation will increase the degree of haemorrhage or precipitate haemorrhage in unstable situations, for example haemophilia.

Tuberculous joints. The increase in temperature will increase the rate of development of the infection, and therefore increase the possibility of joint damage.

Impaired thermal sensation. As the application of a safe level of intensity requires that the patient reports the degree of heat felt, disturbance or loss of thermal sensation could result in high intensities being applied with consequent tissue destruction.

Unreliable patients. For example, very old or very young patients, whose co-operation in monitoring the administration of the level of intensity cannot be guaranteed.

Recent radiotherapy. For a period of up to three months following therapeutic doses of radiotherapy, skin sensation and circulation may be diminished.

Hypersensitivity to heat. Particularly where liniment has been applied, the circulation is already increased by the action of the liniment and may be unable to increase sufficiently further to disperse heat applied.

Acute infection or inflammation. The process is likely to be exacerbated by the application of heat.

Analgesic therapy. If the patient has recently (within the last few hours) taken any analgesic drugs, the thermal sensation may be diminished.

Venous thrombosis or phlebitis. The increase in circulation produced by the heat may dislodge clots.

Pregnancy. Short wave to the pelvis may induce haemorrhage or miscarriage.

Menstruation. Short wave to the pelvis will increase the rate of flow (haemorrhage).

Dermatological conditions. These may be exacerbated by the heat.

Severe cardiac conditions. Heating may require an increase in cardiac output which the diseased heart is unable to produce.

Blood pressure abnormalities. These may be exacerbated by the application of heat to a large area.

TECHNIQUES OF SHORT WAVE DIATHERMY

An advantage of short wave diathermy is its versatility. The variations in the applications available are related to the variations in the field distribution which may be produced.

Six main variations in electrodes are commonly available.

Flexible pads consist of the metal electrode encased in rubber. They are generally available in a variety of sizes. Flexible pads are moderately flexible to allow the electrode to be shaped to the part being treated. They produce an electrostatic field.

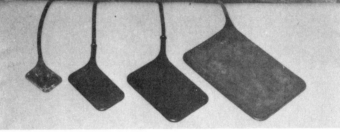

Flexible pads

Space plates consist of a rigid metal electrode encased in a perspex cover. They are generally available in a variety of sizes. The position of the electrode within the cover is usually adjustable. Space plates produce an electrostatic field.

Coil. The coil, or cable, electrode consists of a thickly insulated wire with plugs at either end. It is generally supplied together with wooden or plastic spacers to maintain the position of the coils once they are applied to the part. The coil produces primarily an electromagnetic field.

The **monode** consists of a flat, rigid coil encased in a perspex cover. As it produces primarily an electromagnetic field, it is only suitable for the treatment of superficial lesions.

The **minode** consists of a conical, rigid coil encased in a perspex cover. As it produces primarily an electromagnetic field, it is only suitable for the treatment of superficial lesions.

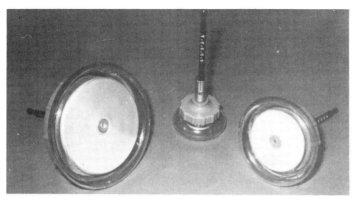

Space plates

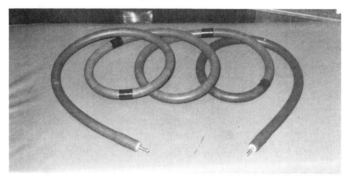

Coil

The **diplode,** or drum electrode, consists of a flat coil electrode encased in a perspex cover with two wings which are attached to a central bar by hinges, allowing adjustment of the angle of each wing independently. It produces an electromagnetic field.

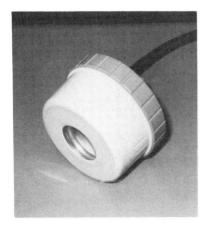

Monode

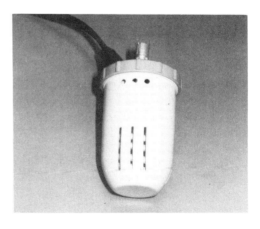

Minode

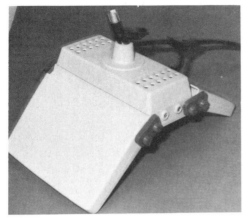
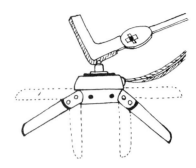

Diplode

FACTORS INFLUENCING FIELD DISTRIBUTION IN SHORT WAVE DIATHERMY

(*a*) **Spacing** allows the lines of force in the electrostatic field to diverge before entering the tissues. This prevents concentration of the heat in the superficial tissues and ensures more even heating through the part. Spacing may be provided by wrapping flexible pads in towelling or by placing felt spacing pads between the pad electrode and the skin. When space plates are used, they are positioned at a distance from the skin so that the air between the skin and the metal electrode provides the spacing.

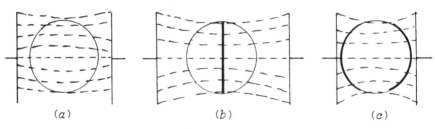

Effects of spacing
(*a*) normal spacing — even field distribution
(*b*) increased spacing — deep field concentration
(*c*) decreased spacing — superficial field concentration

(*a*) **Metal** causes the lines of force to concentrate in the metal, as it has a lower resistance than human tissues. This concentration of the lines of force will result in burning of adjacent tissues.

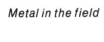
Metal in the field

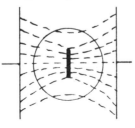

Air in the field

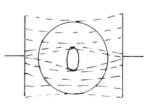

(c)   **Air in cavities,** such as the sinuses or the uterus, causes the lines of force to deviate to avoid the air as it offers a high resistance. As a result only the sides of an air-filled cavity will be heated in a single application.

(d)   **Electrode size** in relation to the size of the area to be treated can be varied to produce different heating patterns in the tissues. For example, if the electrodes are *smaller* than the diameter of the limb to be treated, the lines of force will be concentrated superficially, producing greater heat in those tissues. If the electrodes are *markedly larger* than the diameter of the limb to be treated, some of the lines of force will travel through the air and their effects will therefore be lost. Ideally the electrodes should be *slightly larger* than the diameter of the limb to be treated, ensuring even distribution of the lines of force, and thus of the tissue heating, throughout the tissues.

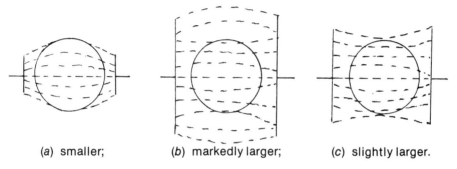

(a) smaller;   (b) markedly larger;   (c) slightly larger.

Effects of electrode size on field distribution

THERAPEUTIC VARIATIONS IN FIELD DISTRIBUTION

(a)   **Applications using two flexible pads or two space plates**

(i) 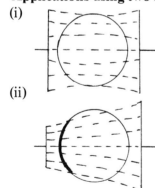 To produce even heating through the tissues, the electrodes should be slightly larger than the diameter of the part, and evenly spaced approximately 25 mm from the skin.

(ii) To concentrate the heat on one aspect of the part, the electrodes should be unequal in size. The smaller one should be placed over the area where concentration of the heat is required, and both electrodes should be evenly spaced approximately 25 mm from the skin.

(iii) 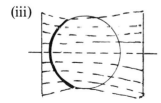 Another method of producing concentration of heating is to apply electrodes of equal size, slightly larger than the part, but to use uneven spacing. Spacing of 25 mm should be used over the aspect where concentration is required, and spacing of greater than 30 mm on the other electrode.

(iv)

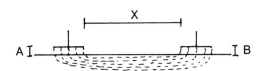

Coplanar applications of short wave diathermy may be used to treat structures on one aspect of the body. The field distribution will be concentrated in the superficial tissues, particularly if minimum (25 mm) spacing is used. Some increase in the depth of heating may be achieved by increasing the amount of spacing used. In this application it is essential that the distance between the adjacent edges of the electrodes (X) must be greater than the sum of the skin-electrode distance (A + B), otherwise the lines of force will pass directly between the electrodes rather than through the tissues.

(*b*)   Applications using a combination of flexible pad and space plate
The applications previously described are suitable for the combination of a flexible pad and a space plate, although the coplanar application is rarely used with this combination.

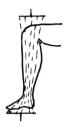

An additional application, particularly useful for treatment of disorders of the ankle, uses a space plate over the top of the knee and a flexible pad under the sole of the foot. Because there is less soft tissue around the ankle joint than elsewhere in the lower leg, the lines of force concentrate at the ankle and the sensation of heat is felt by the patient only in that region.

(*c*)   Applications using a coil electrode
(i)

The most commonly used application is that with the coil wound evenly and firmly around the limb. This application primarily heats the superficial tissues.

(ii)

In some instances a pancake application of a coil may be useful for the treatment of superficial tissues. The coil is wound into a flat pancake which is placed over the area to be treated, producing heat superficially. The advent of the monode and the minode has replaced the use of this application.

(d) Applications using a flexible pad and a coil

(i)

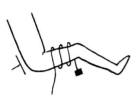

This application is useful for the treatment of a hip or shoulder joint, when pain or a flexion contracture prevents the use of flexible pads or space plates. To localise the heating to the joint, the proximal end of the cable is attached to the machine, together with the flexible pad, and the other end of the cable is insulated. An electrostatic field is produced between the pad and the proximal loop of the coil, and an electromagnetic field is produced around the proximal loops of the coil.

(ii)

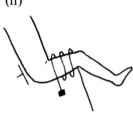

Alternatively, for the treatment of a problem in the hip with referred pain down the thigh, or of a problem in the shoulder with referred pain down the upper arm, the distal end of the cable is attached to the machine and the proximal end of the cable is insulated. An electrostatic field is produced between the pad and the proximal loop of the coil, and an electromagnetic field is produced around all loops of the coil.

(e) Applications using the diplode

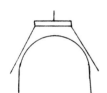

The adjustable wings of the diplode are positioned parallel to the skin of the area to be treated. The effects are those of an electromagnetic field in the superficial tissues.

(f) Application to two limbs

Two knees

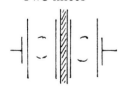

Two flexible pads, two space plates, or a flexible pad with a space plate may be used to treat, for example, both knees or both hands together. It is essential that a thin pad of towelling be placed between the two limbs to absorb any perspiration produced and prevent scalding.

Two hands

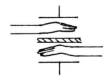

(g) Cross-fire applications

(i)

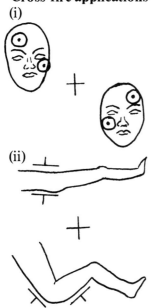

For the treatment of the sinuses, space plates are positioned diagonally over the face, one over the frontal sinus and the other over the opposite maxillary sinus, and after half of the treatment time has elapsed the positions are alternated. This ensures that all aspects of the sinus membrane are heated. Care must be taken to avoid direct placement over the eye.

(ii)

For the treatment of uterine disorders, such as dysmenorrhoea, two applications are used. In the first, two flexible pads or a flexible pad and a space plate are applied anteriorly and posteriorly over the lower abdominal region. In the second, after half of the treatment time has elapsed, two flexible pads are applied, one over the lumbar region and the other over the perineum. This ensures that all aspects of the uterine walls are heated.

DANGERS AND PRECAUTIONS IN SHORT WAVE DIATHERMY

Burns. The greatest potential danger associated with the application of short wave diathermy is that of producing a burn. Therefore the following precautions must be taken in order to avoid such an occurrence:

(*a*) Thoroughly check all *contra-indications* by examining the patient's case history, the area to be treated, and by questioning the patient.

(*b*) A test of *thermal skin sensation* must always be performed.

(*c*) Care must be taken if short wave is to be given over *bony prominences*, as heating will be greater due to the reduced depth of tissue and the heat will be less quickly dispersed as blood flow over bony prominences tends to be less than over muscle tissue. Therefore, if possible, bony prominences should be avoided, or the electrode should be positioned at a greater distance from the skin.

(*d*) *Never* apply short wave over *clothing*, as it will inhibit heat loss from the skin, resulting in excessive heating. In particular, nylon will retain perspiration, resulting in a scald.

(*e*) Ensure that the skin is *dry*. If space plates are being used, watch for any sweat production during treatment. With flexible pad applications, the towelling or felt spacing will absorb any sweat produced.

(*f*) If two skin surfaces are *in contact within the area* which will be affected by the application, they must be separated by a layer of absorbent material, such as towelling or cotton wool, to absorb any perspiration produced, or a scald may result. Common problem areas include the axilla, and between the fingers and toes.

(g)   Care must be taken to ensure that the leads from the machine to the electrodes are not *touching, or within 25 mm* of any part of the patient, the machine or any other conducting material such as metal. An electromagnetic field is produced around the leads which would result in a burn if near the patient, or breakdown of the insulation and a short circuit if near the machine or any other conductor.

(h)   Always apply the electrodes in such a way as to make sure that an *even pattern of heating* will occur.

(i)   Ensure that there is *adequate spacing* between the electrodes and the skin, and fix the electrodes firmly to avoid the risk of electrode contact with the skin.

(j)   Care must be taken to allow *2 to 3 minutes* on each intensity setting so that maximum heat production for that setting is obtained before increasing to the next intensity setting.

(k)   Never resonate the machine on any setting other than the minimum intensity setting.

Shock. The danger of electrical shock is present in the use of short wave diathermy. In this case both the patient and the therapist are potentially at risk. The following precautions must be taken to prevent this occurrence:

(a)   *Do not increase the intensity* unless the leads and electrodes are correctly connected to the machine.

(b)   Ensure that the machine is *correctly earthed.*

(c)   *Do not touch*, or allow the patient to touch, the machine if you are earthed, for example, by also touching another machine which is switched on, or touching a water pipe.

Other precautions which must be taken include:

(a)   Ensure that there is *no metal* within a range of 300 mm of the application as this will distract the field.

(b)   If the patient is wearing a *hearing aid*, it should be switched off, as the high frequency of short wave diathermy produces marked interference.

CONDENSER-FIELD APPLICATION OF SHORT WAVE DIATHERMY

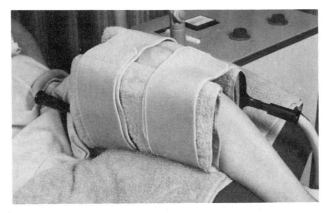

Condenser-field application to the knee using two flexible pad electrodes

Condenser-field applications make use of two flexible pads, two space plates, or a flexible pad and a space plate. An electrostatic field is set up in the tissues to produce heating. The following principles apply to all condenser-field applications:

Equipment required
short wave diathermy unit
electrodes and leads
towelling or felt pads for spacing
test tubes (for skin test) pillows and sheets

The patient should be settled in a position of optimum comfort and support, which allows the area to be treated to be fully exposed.

Explain the procedure to the patient.

Ascertain that there are no *contra-indications* to treatment with short wave diathermy.

Inspect the area to be treated and *palpate* carefully to locate the site of the lesion.

Skin-test the area to be treated for discrimination between hot and cold, using two test tubes, one filled with hot water, the other with cold water.

Select suitable electrodes for the application which would be most effective for the treatment of the patient's problem.

Ensure that there is no metal or moisture within the area to be treated or within 300 mm of the area, for example hairpins or jewellery.

If using flexible pad electrodes, wrap them in several layers of towelling, or place them between felt pads to ensure the required amount of spacing. The minimum safe amount of spacing is 25 mm. It will be necessary to use extra spacing if the electrode is to be placed under any part of the patient, as the amount of spacing will be reduced by the compression of the patient's body weight. Ensure that no part of the pad is protruding from the spacing, and that the pad is firmly encased to prevent it from slipping.

If using space plates, adjust the position of the electrodes within the covers to provide part of the required spacing. The remainder of the spacing will be provided by the air space between the tissues and the outside of the cover.

Test that the machine is operating by placing your hand between the electrodes, resonating the machine and feeling the heat produced. This also serves as a demonstration for the patient.

Position the electrodes according to the application selected, and attach the leads to the machine. In some applications using flexible pads, the electrodes will need to be bound on to prevent them from moving once the machine has been switched on.

Recheck the application —
Is there sufficient spacing?
Are the electrodes positioned so that the treatment will be effective and accurate, without producing unwanted concentration of heating?
Is the patient comfortable and unlikely to move once the machine is switched on?
Are any of the leads touching or within 25 mm of any part of the patient, the machine, or any other conductor?

Check that the machine controls are at zero, then switch the power on at the mains.

Instruct the patient not to move, to avoid touching any part of the machine or the application, and to call out if concerned. If the machine has a patient safety switch, instruct the patient to switch the machine off and call out if concerned.

Warn the patient that he should feel a mild, comfortable warmth and no more, or a *burn* could result. *Note:* The word *burn* must, medico-legally, be used in the warning.

Switch the intensity control to the standby position. If the machine has a separate power switch, this must also be switched on. Most modern machines require only 30 seconds to warm up prior to use.

Turn on the timer to the required treatment time. As there is a circuit breaker on the timer, short wave diathermy cannot be produced unless the timer is switched on.

Turn the intensity control to the *lowest intensity setting*. Never resonate the machine on a higher setting, or the patient could receive a burn.

Adjust the resonator control manually, to adjust a variable condenser, to resonate (or tune) the machine circuit with the patient circuit, ensuring maximum power output to the patient circuit. This will be indicated by either:

(*a*)   an indicator light coming on;

(*b*)   an indicator light changing color;

(*c*)   a power output meter. In this case the machine should be tuned so that the needle reaches and maintains the highest possible setting for the application (similar to a radio tuning meter).

If the machine has an automatic resonator control, it will automatically search and select the adjustment of the variable condenser to ensure maximum power output to the patient circuit.

Wait 2 to 3 minutes on the minimum intensity setting, and ask the patient to describe any sensation of warmth felt. If necessary, increase to the next intensity, waiting a further 2 to 3 minutes before making another increase, until the patient describes the sensation as a *mild, comfortable warmth*.

Once the therapeutic intensity has been reached, adjust the timer to the required treatment time.

After the treatment time has elapsed, the timer automatically cuts out the patient circuit, returning the machine to standby. Return the intensity control to zero.

Remove the application and *inspect* the area treated.

Allow the patient to leave after a brief rest.

If the patient switches the machine off using the patient safety switch, turn all controls to zero, inspect the area and adjust the application as required. Then turn the machine on again in the normal manner.

If the machine will not resonate when it is switched on, recheck the application. There may be too much spacing, leads may be incorrectly attached, or the area treated may be too large for the capabilities of an individual machine.

INDUCTOTHERMY (COIL) APPLICATION OF SHORT WAVE DIATHERMY

This is an application using a coil, monode, minode, or diplode. A combination of an electromagnetic field and an electrostatic field is set up in the tissues to produce heating in the superficial tissues only. The following principles apply to all inductothermy applications.

Equipment required
short wave diathermy unit
coil, monode, or minode
wooden or plastic spacers
towels
test tubes (for skin test)
pillows and sheets
   The patient should be settled in a position of optimum comfort and support, which allows the area to be treated to be fully exposed.

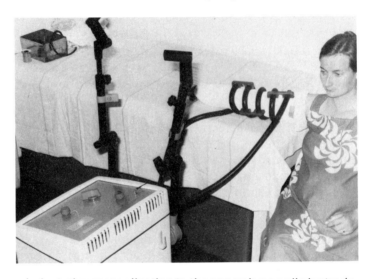

Inductothermy application to the arm using a coil electrode

   Explain the procedure to the patient. Ascertain that there are no *contra-indications* to treatment with short wave diathermy.
   Inspect the area to be treated and *palpate* carefully to locate the site of the lesion.
   Skin-test the area to be treated, for discrimination between hot and cold.
   Ensure that there is no metal or moisture within the area to be treated or within 300 mm of the area, for example, hairpins or jewellery.
   If using a coil, wrap two layers of towelling firmly around the limb, ensuring that there are no creases produced. This is necessary, not to provide spacing, but to absorb any perspiration which may be produced by the heat and result in a scald; and to prevent cross-infection between patients.

Test that the machine is operating by placing 2 or 3 loops of the coil over your arm, resonating the machine and feeling the heat produced. This also serves as a demonstration for the patient.

Loop the coil loosely and slide the loops over the limb. Adjust the loops of the coil so that they are firm against all aspects of the limb and evenly spaced apart. Ensure that no two loops are touching, then hold the loops in place with several wooden or plastic spacers.

Attach the ends of the cable to the machine sockets.

Recheck the application —
Are the loops of the coil evenly spaced and not touching each other?
Is the coil firmly applied?
Are there at least two layers of towelling between the skin and the coil?
Is the towelling smoothly applied?
Is the patient comfortable and unlikely to move once the machine is switched on?
Is any part of the coil touching or within 25 mm of any other part of the patient, any part of the machine or any other conductor?

Check that the machine controls are at zero, then switch the power on at the mains.

Instruct the patient not to move, and to avoid touching any part of the machine or the application, and to call out if concerned. If the machine has a patient safety switch, instruct the patient to switch the machine off and call out if concerned.

Warn the patient that he should feel a mild, comfortable warmth and no more or a *burn* could result. *Note:* The word *burn* must, medico-legally, be used in the warning.

Switch the intensity control to the standby position. If the machine has a separate power switch, this must also be switched on. Most modern machines require only 30 seconds to warm up prior to use.

Turn on the timer to the required treatment time. As there is a circuit breaker in the timer, short wave diathermy cannot be produced unless the timer is switched on.

Turn the intensity control to the *lowest intensity setting*. Never resonate the machine on a higher setting, or the patient could receive a burn.

Adjust the resonator control manually, to adjust a variable condenser, to resonate (or tune) the machine circuit with the patient circuit, ensuring maximum power output to the patient circuit. This will be indicated by either:
(*a*)   an indicator light coming on;
(*b*)   an indicator light changing color;
(*c*)   a power output meter. In this case the machine should be tuned so that the needle reaches and maintains the highest possible setting for the application (similar to a radio turning meter).

If the machine has an automatic resonator control, it will automatically search and select the adjustment of the variable condenser to ensure maximum power output to the patient circuit.

Wait 2 to 3 minutes on the minimum intensity setting, and ask the patient to describe any sensation of warmth felt. If necessary, increase to the next intensity, waiting a further 2 to 3 minutes before making another increase, until the patient describes the sensation as a *mild, comfortable warmth*.

Once the therapeutic intensity has been reached, adjust the timer to the required treatment time.

After the treatment time has elapsed, the timer automatically cuts out the patient circuit, returning the machine to standby. Turn the intensity control to zero.

Remove the application and *inspect* the area treated.

Allow the patient to leave after a brief rest.

If the patient switches the machine off using the patient safety switch, turn all controls to zero, inspect the area and adjust the application as required. Then turn the machine on again in the normal manner.

If the machine will not resonate when it is switched on, recheck the application. There may be too much spacing, leads may be incorrectly attached, or the area treated may be too large for the capabilities of an individual machine.

ADVANTAGES

Versatility due to the wide variety of applications available.
Heat can be applied to deep or superficial structures as required.
Undue skin heat can be avoided.
Operation of the machine is relatively simple.
It is comfortable for the patient.
It is easily adapted to suit body curvature.
It can heat through a joint.

DISADVANTAGES

It requires comparatively complex application.
Accurate measurement of the amount of heat received by the patient is not possible.
Deep tissue burns can occur.

3.2   Pulsed Short Wave Diathermy

Pulsed short wave diathermy is short wave at the frequency of 27.12 MH_z which is pulsed at a rate selected by the therapist. The pulse frequency range is from 15 to 200 H_z. The maximum intensity produced by the machine is 1000 watts, however the mean power delivered to the tissues will be affected by the selected pulse frequency. The pulse duration is constant at 0.4 ms and square pulses are used.

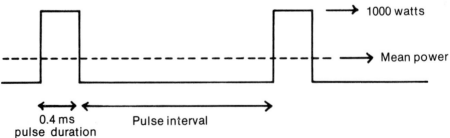

0.4 ms
pulse duration   Pulse interval

The value of pulsed short wave diathermy is that a very high intensity of power can be administered, with no or minimal thermal effects. To achieve this the ratio of the mean power to the pulse power should be as low as possible. By pulsing the output of the machine the thermal effect produced by one pulse is of very short duration, as it is dissipated by the circulation before the next pulse occurs. Thus there are no cumulative thermal effects. However the other biological effects produced are cumulative.

BIOLOGICAL EFFECTS

The effects of pulsed short wave diathermy are the same as those produced by non-pulsed short wave diathermy, with the exception of the increase in temperature in the tissues. The effects are summarised as follows:

increases metabolism by 2 to 4 times
relief of pain
stimulates the peripheral circulation
stimulates the early closure of wounds
decreases the rate of haematoma formation
relaxes muscle spasm

Most of the literature recommends the application of pulsed short wave to the liver and/or the adrenals, in addition to the usual local application. The mechanism behind this rationale is not understood, but it is thought that, as these organs have the highest concentration of reticulo-endothelial cells in the body, a central treatment may stimulate their release into the circulation, increasing the defense mechanisms in the periphery.

INDICATIONS

Pulsed short wave diathermy is particularly useful in the treatment of acute post-traumatic and infective conditions for which non-pulsed short wave would be contraindicated due to its thermal effects. Such conditions include:

sprains
contusions
ruptures
haematoma
bursitis
sinusitis

CONTRAINDICATIONS

Very few contraindications apply to pulsed short wave diathermy. These are listed below.

Pacemakers. The effect of the high frequency current may interfere with the functioning of some pacemakers.

High fever. The effects of increasing the metabolism may not be tolerated in the presence of an increased body temperature when metabolism will already be increased.

Tumours. The increase in metabolism may result in increased growth and metastasis of the tumour.

Metal. Metal is not an absolute contraindication. However, as it will tend to concentrate the field, it may draw the field away from the tissues to be treated, resulting in an ineffective treatment.

TECHNIQUES OF APPLICATION

Pulsed short wave may be applied by either the condenser-field method or by the inductothermy method. Descriptions of these techniques are detailed in the previous section.

DOSAGE

The patient should not feel any heat. The dose is selected as a combination of pulse frequency and pulse power (intensity). In general the pulse power should be as high as possible (up to 1000 watts), though lower for initial treatments and acute conditions.

The pulse frequency should be determined by questioning the patient as to the development of any heat. By reducing the pulse frequency, heat will be reduced.

The manufacturer's literature often details recommendations of specific dosages as a guide to treatment, which may be used as a starting point.

	1	2	3	4	5	6	7	8	9	10	Position of intensity control
Pulse repetition frequency	100W	200W	300W	400W	500W	600W	700W	800W	900W	1000W	Maximum pulse power
15 Hz	0.6	1.2	1.8	2.4	3	3.6	4.2	4.8	5.4	6	
20 Hz	0.8	1.6	2.4	3.2	4	4.8	5.6	6.4	7.2	8	
26 Hz	1.0	2.1	3.2	4.2	5.3	6.4	7.4	8.5	9.5	10.6	
35 Hz	1.4	2.8	4.2	5.6	7	8.4	9.8	11.2	12.6	14	Mean
46 Hz	1.9	3.8	5.6	7.5	9.4	11.3	13.2	15.1	17	18.8	power
62 Hz	2.5	5	7.5	10	12.5	15	17.5	20	22.5	25	in watts
82 Hz	3.3	6.6	10	13.3	16.6	20	23.2	26.5	29.9	33.2	
110 Hz	4.4	8.8	13.2	17.7	22	26.5	30.9	35.3	39.7	44.1	
150 Hz	5.9	11.7	17.6	23.5	29.4	35.2	41.1	47	52.8	58.7	
200 Hz	7.8	15.6	23.4	31.2	39	46.9	54.7	62.5	70.3	78.1	

A mean power of 25 watts is experienced as imperceptible by a patient with normal sensation. Combinations of pulse repetition and pulse power above the line on the table should produce athermal effects, while those below the line will also produce thermal effects.

ADVANTAGES

Pulsed short wave can often be used in conditions where non-pulsed short wave is contraindicated.

In particular pulsed short wave is effective in the treatment of post-traumatic and infective conditions.

DISADVANTAGES

The machines are expensive, though most models also produce non-pulsed short wave so are a dual purpose machine.

Although metal is not a contraindication, its presence may interefere with the effectiveness of the treatment.

3.3   Microwave Diathermy

PHYSICS OF MICROWAVE DIATHERMY

Properties of microwaves. Microwaves are a form of electromagnetic radiation, lying between short waves and infrared waves in the electromagnetic spectrum. Their frequencies are in the range 300 to 30 000 MHz, with wavelengths of 10 mm to 1 metre.

Therapeutic generators most commonly produce microwaves with a frequency of 2450 MHz and a wavelength of 122.5 mm. Generators producing microwaves with frequencies of 915 MHz and 433.9 MHz, and wavelengths of 330 mm and 690 mm respectively, are now also available, as recent trials indicate that these frequencies minimise the heating of the subcutaneous tissues, and produce more effective heating of the underlying tissues, with minimal reflection by bone.

As for all electromagnetic radiations, microwaves travel at the speed of light. They are also governed by the laws of reflection, refraction, absorption, and the inverse square law.

Production of microwave radiation. The magnetron (a diode valve) produces a high frequency alternating current, which is carried by a coaxial cable to the transducer (director).

The transducer contains an antenna and a reflector. The passage of the high frequency current through the antenna energises it and this results in the transformation of the electrical energy into electromagnetic energy.

This energy is then focused by the reflector and beamed to the tissues.

The microwave intensity is varied by altering the amount of power supplied to the magnetron.

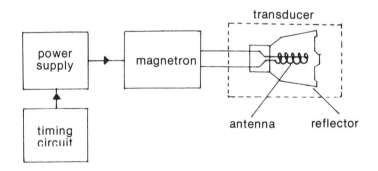

Schematic diagram of microwave diathermy apparatus (from Ward, 1976)

Electromagnetic waves do not require a material medium for their existence and transmission (compare the transmission of sound waves).

BIOPHYSICAL AND BIOCHEMICAL EFFECTS OF MICROWAVE DIATHERMY

The basic events which take place when microwave diathermy is applied to tissues are:

Penetration. The depth of penetration depends on the frequency of the wave and the properties of the medium which it is penetrating. In general, the wave energy decreases exponentially with distance travelled, and decreases as the wave frequency increases. Tissues of low water content are penetrated to a greater depth than tissues of high water content. The *effective* penetration of 2450 MHz microwave is said to be approximately 30 mm.

Absorption. The electromagnetic energy is transformed into heat energy as it interacts with the molecules of different tissues. The non-polar molecules will distort towards the alternating charge in the field; dipolar molecules will rotate back and forth; ions will vibrate in the field direction. The resultant energy losses are converted into heat energy. The differing electrical properties of different tissues determine the amount of absorption which will occur. For example, muscle and other tissues of high fluid content will absorb more electromagnetic energy than tissues such as fat or bone.

Reflection. The proportion of waves reaching the deeper tissues is also dependent upon the amount of energy which is reflected at the air-skin, skin-fat, and the fat-muscle interfaces, back into the air, the skin, and the subcutaneous fatty layer respectively. The relative amount of energy reflected is determined by the electrical properties of the tissues. At frequencies below 1000 MHz most of the energy reaches the deeper tissues, while for frequencies of 2450 MHz the distribution of the energy depends critically on the thickness of the skin and the subcutaneous fat. As much as 50% of the energy may be reflected at the air-skin interface.

Heat conduction. Once the microwave energy has been converted into heat energy, heat exchange will occur with other areas of lower temperature, until a 'steady state' is achieved.

Physiological responses to irradiation with microwave diathermy depend upon the reactions of the tissues to temperature rise and the amount of energy absorbed. Temperature regulation is a function of cardiovascular, hormonal, and nervous control.

Heat applied to the skin (in a restricted area) results in an increased blood flow in the skin, which helps to distribute the heat to other areas. This increase in circulation is accompanied by vasodilatation. The mechanism of these changes is the same as for short wave diathermy.

Mild heat produces reflex reduction of increased muscle tone. It is suggested that increased muscle blood flow plays some part in this mechanism, along with removal of the trigger irritation. Muscle spasm is probably an increased proprioceptor reflex mechanism, and the muscle spindles are the receptor end-organs for this reflex. As it has been shown that temperature increase at the muscle spindle decreases, and in some cases inhibits, the firing of the spindles, this may also contribute to the decrease in muscle spasm produced.

When the temperature at a nerve, or in subcutaneous tissues with a high proportion of cutaneous nerve fibres, is elevated to above 45°C, then neural stimulation resulting in various reactions, and blood pressure and vascular responses are seen.

Mild heating causes an analgesic effect in the underlying tissues, though the mechanism of this effect is not understood.

THERAPEUTIC EFFECTS OF MICROWAVE DIATHERMY

The therapeutic effects of microwave diathermy are similar to those of short wave diathermy, but since the penetration of microwave is only superficial, it is only likely to be effective in the treatment of superficial structures. As only one aspect of the body can be irradiated at a time, it is more suitable for the treatment of localised rather than widespread conditions.

Pain. The relief of pain by microwave diathermy is useful in the treatment of traumatic and rheumatic conditions affecting superficial muscles, ligaments, and small superficial joints. Relief of pain may also be helped by the relief of associated muscle spasm.

Muscle spasm may be reduced directly by microwave diathermy, or may be reduced by relieving the pain which is contributing to it.

Inflammation. Resolution of chronic inflammation may be accelerated by treatment with microwave diathermy as a result of the increase in blood supply. This increases venous return from the area and aids the resorption of the oedema exudate.

Delayed healing. To promote the healing of open skin areas, an increase in the cutaneous circulation may be of assistance, provided the vascular responses to heat are normal. If the arteriolar and capillary dilatation does not allow sufficient increase in blood flow, heat should not be applied directly but may be applied proximally to an area with a good blood supply. This is done in an attempt to achieve reflex vasodilatation in the required area.

Infection. Treatment with microwave diathermy may assist in the control of chronic infection by increasing the circulation. This will increase the number of white blood cells and antibodies brought to the area to fight the infective organism, thus reinforcing the body's normal defence mechanism.

Fibrosis. Heat has been found to increase the extensibility of fibrous tissues, such as tendons, joint capsules, and scars, by from 5 to 10 times. The effect is produced by temperature increases within the therapeutic range.

DOSAGE

Duration of treatment. It is accepted that 20 minutes is the optimum treatment time since the tissue temperature will usually reach a 'steady state' in this time and the increase in circulation will have reached its maximum. Shorter durations will not achieve maximum physiological effects, though they may be useful as a test dose to ascertain any untoward effects of microwave diathermy.

Intensity of microwave. The only safe measure of the intensity of treatment is the sensation of warmth described by the patient. The patient should feel no more than a 'mild, comfortable warmth' — anything hotter could result in a burn.

Although most machines have a power output meter, the power reading does not give an indication of the level of temperature increase in the tissues, since it cannot adjust for varying reflection at the air-skin interface, or for different skin and subcutaneous fat thickness.

Frequency of treatment. Treatments may be given daily or on alternate days as indicated. The factors which determine the frequency of treatment include the response to treatment and the availability of the patient for treatment. Ideally treatment would be most beneficial if given once or twice each day.

INDICATIONS

Microwave diathermy is generally indicated for the treatment of superficial structures. However the development of lower frequency microwave should allow deeper heating if there is only a thin subcutaneous fat layer.

In summary, microwave could be indicated in the treatment of:

disorders of the musculo-skeletal system
sprains
strains
muscle and tendon tears
capsular lesions
degenerative joint disease
chronic rheumatoid arthritis
joint stiffness in superficial joints
haematoma

superficial inflammatory or infective conditions
tenosynovitis
bursitis
synovitis
infected surgical incisions
carbuncles
abscesses

CONTRA-INDICATIONS

The contra-indications, as distinct from precautions, for microwave diathermy are specified as follows:

Over malignant tissues. The increase in metabolism resulting from the increase in temperature would accelerate the rate of growth and metastasis of the malignancy.

Over ischaemic tissues. The inability of the circulation to disperse the heat could result in temperature elevation to a level which would produce tissue destruction (a burn). Also the inability of the circulation to provide the increased oxygen required by the resultant increase in metabolism could result in the development of gangrene.

Moderate and excessive oedema. Particularly non-inflammatory oedema is likely to be aggravated by the administration of any form of heat.

Over wet dressings and adhesive tape. Microwave will be more readily absorbed, and a burn or scald could result.

Metallic implants. Any metal within the range of penetration of microwave will concentrate the microwave and result in the production of temperatures in the destructive range in adjacent tissues.

Pacemakers. The high frequency of microwave has been demonstrated to interfere with or even inhibit the function of some pacemakers. Therefore it is advisable not to use microwave in the presence of any pacemaker, because the type is not always known.

Over growing bone. High doses of microwave have been shown to limit bone growth.

Male gonads. Repeated irradiation with microwave is said to produce sterility. If an area near the gonads is to be treated, for example the hip, the gonads may be shielded by fine wire mesh.

Haemorrhagic areas. The increase in circulation will increase the degree of haemorrhage or precipitate haemorrhage in unstable situations, for example, haemophilia.

Tuberculous joints. The increase in temperature will increase the rate of development of the infection, and therefore increase the possibility of joint damage.

Impaired thermal sensation. As the application of a safe level of intensity requires that the patient reports the degree of heat felt, any disturbance in, or loss of thermal sensation could result in high intensities being applied and consequent tissue destruction.

Unreliable patients, for example very old or very young patients, whose co-operation in monitoring the administration of the level of intensity cannot be guaranteed.

The eyes. The development of lenticular opacities (cataracts) has been demonstrated in subjects exposed to microwaves at comparatively low dosages, and these may or may not result in visual disturbance.

Recent radiotherapy. For a period of up to three months following therapeutic doses of radiotherapy, skin sensation and circulation may be diminished.

Hypersensitivity to heat. Particularly where liniment has been applied, the circulation is already increased by the action of the liniment and may be unable to increase enough to disperse heat applied.

Acute infection or inflammation. The process is likely to be exacerbated by the application of heat.

Obesity. Particularly with 2450 MHz microwave, there is a danger of producing an excessive level of heat in the subcutaneous fat layer.

Analgesic therapy. If the patient has recently (within the last few hours) taken any analgesic drugs, the thermal sensation may be diminished.

Venous thrombosis or phlebitis. Heat applied to the affected area may result in embolus formation.

Pregnancy. Heat applied to the pelvis or hip in pregnancy may cause haemorrhage or miscarriage.

Menstruation. Heat applied to the pelvis or hip may increase the volume of blood lost.

Acute dermatological conditions. Heat may exacerbate these conditions.

Severe cardiac conditions. The increase in cardiac output required when heat is applied, particularly to large areas, may not be possible in patients with severe cardiac conditions.

Blood pressure abnormalities. Changes in blood pressure produced by the application of heat, particularly in large areas, may exacerbate problems with blood pressure.

TECHNIQUES OF MICROWAVE DIATHERMY

An advantage of microwave diathermy is the ease of application with the apparatus. The variations in the applications available with microwave diathermy are related to the sizes and heating patterns of the directors available.

Three main variations in directors are commonly available.

Large circular field director. The effective diameter is 200 mm. The heating pattern is more intense around the outer portion than in the centre. The power output range used is up to 250 watts.

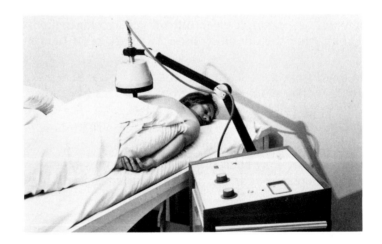

Large circular field director

Small circular field director. The effective diameter is 100 mm. The heating pattern is more intense around the outer portion than in the centre. The power output range used is up to 25 watts.

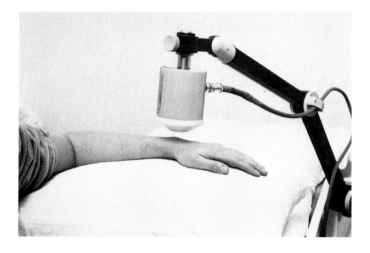

Small circular field director

Longitudinal director. The effective treatment area is 500 mm by 100 mm. The heating pattern tends to be more concentrated in the centre of this area. The power output range used is up to 250 watts.

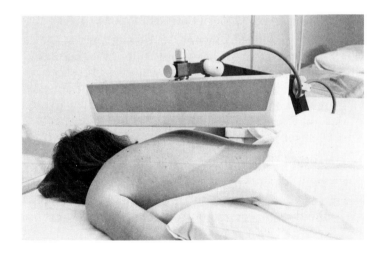

Longitudinal director

Some microwave machines also have focusing directors for defined areas.

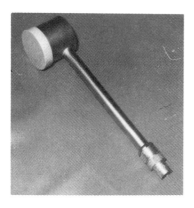

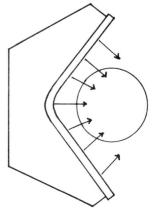

Focusing director   *Large-field director showing direction*
                                                     of travel of waves produced

Recently directors with curved surfaces have been developed for the treatment of larger areas.

The operating manual for each machine should give guidelines as to the optimum distance between the patient and the director, as this will vary to some extent.

Although some manufacturers state that their directors can be positioned in contact with the skin, this is not recommended since it could result in sweat being trapped against the skin, thus overheating it, and causing a scald. An air space between the director and the skin will allow the sweat to evaporate, rather than reaching scalding temperatures. Another consideration is the prevention of cross-infection between patients.

DANGERS AND PRECAUTIONS IN MICROWAVE DIATHERMY

Burns. The greatest potential danger associated with the application of microwave diathermy is that of producing a burn. Therefore the following precautions must be taken in order to avoid such an occurrence:

(*a*)   Thoroughly check all *contra-indications* by examining the patient's case history, the area to be treated, and by questioning the patient.

(*b*)   A test of *thermal skin sensation* must always be performed.

(*c*)   Care must be taken if microwave is to be given over *bony prominences*, as heating will be greater due to the reduced depth of tissue and the reflection of the microwave by the bone, giving a double heating effect. Heat will be less quickly dispersed as blood-flow over bony prominences tends to be less than over muscle tissue. Therefore, if possible, bony prominences should be avoided, or the director should be positioned at a greater distance from the skin.

(*d*)   Care must be taken when applying microwave over areas where the *subcutaneous fat layer is thicker* as 'hot spots' may occur. In some cases, microwave may not be the treatment of choice for this reason.

(e)   Ensure that *the skin is dry,* and watch for any sweat formation during treatment.

(f)   *Never* apply microwave over *clothing*, as it will inhibit heat loss from the skin, resulting in excessive heating. In particular, nylon will retain perspiration, resulting in a scald.

(g)   Always *align the director accurately* to ensure an even pattern of heating.

Shock. The danger of electrical shock is present in the use of microwave diathermy. In this case both the patient and the therapist are potentially at risk. The following precautions must be taken to prevent this occurrence:

(a)   *Do not increase the intensity* unless the coaxial cable is correctly connected both to the machine and to the director.

(b)   Ensure that the machine is *correctly earthed*.

(c)   *Do not touch*, or allow the patient to touch, the machine if you are earthed, for example by also touching another machine which is switched on, or touching a water pipe.

Other precautions which must be taken include:

(a)   Do not position the director in such a way that the *eyes* could receive radiation. Mesh goggles are available to protect the eyes.

(b)   Avoid irradiating the *male gonads*.

(c)   Do not position the director over any *metal surfaces* or reflection may result in damage to the magnetron.

(d)   If the patient is wearing a *hearing aid*, it should be switched off, as the high frequency of microwave produces marked interference.

METHOD OF APPLICATION OF MICROWAVE DIATHERMY

Equipment required

microwave diathermy unit
director
pillows and sheets
test tubes (for skin test)
towels

The patient should be settled in a position of optimum comfort and support, which allows the area to be treated to be fully exposed.

Explain the procedure to the patient.

Ascertain that there are no *contra-indications* to treatment with microwave diathermy.

Inspect the area to be treated and *palpate* carefully to localise the site of the lesion.

Skin-test the area to be treated, for discrimination between hot and cold.

Check that all controls are at zero, then switch the power on at the mains.

Switch on the machine power control.

Check that the mains pilot lamp has come on.

The machine now requires approximately 4 minutes warming-up time in order to bring the filament of the magnetron to operating temperature. This may be indicated by a pilot lamp switching on, either automatically, or when the timer is turned on.

Select a suitable director and attach it to the arm of the machine. Recheck the connections.

Attach the coaxial cable to the director.

Test the machine by placing your hand under the director, about 20 mm away from the surface, and turning the intensity up slowly until heat is felt. Watch the meter to ensure that the needle rises smoothly, without any surges of power.

Ensure that there is no metal or moisture within the radiation field.

Position the director so that the radiation will strike the skin surface at 90°. The rim of the director will then be parallel to the part to be treated. The distance of the director from the part varies, and the manufacturer's guidelines should be observed.

Instruct the patient to avoid looking at the director, keep still, avoid touching the machine, and to call out if concerned. If the machine has a patient safety switch, instruct the patient to switch the machine off and call out if concerned.

Give the patient protective goggles to wear if there is any chance of the microwaves irradiating the eyes.

Warn the patient that he should feel a mild, comfortable warmth and no more or a *burn* could result. *Note:* The word *burn* must, medico-legally, be used in the warning.

Turn the timer fully clockwise to 30 minutes and from there back to the required treatment time. (This winds mechanical timers.) As there is a circuit breaker in the timer, microwave cannot be emitted unless the timer is switched on.

Slowly turn up the intensity control, asking the patient to tell you the moment a sensation of warmth is felt. Depending on the type of director used, the relevant power range (0 to 25 watts or 0 to 250 watts) is selected automatically. *Note:* The meter only records the output from the machine and *not* what the patient is feeling. The patient's description of warmth is essential.

After the treatment time has elapsed, the timer turns off, automatically switching off the power, or the patient may terminate the treatment using the patient safety switch. Turn the intensity control to zero and, if the patient has terminated the treatment, set the timer to zero.

After the termination of treatment the machine remains in the standby position so that another treatment can follow without incurring the 4-minute warm-up time.

Unless doing consecutive treatments, the machine should be switched off completely, because the life of the magnetron depends upon the number of hours for which the filament is on.

Remove the machine and *inspect* the area treated.

Damage to the magnetron may occur if the machine is switched on with the director facing metal, due to reflection of the waves back to the antenna.

Before changing directors, the intensity control and the timer must be turned to zero.

ADVANTAGES

Simplicity of application.
Heat can be localised accurately.

Undue skin heating need not occur if all precautions are taken.
Operation of the machine is simple.
The machine is comfortable for the patient.
Using low frequency microwave, selective heating of muscle is possible.

DISADVANTAGES

It cannot be used for heating of deep structures.
It can only heat one aspect of a joint at a time.
Accurate measurement of the amount of heat received by the patient is not possible.
Skin burns may develop very rapidly.

3.4 Pulsed Microwave Diathermy

In recent years some manufacturers have realised that the principles of pulsed short wave diathermy could also apply to microwave, and machines have been developed which produce pulsed microwave diathermy. The effects of pulsed microwave are the same as those of non-pulsed microwave with the exception of the production of a rise in temperature in the tissues. Thus many of the conditions which contraindicate treatment with microwave diathermy can be effectively treated by pulsed microwave. However, as with non-pulsed microwave, the depth of penetration is comparatively superficial and only one aspect of the part can be treated at a time.

Pulsed microwave machines are not seen as frequently as pulsed short wave machines. They are expensive and the purchase of a pulsed short wave machine allows a wider range of usage because of the greater versatility of short wave diathermy.

3.5 Infrared Radiation

PHYSICS OF INFRARED RADIATION

Infrared radiations and visible light are a small segment of the electromagnetic spectrum of radiant energy. Infrared has a frequency of 7×10^{14} to 400×10^{14} Hz and wavelengths from 700 to 15 000 nm. Visible light has wavelengths from 390 to 770 nm.

Infrared radiations are further classified according to their distance from the visible spectrum.

Near or short infrared rays	770 nm to 4 000 nm
Far or long infrared rays	4000 nm to 15 000 nm

For centuries heat has been obtained from radiant energy sources such as sunshine, open fires, heated stones and irons. During the late nineteenth century in North America and Germany, interest was shown in the Edison light lamps as a source of heat for medicinal purposes. In 1891 the radiant heat tunnel or baker was the first medical luminous heat source to be used. It is still in use in some parts of the world today.

In 1802 Herschel generated infrared rays by the motion of valence electrons in atoms, and of atoms in molecules. In the early twentieth century, the infrared burner was manufactured for medical purposes, and today infrared lamps are used for specific clinical purposes.

Production of infrared radiation. Infrared rays are produced when an object has a temperature above that of absolute zero. At a given temperature the body heat will emit a continuous spectrum of radiation. The wavelength and frequencies of the radiation will depend on the absolute temperature of the part. The frequency of the radiation will be directly proportional to the absolute temperature of the source. Wien's Law states that the wavelength of the maximum production of radiations is inversely proportional to the absolute temperature of the source.

Luminous and non-luminous sources of infrared rays. All *incandescent* bodies, such as tungsten or carbon filament lamps, produce visible and infrared rays which are termed luminous radiations. An electric current passed through resistance wire covered with copper tubing or refractory material generates mostly infrared rays. This is the principle of production of infrared rays from a *non-luminous generator*.

Heat production. Infrared rays with wavelengths of 770 to 4000 nm, which represent the short infrared rays, have sufficient energy to cause thermal agitation by molecular and atomic motion. *This thermal agitation is heat.* Shorter wavelengths can cause electron displacement and produce electronic and vibrational changes, causing chemical changes in the tissues of the body. The degree of elevation of temperature will depend upon the ability of the tissue to dissipate heat, and also depends on the specific heat, the thickness and absorptivity of the tissues through which the infrared rays pass. There is generally no more than a 1° to 2°C rise in temperature.

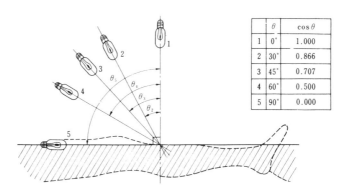

	θ	$\cos\theta$
1	0°	1.000
2	30°	0.866
3	45°	0.707
4	60°	0.500
5	90°	0.000

Relative intensity for different values of θ ($\cos\theta$ = relative intensity)

ABSORPTION AND PENETRATION OF INFRARED RADIATION

All radiant energy when it strikes the body must be reflected, absorbed, or transmitted. The absorption of infrared radiations and the maximal penetration of the rays will depend upon the following variables:

    frequency or wavelength of the rays
    thermal conductivity of the tissues
    density of each tissue

specific heat of each tissue
angle of incidence of the rays
distance from the source of infrared
patency of the circulation
source of the infrared

It is important to ensure that all rays *fall perpendicular to the surface in order to be maximally absorbed*. Reflection is minimal if the angle of incidence is 0°. As the angle of incidence increases, the amount of reflection is increased. The human skin absorbs 95% of the energy if the rays are perpendicular to the surface. If the angle of incidence is 15° the intensity is reduced by 3%. The long infrared rays are absorbed in the superficial 0.1 mm. Wavelengths longer than 3000 nm are totally absorbed by the moisture of the skin, except for the very long waves from 15 000 to 40 000 nm that can penetrate into the deeper tissues by several centimetres.

The maximal penetration of the short infrared rays is about 3 mm, and then only a small proportion of the rays penetrates to that depth. Authorities still differ on the relative depth of penetration of the short and long infrared rays. *Depth of penetration is a relative term*, as the intensity of radiation is reduced to one-tenth or one-thousandth of the incident rays on penetration. Thus the rays that penetrate deeper may be too few to produce an effective biological reaction. It is important to consider all factors governing absorption of infrared rays before considering the biological effects of infrared rays.

The relative thickness of the layers of the skin, the patency of the skin circulation, and the quantity of fat will affect heat conduction. Any impairment of the heat-dissipating mechanism will produce adverse effects. The density of connective tissue and fat will impede thermal conductivity. The resulting temperature rise in the tissues will depend on the specific heat of the substance and the initial transient period of rise and fall in temperature.

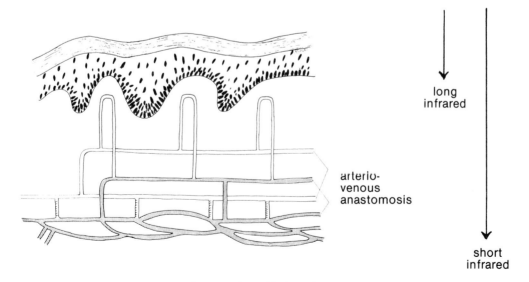

long
infrared

arterio-
venous
anastomosis

short
infrared

Penetration of infrared rays

One also considers the angle of the incident ray when it strikes the body, the temperature of the body, and the complex heat exchange characteristics. If a hand is immersed in a hot bath of 40°C, the skin temperature rises to bath temperature within 0.5 seconds. It then decreases rapidly in the next 5 seconds. Pain is reported in the first 5 seconds, and then the tissues adapt to pain in the next 2 to 6 seconds. Infrared rays produce a slow rise in temperature, the thermal gradient is slow, and pain is only registered if the temperature reaches 45°C.

Measurement of intensity. The intensity of radiant heat can be measured by radiometers. Apparatus in therapeutic use does not have radiometers. The subjective feeling of warm, hot, and very hot is all that the therapist has as an indication of the intensity of the heat. A radiometer is useful only for comparing sources of radiations, but is not a useful guide for treatment. Skin temperature can be measured by means of an insulated fine wire copper constantan thermocouple (No. 40 gauge).

APPARATUS FOR INFRARED HEATING

Generators in use today are classified as luminous or non-luminous. They are all generally portable and come in varying sizes and energy output, from 250 to 1000 w.

The reflectors of the lamps are shaped like a *parabola* to give a floodlight beam or a spotlight beam.

Non-luminous infrared generators consist of a resistance wire coiled on a cylinder of insulating material such as fireclay or porcelain, or on a plate or cylinder of resistant metal. The resistance wire serves as the heater, and the cylinder or plate becomes the radiation source. Infrared rays are emitted from the heated wire and the cylinder or plate, which is heated by conduction. Sometimes the resistance wire is covered with copper tubing or other metal, or with carborundum or some other refractory material.

Another method of producing non-luminous infrared is by using a 10 mm steel tube, within which there is a spiral wire embedded in an insulator. Current is passed through the central wire which is heated. Heat is conducted to the steel tube by the insulator, and infrared rays are emitted from the tube. The tube is bent into 'U' turns and mounted on a reflector. The elements of the non-luminous lamps take about 5 to 10 minutes to heat up and emit their maximum intensity. In all radiators there are always some visible light rays emitted, as a red glow is visible when the element is hot. So they are not completely non-luminous.

The small elements consume from 250 to 500 w. The large elements consume 750 to 1000 w. Large lamps have now been constructed and designed to have a wide range of adjustments and possess a long-lasting element.

The lamp must have a steady base and a stand which is adjustable for varying height and angle of the reflector. The control knobs must have a safe locking device.

Energy emission and penetration. Non-luminous infrared generators emit rays with wavelengths of between 15 000 and 770 nm. Maximum emission is between 3500 and 4000 nm. There is a minimal emission of short infrared rays.

About 34% of the longer infrared rays are reflected, 59% absorbed in the superficial epidermis and about 6.4% may enter the deep part of the epidermis. The long infrared rays generally convert to vibrational energy when they are absorbed by the skin.

SPECTRAL REGION	WAVELENGTH	PENETRATION OF RAYS	PHYSIOLOGIC ACTION
90% long infrared rays	1500 nm – 15 000 nm (mainly 3500 – 4000 nm)	0.5 mm – 1 mm	vibrational energy heat production nerve stimulation capillary hyperaemia
10% short infrared	770 nm – 1500 nm	1 mm – 3 mm	minimal action

Luminous generators. Ionised gases and very hot bodies emit visible rays with wavelengths of from 392 to 800 nm. Incandescent lamps containing tungsten or carbon filaments emit these visible rays plus a large proportion of infrared rays. Lamps that produce both visible and infrared rays are called luminous infrared lamps.

A luminous lamp consists of a coil of fine wire made of tungsten enclosed in a glass bulb, which is evacuated of air or contains an inert gas. The glass bulb is mounted on the center of a parabolic reflector. Carbon filaments are sometimes used, however tungsten is usually selected, as it tolerates repeated heating and cooling.

Lamps come in varying sizes. The power varies from 100 to 1500 w. Large wattage bulbs must have a firm screw cap connection. Small luminous generators are generally fitted with 250 or 500 w bulbs and are useful for small area treatments such as the hand, shoulder or foot. Large luminous generators are fitted with 600 to 1500 w bulbs. These lamps may be used for larger areas, such as the lumbar spine, thoraco-lumbar area, hips, and two knees. With large lamps, care must be taken that the lamp is fitted with a wire guard across the reflector to contain broken glass in case the bulb explodes. Special pyrex glass is now used to eliminate explosions, particularly in the high wattage bulbs.

Energy emission and penetration of luminous infrared generators. The luminous generators emit 70% of short infrared rays of wavelength 770 to 4000 nm, 4.8% of visible rays of wavelength 390 to 770 nm, 1% of ultraviolet rays, and 24% of long infrared rays of wavelength 4000 to 15 000 nm.

Visible rays. About 11% is absorbed by the bulb glass, 33% is reflected from the skin, and 56% is absorbed. From the absorbed rays, about 36% is absorbed in the epidermis, about 10% goes deeper into the dermis, and the remainder is scattered in the epidermis.

Short infrared rays. 34% is reflected, 20% is absorbed in the superficial epidermis, while 16% reaches the deep epidermis, 19% penetrates to the dermis, and 11% is transmitted into the subcutaneous regions. The deep penetration is mainly by the rays of wavelength 700 to 1000 nm. The measurement of the depth of penetration cannot be gauged by increased circulation or a feeling of heat, as some of the deeper effects are reflex in character, and deeper radiations are less effective than superficial rays.

Ultraviolet rays are mainly absorbed by the glass of the globe.

SPECTRAL REGION	WAVELENGTH	PENETRATION OF RAYS	PHYSIOLOGIC ACTION
1% ultraviolet rays	10 nm – 390 nm	—	absorbed by glass
4.8% visible rays	390 nm – 770 nm	1 mm – 10 mm	electronic energy and vibrational energy producing heat; sensory nerve stimulation; capillary hyper-aemia; reflex vasodilatation
70% short infra-red rays	770 nm – 4000 nm	1 mm – 10 mm	as above
24% long infra-red rays	4000 nm – 15 000 nm	0.05mm—1mm	vibrational energy producing heat; sensory nerve stimulation; capillary hyper-aemia and reflex vasodilatation

PHYSIOLOGICAL RESPONSES TO INFRARED AND VISIBLE LIGHT

Infrared rays have the immediate effect of producing heat wherever they are absorbed. The amount of temperature rise will be governed by various factors. It is important to analyse the underlying pathophysiology, and to examine particularly the patency of the skin circulation, whose function is to dissipate heat, and to observe any alteration in osmotic or hydrostatic pressure of the fluids.

The main effects of infrared rays are due to the moderate temperature rise at superficial levels. It is a slow rise with a minimal thermal gradient. The temperature rise at deeper dermis levels is not more than 2°C, and about 1° to 2°C rise in the superficial dermis.

Nerve stimulation. Both the long and the short infrared rays stimulate the sensory nerves, and can thus reduce pain and muscle spasm. The underlying physiological mechanism to explain this is not fully known. Perhaps the raised temperature decreases gamma fibre activity. Usually a fast warming of the muscle spindle causes a temporary inhibition of its activity.

Vasodilatation. If skin temperature is raised above core temperature, cutaneous vasodilatation occurs to help distribute the heat more evenly. There is some conduction of heat to the deeper levels, but unless muscle is very superficially placed there is no vasodilatation in muscles. Even if muscle is superficially placed, no effective vasodilatation occurs. Circulation in superficial joints may be increased reflexly.

Heat causes the liberation of histamine-like substances which act on the capillaries causing them to dilate. The heat-regulating center in the medulla also signals the capillaries to vasodilate when the temperature rises. An increase of temperature to 43°C produces vaso-depression of the vasomotor reflexes. If the leg is heated and then the calf muscle pump exercised to cause circulatory changes, the pumping mechanisms may not be effective, as the cutaneous veins are fully relaxed.

Phagocytosis. This process increases with temperature, and if there is superficial inflammation, heating will promote phagocytosis. In cases of suppurative inflammation, heat can help in the draining of the suppurative material, as in carbuncles and abscesses.

Reflex heating. Infrared rays can be applied to the abdominal area to promote peripheral circulation. The physiological basis of this mechanism is that heating of the large splanchnic vessels in the abdomen stimulates the heat-regulating center in the medulla, which then reflexly opens up the peripheral vessels in an endeavour to regulate the body temperature quickly.

Pigmentation and erythema. Infrared rays cause a reddening of the skin, which is a gentle erythema that disappears rapidly. If irradiations are given frequently, the skin pigments in a mottled fashion, quite unlike ultraviolet rays, and this is termed *erythema ab igne*. This is due to the destruction of red blood corpuscles.

Sweating. There is increased activity of the sweat glands by reflex stimulation from the heat-regulating centre.

Blood pressure. If heating is given to a *large area of the body for a prolonged period*, as in the use of the infrared baker, there will be a fall in blood pressure due to the generalised vasodilatation, and reduction of peripheral resistance in the arterioles. The normally prescribed time of 15 to 20 minutes will not generally alter blood pressure.

INDICATIONS

Pain and muscle spasm. The use of short and long infrared will cause a reduction of pain and muscle spasm in superficial areas. It should not be used in acute trauma in the first 24 hours, but it can be effective later. The luminous lamp is more effective than the non-luminous lamp. Increased vasodilatation will also remove pain metabolites and break the cycle of pain and muscle spasm.

Oedema. In cases of chronic oedema of the hand and foot, if the exudate is mild and not tenacious, infrared in elevation will increase absorption of the exudate as a result of the capillary vasodilatation produced.

Healing of wounds and chronic suppurative areas. Infrared aids the healing of indolent wounds by its vasodilatatory effect. For cases of slow-healing post-operative wounds in the abdominal and perineal regions, infrared can be effectively used. It is also used in the treatment of infected hands, carbuncles and abscesses to accelerate drainage to the exterior.

CONTRA-INDICATIONS

Impaired sensation. Patients with impaired sensation in the area to be treated will not be able to determine if excessive heating is occurring. As there are no meters to register the intensity delivered to the patient, it is essential to assess sensation prior to treatment. Large areas of scar tissue with impaired sensation will also be a contra-indication.

Impaired circulation. When there is a history of defective circulation from any circulatory disease, such as atherosclerosis, deep vein thrombosis, and Beurger's disease, care must be taken not to administer heat over the area with impaired circulation. The function of skin circulation is to dissipate heat, and if this heat-regulating mechanism is defective then it would be quite easy to cause a burn. Heating of thrombi will also cause dislodgement of the thrombi with severe consequences.

Dermatological conditions. Heat must not be given over any dermatological dysfunction. Skin lesions such as fungus, dermatitis and eczema are some of the lesions to look for. Heat tends to irritate skin lesions.

Metal. There should be no metal in the area that is irradiated with radiant heat. Metal retains the heat and will cause a burn to the underlying tissue. Metal implants are not a contra-indication. Superficially placed implants can be irradiated, provided the circulation is intact and functioning normally.

Eyes. It is important that the eyes are protected from the infrared rays, as it is thought that the radiations can cause radiation cataracts. This will occur if infrared is given over a long period. It can also cause iritis.

Age. Elderly patients generally have impairment of sensation and circulation. In addition, lack of normal cardiovascular and respiratory reserves may lessen the tolerance of thermal stress of a mild degree. It is important not to give radiant heat if the room is hot and humid. Large areas must not be irradiated in elderly patients. Additional dangers in elderly patients include unreliable reporting of the intensity of the heat, and the tendency to fall asleep.

Analgesic and narcotic drugs. If patients have had strong analgesic or narcotic drugs just prior to treatment, infrared radiations must not be given. These drugs will raise the pain threshold and the patient will not be able to determine whether the infrared rays are of too great an intensity.

Deep X-ray therapy. Patients who are on deep X-ray therapy or who have had it in the past 3 months, must not be given infrared, as deep X-ray therapy reduces sensory appreciation.

Topical creams and oils. All topical applications must be removed before giving infrared rays or the creams and oils will cause a burn.

Skin tumors. Patients with skin tumors or melanomas must not receive infrared, as tumor growth may be increased.

Acute infections. All acute infections are a contra-indication to infrared rays, as the increase in temperature is likely to exacerbate the infective process.

Blood pressure abnormalities. Infrared radiation should not be given to large areas for a prolonged time, as the patient may be unable to tolerate the change in blood pressure which may be produced.

Severe cardiac conditions. Heating a large area will cause an increase in cardiac output which may not be tolerated by patients with severe cardiac conditions.

TECHNIQUE FOR INFRARED THERAPY

Equipment required
luminous or non-luminous infrared generator
test tubes
pillows
sheets
towels

Selection of infrared source. A non-luminous source produces a smaller and gradual rise of temperature in the skin and subcutaneous tissues, with reflex heating of the superficial joints. A luminous source produces a more vigorous rise of temperature in the skin and superficial fascia, a small rise of temperature in superficial muscle, and reflex heating of superficial joints. Infrared tunnels or bakers produce a higher rise of temperature in skin, superficial fascia and muscle.

Position the patient with pillows and a towel under the area to be treated. Make sure that the limb, trunk or head is supported in a pain-free position with *the area to be treated adequately exposed*.

Remove all metal objects such as rings, jewellery, safety pins and metal hooks from the area to be treated.

Ensure that there is ample room around the patient to position the lamp.

Inform the patient regarding:

the choice of modality	— luminous or non-luminous source of infrared;
rationale for treatment	— relief of pain and muscle spasm; promotion of healing;
sensation to be experienced	— a comfortable warm sensation which must not feel hot;
frequency and duration of treatment	— 10 to 20 minutes daily or a specific number of times per week.

Check for any contra-indications to heat.

Assess the clinical symptoms or cause to be treated by the infrared rays.

Examine the area for cuts, skin lesions, scars, inflammation and infection.

Test thermal sensation, using one test tube filled with hot water and the other filled with cold water.

Check the patency of the circulation in the underlying areas.

NEVER position the lamp directly over the patient. The position should ensure that all rays strike the body at right angles to obtain maximum absorption. This means that the rim of the reflector must be parallel to the part treated. Adjust to the distance required for the particular lamp by measuring from the front and back of the rim and the lateral sides. The distance is usually 0.45 to 0.6 m.

Do not let the lamp touch the plinth or bed on which the patient is lying.

Make sure the lamp is steady and not likely to fall. The head of the lamp must be over one leg of the lamp base for balance.

Protect the eyes from the rays by a localiser, towel or pads of cotton wool.

Watch that the lead from the lamp does not touch any part of the metal reflector.

Make sure that the lead to the mains terminal is not in anyone's path.

Check the knobs and screws of the lamp that control the height and angle of the reflector. Only switch on the heating element of the lamp prior to positioning if the element takes longer than 5 minutes to reach its maximum output of infrared rays. Position the generator directly opposite the center of the area to be treated. Cover the area to be treated before positioning the lamp, if the element is switched on.

Warn the patient of the danger of a BURN if the treated part becomes very hot or if the pain increases.

The patient must not MOVE, TOUCH the lamp or LOOK at the generator.

Advise the patient not to sleep or read during the treatment.

Give the patient an adequate method of calling for attention.

Switch on the lamp and stay with the patient (or intermittently supervise the application).

As the lamp warms up, put your hand between the lamp and the patient to check that it is producing heat.

Ask the patient to tell you when heat is felt and to describe the intensity. Adjust the distance of the lamp to produce a mild comfortable warmth — move the lamp closer to the patient to increase the intensity, further away to decrease the intensity. Give the patient a means of calling you if concerned.

Large generators with over 500 w output can be used at a distance of 0.6 m for a 20-minute period to obtain a more vigorous heating of the superficial regions.

Small generators with an output of 250 or 500 w can be used at a distance of 0.45 to 0.5 m for a period of 20 minutes. This will give moderate heating effects.

A luminous source with red filters can be used for mild analgesic and circulatory effects at a distance of 0.6 m for 20 minutes.

At the end of the treatment time, switch the lamp off and remove it before assessing the area for any excessive erythema and for relief of symptoms.

ADVANTAGES

Infrared can be used to treat large areas.
Patients may be taught to apply infrared for home use.

DISADVANTAGES

Heating is only very superficial.
Equipment is often rather unstable.

It is often difficult to position the patient and the lamp so that the lamp is not directly over any part of the patient.

CARE OF EQUIPMENT

Non-luminous generators must be kept dust-free and the inside of the reflector must be shiny. The reflector must be free of dents, as these alter the reflection of the rays to the patient.

Luminous generators must be kept dust-free.

3.6 Summary of Conversive Heating Techniques

Three methods of applying conversive heating to the tissues have been described. They differ in the method by which the heat is produced in the tissues, and the depth to which the effects of the heat will penetrate.

Short wave diathermy is a means of applying heat to the tissues at any depth. The variety of methods of applying short wave diathermy makes it versatile, not only in respect of the depth of heating, but also in terms of the structures which may be treated. Heat is produced by the effect on the tissues of an electromagnetic field, an electrostatic field, or a combination of both. In order to produce these fields in the tissues, the patient is incorporated into the circuit from the machine. Because of this, and also because of the depth of heating which can be produced, certain precautions must be taken with all applications of short wave diathermy to prevent the dangers of shock or burns occurring.

Pulsed short wave diathermy has the same effects as non-pulsed, with the exception of producing an increase in temperature in the tissues. Thus the contraindications are few, enabling many more patients to receive effective treatment.

Microwave diathermy is also a means of applying heat to the tissues. Whilst microwaves do not penetrate as deeply as short wave diathermy, they penetrate more deeply than infrared rays. Heat is produced on absorption of the electromagnetic waves by the tissues and the effects are mainly in the area of absorption, although some dispersal to deeper areas also occurs. The variety of directors available for the application of microwave diathermy allows the beam to be focused for the treatment of small areas, or spread in circular or rectangular patterns to suit larger areas. The ease of application of microwave diathermy makes it an efficient as well as effective form of heating for the treatment of superficial structures.

Pulsed microwave diathermy is now also available, though not frequently seen. It has the advantage of producing the biological effects of microwave without the thermal effects, so reducing the number of contraindications to treatment.

The application of infrared rays to produce a fairly vigorous form of heat in the superficial regions of the body is based on the absorption of infrared rays from 770 to 15 000 nm. The penetration depth of the various rays is variable. The short infrared rays penetrate to the level of the dermis and subcutaneous tissues, while the long infrared rays penetrate only to the epidermis level. It is a useful method of superficial vigorous heating for large areas. There is some reflex vasodilatation in deeper regions and distal areas, but in the main it is the superficial heating effects that can be utilised appropriately for superficially placed lesions. The beam of the lamp is divergent and hence the intensity of radiation varies inversely with the square of the distance from the lamp. The rise in temperature is maintained as long as the lamp is on the patient, and quickly subsides on removal. It produces the same rise in temperature as hot packs, but it is a dry form of heat which is more conducive for the various effects than moist heat for some patients, and penetrates slightly deeper than hot packs.

References

Abrahamson, David J, 1962, Use and abuse of physical therapy in industry, *J of Occ Med*.

Cameron, B M, 1961, Experimental acceleration of wound healing, *The American Journal of Orthopaedics*, 336-343.

Crosby, P A, 1979, Microwaves and ocular pathology:— a review, *Aust J of Ophthal*, 7, 163-166.

Ducker, Howard G E, 1968, The effects of metal on short wave field distribution, *Physiotherapy*, 54, 7, 244-246.

Hardy, J D, 1966, Thermal pain, *Ciba Foundation Symposium*, J & A Churchill Ltd.

Health Equipment Information, 1981, Microwave diathermy: Safety in normal use, *Physiotherapy*, 64, 4, 108-109.

Huang, Z et al, 1980, Rewarming with microwave irradiation in severe cold injury syndrome, *Chin Med J (Engl)*, 93, 2, 119-120.

Lehmann and others, 1974, Therapeutic heat and cold, *Clin Orthop and Rel Res*, No 99.

Lehmann, J F et al, 1979, Microwave therapy: Stray radiation, safety and effectiveness, *Arch Phys Med Rehabil*, 60, 578-583.

Licht, Sydney (Ed), 1965, Therapeutic heat and cold, *Maryland: Waverley Press*.

Peyton, Mary Fouse, 1961, Biological effects of microwave radiation, *New York: Plenum Press*.

Rajamaku, 1971, Healing of open wounds, *Acta Chir Scand*.

Scott, Bryan O, 1957, The principles and practice of diathermy, *London: William Heinemann*.

Scott, Pauline M, 1975, Clayton's electrotherapy and actinotherapy, *London: Balliere Tindall*.

Thom, Harald, 1966, Introduction to short wave and microwave therapy, *Springfield*.

Wadasdi, M, Inhibition of experimental arthritis by athermic pulsating short waves in rats, *Orthopedics*, 2, 5.

Ward, A R, 1976, Electricity fields and waves in therapy, *Sydney: Science Press*.

Wareham, T, 1968, The hazards of electrical and allied treatments, *Physiotherapy*, 54, 7, 230-231.

Wilson, D H, 1974, Comparison of short wave diathermy and pulsed electromagnetic energy in treatment of soft tissue injuries, *Physiotherapy*, 60, 10, 309-310.

Wright, G G, 1973, Treatment of soft-tissues and ligamentous injuries in professional footballers, *Physiotherapy*, 59, 12, 385-387.

Wyper, DJ and McNiven, D R, 1976, Effects of some physiotherapeutic agents on skeletal muscle blood flow, *Physiotherapy*, 62, 3, 83-85.

Young, R G, 1965, Value and limitations — pulsed high frequency, *Diapulse Corp of America*.

4 Cryotherapy

4.1 **Treatment by Cooling**
4.2 **Summary of Ice Techniques**
References

Some Key Points in this Unit

Cryotherapy is the treatment of pathological lesions by the use of low temperatures.

Cryogel is a polyvinyl alcohol gel which maintains a low temperature for over 30 minutes.

4.1 Treatment by Cooling

Cryotherapy is the local or systemic application of cold for clinical and diagnostic uses. The use of cold in medicine dates back to Hippocrates who recommended cold for recent trauma. Cold compresses for sprains is an age-old remedy. Ice cubes, evaporating sprays producing rapid cooling, and ice baths are some forms of ice therapy used. The treatment of patients with various neurological and musculo-skeletal conditions has been largely empirical. New techniques are being tried in an effort to obtain more effective care for the patient.

The therapeutic value of cold is still controversial. Many physiotherapists prescribe cold for the relief of pain, muscle spasm, and oedema, but this usage continues to be based on the subjective feeling of the patient, with some relation to pathology, rather than on specific data and well-controlled studies. Recent research is beginning to give us better information.

PROPERTIES OF COLD

When cold is applied to the body, the skin temperature changes. The speed at which the changes occur depends on various factors:
(*a*) application temperature, and the temperature of the part receiving the treatment;
(*b*) ability of the tissue to recover from the lowered temperatures;
(*c*) specific resistance of the tissues to low temperatures;
(*d*) duration of the cold application;
(*e*) density of the skin, fat, subcutaneous fascia, and muscle;
(*f*) water content of the tissues;
(*g*) patency of the circulation;
(*h*) region to which it is applied;
(*i*) existing pathophysiology of the lesion.

The speed at which the skin temperature will change depends on the ability of the skin to regulate skin temperature and dissipate heat. The water content of skin in adults is about 60% greater than in infants and the elderly. Water content varies from hour to hour and accounts for variations in the spread of cold areas. The physical properties of subcutaneous fat, in particular its low thermal conductivity, allow it to act as a barrier to heat exchange. This means that short applications of cold do not lower muscle temperatures. If cold is applied for over 20 minutes, it can be anticipated that the skin will return to its previous temperature more rapidly than deep muscles, especially since vasoconstriction will occur in the cooled muscle.

METHODS OF COOLING TISSUES

Convective cooling. For reduction of hyperthermia, using an electric fan to blow air over the skin.

Evaporative cooling. The use of volatile fluids for evaporation from the skin. When the volatile fluid evaporates from the skin, thermal energy is removed, and the skin temperature may be reduced to as low as –4°C. Fluids used are ethyl chloride, and non-flammable chlorofluoromethane, and fluoromethane.

Conductive cooling. Therapeutic application of cold, using methods that will cause a direct conduction of heat from the tissues of the body, includes crushed ice packs, frozen gel packs, ice baths, wet iced towels, and ice cubes. Temperatures are reduced to 10°C in most cases.

PHYSIOLOGICAL EFFECTS OF COLD

A large number of physiological responses to cold have been investigated and found to have therapeutic significance. They include a decrease in circulation, decrease in haemorrhage following trauma, decrease in the formation of exudate, decrease of muscle spasm and spasticity, decrease in pain, a reflex stimulation of muscle, a delayed vasodilatation in tissues, and a reduction of muscle fatigue.

Normal temperature regulation. When exposed to a change in temperature, man responds by adjusting his heat balance so as to maintain his core temperature at or near its constant level. This involves the integration of an extremely sensitive and complex thermoregulating system. The system maintains an appropriate heat gradient between the core and the skin surface, so that the body is at a suitable temperature for its metabolic activity whether the surface is losing or absorbing heat.

Heat loss is increased by peripheral vasodilatation and heat is conserved by peripheral vasoconstriction. Temperature is controlled by the skin receptors regulating skin reflexes, which are short latency reactions by the axon reflex, reflex vasoconstriction and counter-irritation. Longer latency reactions involve the posterior hypothalamus, the vasomotor center of the medulla, the gamma system and the 'hunting' response of Lewis.

Primary thermal receptors in the skin are simple unencapsulated nerve endings found abundantly throughout the skin. There are 7 to 8 times as many cold receptors as hot receptors. A cold receptor responds to cooling by a proportionate, sharp but transient increase in discharge, and to warming by an inhibition of discharge. The warm receptor acts in the opposite way.

The application of cold produces the short latency response of vasoconstriction of the superficial skin vessels by the axon reflex and through the spinal segmental reflexes, causing vasoconstriction of adjacent areas, such as muscles and joints in the region. Long latency thermoregulation takes place by reflex action through the central nervous system involving the posterior hypothalamus, and the vasomotor center of the medulla. The adequate stimulus for the hypothalamus is a diffuse heat loss over a large area of the body, and a decrease in blood temperature or core temperature.

The hunting response. In 1930 Lewis stated that, following the application of intense cold to the body, there was a vasoconstriction with the liberation of histamine-like ('H') substances produced by the intense cold and noxious stimuli. When there were sufficient 'H' substances, vasodilatation occurred for a brief period of time, about 4 to 6 minutes, and this vasodilatation removed all the 'H' substances.

Vasoconstriction was established again, with vasodilatation occurring at further intervals of 15 to 30 minutes. The sudden vasodilatation due to an *intense cold application* is termed the *hunting response*. The initial vasoconstriction lasts about 9 to 16 minutes. Lewis also stated that the 'after-effect' following removal of intense cold for a prolonged period was vasodilatation, which increased greatly for 20 minutes, and then subsided slowly.

Prolonged ice applications. Hartvicksen (1962) and Bierman state that, if iced towel applications are placed on a limb for a period of 20 minutes, the temperature drops for a period of 40 minutes, even after removal of iced towels, to a temperature of 28°C. The deeper muscles go down to 30° to 33°C following the application of iced towels for 20 minutes. The response of joint and ligamentous structures is less defined. Hollander and Harvatt (1950) found increased temperatures of the joint after 20 minutes of ice application. Initially blood flow to joints shows vasoconstriction and lowered temperatures.

Cold applied to the abdominal wall has the effect of increasing gastric mobility and increasing acid secretions in the stomach by reflex activity, whereas direct application of cold to the stomach by drinking an iced cold drink causes decreased gastric mobility and secretions. Unlike heat applications, the after-effect of vasodilatation with prolonged ice applications remains for 2 to 3 hours.

Effects of varying reductions of temperature on the tissues of the body. Therapeutic applications of ice drop the temperature down by 5° to 28°C. Ethyl chloride causes the biggest drop, to –5°C, while ice massage and ice immersion can bring the temperature of skin down to 14°C. Long-duration ice packs and iced towels reduce the skin temperature to 18° to 20°C, and the muscles between 30 and 50 mm from the skin are lowered to 30° to 33°C.

At temperatures less than 10°C, there is initial vasoconstriction of the superficial vessels, followed by a general vasoconstriction. Involvement of more generalised reactions would depend on the period of the cold application. The oxidative processes of the tissues are depressed, and oxyhaemoglobin undergoes little dissociation. Redness of the skin occurs from the periodic dilatation of the arterioles (the 'hunting' response of Lewis), and this occurs with temperatures of between 5° to 10°C. In addition, there is delayed vasoconstriction as a result of the activation of the hypothalamus by the return of cooled venous blood. There are also cyclic phases of vasodilatation as a protective mechanism to maintain the body's heat balance.

At −5 °C (below freezing point) there is extensive cellular damage and liberation of histamine-like substances, causing frostbite and ice burns.

Cooling under 18 °C increases the viscosity of muscle, and there is greater utilisation of energy for the same amount of work. This causes a lowering of muscle tone and efficiency. Changes in joint and tendon viscosity at this temperature range also account for diminution of function at low temperatures. Cooling of muscle under 18°C reduces both the contraction time and latency considerably.

At temperatures of 20° to 29°C, muscles can sustain their activity for longer periods of time without fatigue. Isometric muscle endurance can be improved when iced towel applications are applied for 15 to 20 minutes, bringing the temperature of the muscle to 20° to 29°C.

Effects on nerve conduction. Many physiologists have experimented with the effects of local cooling on the nervous system. The effects are determined by the duration of the cold application, the temperature reduction, the rate of reduction, and the specific nerve fibre cooled.

Selective inhibition

NERVES	FIBRES	DIAMETER	NERVES AFFECTED
Group I	A	20 μm – 12 μm	motor fibres in extra-fusal muscle fibres highest resistance to cold
Group II	A	12 μm – 8 μm 8 μm – 5 μm	fusimotor nerves of muscle spindle and the afferent secondary windings to muscle spindle easily affected by cold; conductivity readily diminished
Group III	A	5 μm – 2 μm	some pain fibres are in this group susceptible to cold
Group IV	C	0.5 μm – 1 μm	least susceptible; low temperatures needed to reduce conductivity

Brief icing with ice colder than 0°C, over a skin area which has the same nerve supply as the underlying muscle will facilitate reflex contraction. A cooling of 1°C raises the impulse frequency of non-specific C fibres by 30 impulses per second immediately. Selective peripheral nerve inhibition occurs if rapid and large temperature changes to below 10°C take place. If the temperature drops below 20°C, there is a decrease of endplate potential, reduction in the production of acetylcholine, reduced rate of nerve conduction (depending on the type of nerve fibre), and selective reduction of action potential. This causes an asynchrony of impulses (Clarke, Lind and Hellon).

Effect on muscle spasm and spasticity. Cooling has been found effective with muscle spasm and spasticity. *Spasticity* is a state of hypertonicity of muscle, with hyperactivity of the phasic and tonic stretch reflexes, and loss of inhibitory mechanisms from the suppressor areas of the brain through the medial reticular system.

Spasm of a muscle is an involuntary sustained contraction utilising large amounts of nutrient substances, while simultaneously creating ischaemia because of compression of intramuscular blood vessels. The muscle ischaemia results in tissue damage and more liberation of metabolites that excite pain fibres and produce additional pain and muscle spasm.

Cold decreases nerve conduction velocity of the gamma motor neurons, and at the same time, when there is pain and muscle spasm following trauma, the initial vasoconstriction which occurs reflexly is thought to control the bleeding of the lacerated blood vessels, and the uncontrolled oedema fluid. It promotes absorption of the exudate and prevents further bleeding and exudate formation. This will remove the factors causing pain.

The cold also bombards the central pain receptor areas with a barrage of cold impulses so that pain impulses are negated, causing a break in the vicious cycle of pain-metabolites-muscle spasm-pain.

The influence of the gamma bias in the neural control of muscle tone is disturbed in spasticity. Lowering the temperature of the muscle spindle nerve fibres causes a reduction in their over-activity, while also increasing the excitability of the alpha motor neurons. The therapeutic effectiveness of cooling in any given spastic patient is not always predictable. If cooling does reduce spasticity, it then becomes a useful tool. However it is only a temporary cessation of spasticity.

Apparatus for Ice Techniques

An automatic ice machine is essential apparatus in any physiotherapy department or treatment rooms. There are many commercial machines available today, varying in output. A machine which makes suitable flaked ice and ice cubes is essential. The small machines supplied to hotels for the production of crushed ice for drinks are suitable for small departments.

Commercial ice machines vary in size and produce from 40 kg to 250 kg over 24 hours. They have a built-in storage bin, thermostatically controlled, to control the output of the icemaker. The machine has to be installed with adequate plumbing with a water inlet and a drainage outlet. It takes up about one square metre of floor space.

Cryogel cold packs. A Cryogel cold pack consists of a polyvinyl alcohol gel which is enclosed in a poly-ethylene-vinyl acetate bag. The gel consists of a water-soluble solution of polyvinyl alcohol in a solution of sodium borate which remains flexible down to a temperature of $-20°$ to $-23°C$. The poly-ethylene-vinyl acetate bag is soft and light, but strong. The gel in its bag remains entirely flexible, which makes it conformable to each body contour and provides maximum efficiency of cooling of tissues. Cryogel, cooled to $-1°C$ for 2 hours, remains under $4°C$ for 1 to 2 hours.

There is a cooling effect of the skin of significant degree for about 20 minutes. The application temperatures are variable unless the freezing temperature is known. It is important to wrap the Cryogel packs in a cold, wet towel to prevent the occurrence of a burn. In the sports medicine field, some trials have shown that they do not maintain their temperature long enough to produce the desired effects (Laing, 1975), yet other users are satisfied with the results.

INDICATIONS

Pain and muscle spasm. The use of ice packs or iced towels is useful for the relief of pain and muscle spasm. The iced towel is used for the whole muscle which is in spasm, from origin to insertion, in an endeavour to obtain a 10°C reduction of temperature, to reduce the conductivity of the fusimotor fibres of the muscle spindle. The iced towel must remain on the muscle for at least 10 to 15 minutes.

Pain in joints due to arthritis is readily reduced. In rheumatoid arthritis there is an increase in joint temperatures. Normal joint temperatures (31°C) are lower than body temperatures. Increased temperature in joints causes cartilage destruction, as there is enzymatic lysis of human cartilage collagen by the rheumatoid synovial collagenase. If the temperature of the joint is reduced to 30°C, then the enzymatic collagenolysis appears negligible (Hollander, Castor and Yaron).

Does an ice pack to a joint increase joint temperature? There have been conflicting reports on the effect of ice on joints, and so an ice pack for 10 minutes, to cause a marked vasoconstriction and reduction in nerve conduction velocity of pain fibres, would be the rationale for the use of ice. The temperature of the ice pack must be cold enough to reduce the temperature by 10°C at least.

Acute ligamentous or tendon lesions or tenosynovitis with pain and in-flammation are best treated with *ice cube massage* for the relief of pain and vasoconstriction to combat the inflammation.

Acute inflammation following trauma. Following trauma, the injured tissues secrete 'H' (histamine-like) substances which cause vasodilatation of arterioles and capillaries. There is also bleeding from the lacerated tissue, and extravasation of tissue fluid producing oedema. Vasodilatation is followed by plasma fluid release from capillaries and movement of leucocytes, and there is increased hydration of tissue fluid. These processes take place in the first 48 to 72 hours. Uncontrolled vasodilatation and oedema will lead to contractures, chronic swelling and impaired function of muscles and joints. If ice applications are placed on the injured tissues, then the intense vasoconstriction will limit bleeding and the formation of haematomas. Indirectly vasoconstriction increases ab-sorption of oedema, and prevents it from occurring.

For injuries of the lower leg or lower arm, ice immersion techniques can be used. Following immersion, the cyclic phase of vasoconstriction for 10 to 16 minutes is followed by 4 to 6 minutes of vasodilatation.

At the Sports Injury Center in Western Ontario, and in Tokyo, the following regime based on Lewis's assumptions has proved successful. In the immediate 24-hour period following injury, the affected part is immersed for 10 minutes to allow vasoconstriction only, and then elevated with a compression bandage applied firmly to the part for a further 10 to 15 minutes. This is to prevent any vasodilatation occurring. The whole procedure is repeated for up to one hour. This may be done frequently for the first 48 to 72 hours after injury.

Alternatively, Laing, New Zealand, suggests that for the first 48 to 72 hours after injury the affected limb is placed in elevation, and an ice pack, made with ice chips in terry-towelling, is placed on the affected area. Prior oiling of the skin with olive oil reduces the incidence of ice reactions. The pack is bandaged with a crepe bandage and towels and a basin kept nearby to catch any dripping water. The pack is kept on for 20 minutes. With ice packs, the temperature change is not so dramatic or noxious as immersion icing, hence the cyclic phases do not operate as much. There is primarily vasoconstriction.

Both these methods conform to the principle expressed as

I = ice
C = compression
E = elevation.

Ice packs are useful for acute neck pain, such as in a whiplash injury, all the affected muscles being treated.

Chronic inflammation following trauma. Ice on its own is not useful for the healing process after injury. Heat is more useful, but in cases of chronic oedema and pain, alternate application of hot packs and ice packs of 20 minutes duration has been found useful.

The prevention of injury. Brief immersion icing is done after vigorous sports in order to prevent the after-effects of minor injuries or strains being allowed to take hold of the player or athlete. Following vigorous arm sports, the whole arm is immersed in ice following the immersion icing technique. Immersion icing done after every injury, including minor fractures, will reduce the incidence of large haematoma formation.

Spasticity. As discussed earlier, ice may or may not be effective for spasticity. But ice immersion for up to 5 minutes can reduce the spasticity temporarily. It must be followed immediately by rehabilitation techniques.

Facilitation of movement. Weak muscles, such as are seen following a Guillain-Barre Syndrome, Bell's Palsy, or paresis of any form, are successfully stimulated with brief icing as part of the total facilitatory treatment. Sensory input to stimulate movement is proving to be a valuable technique to all physiotherapists. Re-education of orofacial function with brief icing as part of the regime has been found effective.

Increase of isometric strength. If an ice pack or iced towels are placed on a muscle to reduce its temperature to 20° to 29°C, then the muscle readily increases its endurance power in an isometric endurance exercise program performed immediately after the icing.

CONTRA-INDICATIONS

Peripheral vascular disease. Patients with mild vascular conditions could develop a histamine reaction. In patients with advanced conditions it could cause an episode of paroxysmal haemoglobinurea. Even gangrene can be precipitated in advanced cases.

Cardiac disease or cerebrovascular insufficiency. Large areas should not be treated because of the possible effects on the general circulation.

Ice packs on the left shoulder in patients with coronary artery disease, or a history of myocardial infarct has been a contra-indication in the past, as cooling of the vagus occurs, but this has not been upheld by further research. An ice pack could be applied to the left shoulder with the towel wrung out in warm water and then packed with ice chips, to reduce the first impact of intense cold on the tissues.

Loss of sensation. Ice should not be applied to any anaesthetised areas as there is a danger of ice burns. Any area that has had deep X-ray therapy should not be iced. Tests of hot/cold and pain sensitivity should be performed.

Cancer and sickle-cell anaemia. Ice should not be applied to large areas as it could upset the general circulation.

Brief icing over the posterior primary rami of the trunk. Brief icing to the skin supplied by the posterior primary rami of the thoracic nerves can stimulate the deep viscera and cause a chain of adverse reactions.

Emotional subjects and mental instability. Some patients are apprehensive and nervous, and dislike cold intensely. These subjects are best not treated with cold, as they would not allow a satisfactory treatment to be carried out, and this will negate the results. Ice to the sole of the foot or palm of the hand is harmful to the neurotic patient.

Patients who are hypersensitive to cold. The patient may react adversely or show an abnormal response to cold. The patient's reaction to ice should be tested.

Throat, ear or side of the neck. These areas should be avoided as adverse visceral or cerebral reactions may occur.

Unreliable patients. Patients who are too old, too young, or who are unable to understand the potential dangers of ice.

Severe blood pressure abnormalities. Alterations to the blood pressure produced by the ice may not be tolerated.

APPLICATION OF ICE TECHNIQUES
ICED TOWEL TECHNIQUE

Equipment required
twice as many towels as are needed to cover the affected area
large basin or baby bath to hold the ice flakes, water and towels
test tubes to test thermal sensation
protective plastic sheets
oil
towels for drying the area
bucket with ice flakes

Explain the procedure to the patient. Check that there are no conditions present which may contraindicate treatment with ice. Examine the signs and symptoms of the condition being treated.

Examine the affected area for cuts, abrasions and skin conditions, or use of liniments and creams. Place the patient in a suitable position with the part to be treated supported and relaxed. Test the thermal sensation of the affected part and also the pain sensation.

Place plastic sheeting under the part and around the clothes closest to the region.

Test the patient's reaction to ice by placing a small ball of ice on oiled skin in an area similar or adjacent to the area to be treated. Leave this in place for 5 minutes, then examine the area for any signs of an abnormal reaction to the ice, for example the development of a raised wheal. This test should be done on a previous visit so that any delayed abnormal response can be observed and reported by the patient. Approximately 5% of patients may demonstrate an abnormal response to ice.

Apply oil to the skin to which the ice will be applied. This slows the conduction of the cold and reduces the danger of an ice burn.

Some patients may be unable to bear the immediate discomfort of the noxious cold stimulus, so it is important to warn the patient of the discomfort that will be first experienced and which will be followed by numbness and then a warm glow.

Warn the patient not to tolerate excessive discomfort as there is a danger of an ice burn.

Place ice flakes and a little cold water in the container. Soak half the number of towels needed in the container. The towels are folded lengthwise and then soaked. Wring out the towels, making sure that there are sufficient ice chips in the towels, and place them on the patient to cover the entire area.

Change the towels every minute, making sure that the iced towels are always at the same temperature. The iced towels should be at a temperature of 10° to 14°C. The whole treatment should be given for at least 15 to 20 minutes.

Assess the area after the application for any excessive erythema. Check that numbing of the area has occurred and assess the degree of symptomatic relief produced.

Iced towels and isometric exercises

If limitation of movement is purely muscular and not a joint or mechanical dysfunction, then an iced towel can be placed along the whole of the muscle from its origin to its insertion. While the iced towels are in place, isometric contractions of the muscle in a functional pattern of facilitation are given. There should be no movement of the joint. If there is difficulty in exercising and holding the iced towel in position, then isometric contractions are given after icing the part with 3 or 4 towel applications, and the process repeated until relaxation is obtained.

ICE PACKS

Equipment required
ice chips
terry-towelling bag or towel
protective plastic sheets
towels to dry the part
test tubes to test thermal sensation
oil

Place the patient with the part to be treated relaxed and comfortable. If the part is oedematous, then elevation should be obtained.

Prepare the patient as described under 'iced towel technique', performing an assessment, checking contraindications, skin testing for thermal and pain sensitivity and for the reaction to ice, and warning the patient of the dangers of the treatment.

Place the ice chips in a wet terry-towelling bag, which has been completely moistened and wrung out. Rub a thin layer of oil around the part to be treated.

Gently mould the pack around the area to be treated. Ensure that there is firm and even contact. Leave the pack on for 10 to 20 minutes.

In cases of swelling, ice packs can be bandaged with a crepe bandage to obtain compression. Care must be taken not to bandage too firmly and unevenly for fear of causing an ice burn.

If there are no terry-towelling bags, then ice chips can be placed in a terry-towel which has been moistened and wrung out, and then folded into a pack the size of the area to be treated.

CRYOGEL PACKS

Cryogel packs must be wrapped in a wet towel that has been wrung out to ensure an even application of cold. The temperature of the pack must be ascertained. If kept in a freezer compartment, then there will be a greater temperature difference between the pack and part treated. The packs are useful for the treatment of pain. Conolly reports success as a post-operative measure for the treatment of pain following hand surgery. Cryogel packs kept in a refrigerator at a lower temperature are useful for pain and swelling. They can be used in the same manner as ice packs in terry-towelling.

ICE IMMERSION

Equipment required
bath that will contain the affected area
ice chips and water
towel for drying the area
oil
protective plastic dressing
test tubes to test thermal sensation

Prepare the patient as described under 'iced towel technique', performing an assessment, checking contraindications, skin testing for thermal and pain sensitivity and for the reaction to ice, and warning the patient of the dangers of the treatment.

Fill the bath with water to the desired level, immerse the oiled hand or foot and add ice chips slowly to allow the patient to adjust more gradually to the drop in temperature.

For pain and swelling immerse the hand or foot in the bath, withdraw when it becomes uncomfortable, and wipe dry with a towel. This is repeated for up to 10 minutes.

For spasticity, the affected limb is maintained for as long as possible in the water. The problem of immersion icing of spasticity is the onset of shivering and hypothermia that can increase spasticity. Bilateral application of heat and cold has been tried to counteract this. Heat applied to a large area such as the abdomen using a hot pack, while ice was applied simultaneously to the spastic part, was found to be effective by Don Tigny and Sheldon. Another method tried was to apply an ice pack over the spastic muscle groups, and place warm towels around it.

Ice bath to the whole body for spasticity

The bath must have a larger proportion of ice than water. Lower the patient into the bath and pack the ice chips firmly around the affected areas. More cold water is then slowly added. Ensure that the bathroom temperature is warm and that there are no draughts. Patients with flexor spasms must let their buttocks first touch the water. Passive stretchings are done while the patient is in the bath. Generally in 5 to 7 minutes a release of spasticity can be felt. The patient is removed from the bath and taken to the gymnasium for further treatment.

ICE CUBE MASSAGE

Equipment required

ice cube or ice lolly on a stick
small towel to wrap around the ice cube or ice lolly stick
towel to dry the patient
test tubes to test thermal sensation
oil

Prepare the patient as described under 'iced towel technique', performing an assessment, checking contraindications, skin testing for thermal and pain sensitivity and for the reaction to ice, and warning the patient of the dangers of the treatment.

Apply oil to the area to be massaged.

The ice cube or ice lolly is wrapped with a towel, leaving one surface free. It is important that the ice cube must contact the tissues directly, and there should be no water around the edges, as this will upset the temperature difference needed for the required physiological effects.

Ice cube massage is given for painful areas and swelling. The painful area is massaged slowly with a constant motion, care being taken not to allow any water to drip. The massage is continued while the patient feels a burning sensation, followed by aching and then numbness. When the pain is reduced, other mobilisation techniques or exercises may follow. The ice massage produces a counter-irritant effect for pain.

BRIEF ICING FOR STIMULATION

Rood has advocated brief icing of muscles to reflexly stimulate the fusimotor fibres to the muscle spindle. Applications by quick stroking with a dry cube of ice, colder than 0°C so that it does not drip around the adjoining skin area, is used on dermatomes that have the same nerve supply as the underlying muscle. The myotome and the dermatome of the skin over the affected muscle must be the same.

There is no delay in the response of brief ice, so it is used immediately prior to other stimuli to activate the muscles required. Brief icing is part of the total facilitatory techniques used.

The following table summarises the areas which should be iced to facilitate various movements.

Brief icing for stimulation

FACILITATION AREA	ICED AREA
to facilitate extensor muscles to obtain knee stability if extensor lag is present	skin over vastus medialis and lateralis
swallowing and speech	area over supra sternal notch lips, tongue, inside cheek (teeth must be avoided); suck ice lolly
to initiate micturition by relaxing the internal sphincter of urethra and contracting bladder wall and transversus abdominis	over the skin of gluteus maximus; front and side of lower trunk — (L1 and 2 region of ilio hypogastric nerve supply)
to facilitate manual skilled movements	ice finger tips
as a preventive measure for the occurrence of decubitus ulcers	icing over the affected area
to facilitate diaphragmatic breathing	T7 to T12 in the anterior part of the trunk; avoid rectus; right side first

DANGERS AND PRECAUTIONS WITH ICE TECHNIQUES

The main complication following ice treatments is injury to the skin or soft tissue. Ethyl chloride sprays can reduce the temperature to -5°C and must be used carefully. The eyes must be protected when spraying with ethyl chloride. Ice cube massage does not reduce the skin temperature to below 14°C, so there should be no danger of a burn, though histamine reactions appear with some fair or obese patients. If ice burns occur, they develop as painful red blotches which are uncomfortable and remain so for about 3 days. More severe cold injury includes tenderness and thickening of the subcutaneous tissues due to fat necrosis, and this may persist for 3 weeks.

Intensive ice treatments done 3 or 4 times per day make the patient more susceptible to ice damage. Ice around the whole of the knee joint predisposes to fat necrosis and should be avoided. The danger of undue pressure of an ice application on a bony prominence or subcutaneous area with poor blood supply is that it will cause an ice burn.

In older patients it is possible to cause a venous thrombosis, and some patients in the older group complain of persistent pain in the lower leg following ice application to the anterior tibial compartment (Laing).

Young people who are fair and do not react to the cold well could develop a blotchy skin immediately after icing. All patients should have prior application of olive oil to the skin.

The treatment of ice burns is to rest the part and prevent any skin breakdown and risk of infection. Analgesics for the relief of pain may be given.

4.2   Summary of Ice Techniques

The physiological effects of cold are based on the manipulation of the extremely sensitive and complex thermostatic system of the heat-regulating centers of the body. The body uses physical phenomena of conduction, convection and radiation to maintain heat balance, and neural and chemical phenomena to maintain a favorable heat gradient between its core temperature and skin temperature. The neural phenomena, which brings about vasoconstriction and vasodilatation as short and long latency reactions, are used to combat the problems of swelling and inflammation. The effect of cold on the various nerve fibres has been used to either combat pain or to stimulate a muscle response.

The list of responses which have been valuable for therapeutic purposes are the short-latency and long-latency vasoconstriction period, the hunting response to intense, noxious cold stimuli — cyclic phases of vasodilatation and vasoconstriction, after-effect vasodilatation, gamma spindle receptivity alteration facilitating alpha motor neurons, decreased conductivity of pain receptors and fibres, increased adrenalin production, and increased muscle metabolism at specific temperatures.

The physiological effects of ice depend on various factors. The application temperature, duration of the application, the ability of the tissues to conduct heat, the patency of the circulation, and the method of application are the main variables.

Physiological evidence suggests that cold is effective in decreasing the degree of haemorrhage and oedema which complicate acute trauma; in relief of pain and muscle spasm following acute trauma, and sometimes for chronic traumatic injuries; in reduction of pain and inflammatory processes in rheumatoid arthritis; in reduction of pain and swelling in osteoarthrosis; in reduction of spasticity (temporarily); in hemiplegia, multiple sclerosis, and spinal cord injuries; in the re-education of weak muscles as part of the neuromuscular facilitation techniques; in improving the isometric endurance of muscles; and in preventing bleeding and swelling in sports injuries.

To use cold effectively, the physiotherapist must understand the physiological effects of each method of ice application, and must be able to apply it effectively to the patient's pathology, taking into account the patient's ability to tolerate the application of cold. In view of current knowledge the use of cold is a valuable adjunct to treatment in physiotherapy.

References

Abrahamson, D I, 1962, Use and abuse of physical therapy in industry, *J of Occ Med, 4,* No 11.

Arnell, P and Beattie, S, 1972, The physiological basis for, and clinical application of heat and cold in the treatment of hypertonicity, *J of Can Physio Assoc, 24,* 61.

Barcroft, H and Edholm, O G, June 1943, The effect of temperature on blood flow, *J Physiol, 102,* 5-19.

Basmajian, Wolf and Shine, 1973, Device for controlled rapid localised cooling, *Am J of Phys Med, 52,* 65.

Bassett, S W and Cake, B, May 1968, Use of cold application in the management of spasticity, *P T Rev, 58,* 333.

Benson, T B and Copp, E P, 1964, The effects of therapeutic forms of heat and cold on the pain threshold of the normal shoulder, *Rheum and Rehab, 13,* No 2, 101.

Bierman, W, 1955, Therapeutic use of cold, *J Am Med Assoc, 157,* 1189-1192.

Bierman, W and Friedlander, M, 1940, The penetrative effects of cold, *Arch Phys Ther, 21,* 585-591.

Denny-Brown, D, Adams, R D, Brenner, C and Doherty, M M, 1945, The pathology of injury to nerve induced by cold, *Neuropath Exp Neurol, 4,* 305-323.

Don Tigny, R L and Sheldon, K W, 1962, Simultaneous use of heat and cold in the treatment of muscle spasm, *Arch Phys Med Rehab, 43,* 235-237.

Downey, J A, 1964, Physiological effects of heat and cold, *Phys Ther, 44,* No 8, 713.

Fischer, E and Solomon, S, 1965, Physiological responses to heat and cold, S Licht, Ed, Therapeutic heat and cold, *Baltimore: Waverley Press Inc,* 126-169.

Goff, B, 1969, Excitatory cold, Congress Lecture, *Physiotherapy, 55,* 467.

Grant, A E, 1964, Massage with ice (cryokinetics) in the treatment of painful conditions of the musculoskeletal system, *Arch Phys Med Rehab, 45,* 233-238.

Guyton, A C, 1968, Textbook of medical physiology, *Philadelphia: W B Saunders Co.*

Haines, J, 1967, A survey of recent developments in cold therapy, *Physiotherapy, 53,* 222-229.

Hartviksen, K, 1962, Ice therapy in spasticity, *Acta Neuro Scandinav, 38,* Suppl 3, 79-84.

Hayden, C, 1964, Cryokinetics in an early treatment programme, *P T, 44,* 990.

Hollander, J L and Horvath, S M, 1949, The influence of physical therapy procedure on the intra-articular temperature of normal and arthritic subjects, *Am J Med Sci, 218,* 543-548.

Kirk, J A and Kersley, G D, 1968, Heat and cold in the physical treatment of rheumatoid arthritis of the knee, *Ann Phys Med, 9,* 270-274.

Lewis, T, Hagnal, I, Kerr, W, Stern, E and Landis, E, May 1930, Observations upon the reactions of vessels of human skin to cold, heat, *15,* 177-208.

Mead, S and Knott, M. The use of ice in the treatment of joint restriction spasticity and certain types of pain, *Calif Rehab Center, Vallejo.*

Miglietta, O E, 1962, Evaluation of cold in spasticity, *Am J of Phys Med, 41.*

Murphy, A, 1960, Physiological effects of cold application, *Phys Ther Rev, 40,* 112-115.

Olsen, J E and Stravino, V D, August 1972, Review of cryotherapy, *Phys Ther, 52,* 841-845.

Pegg, S M H, Littler, T R and Littler, E N, 1969, A trial of ice therapy and exercise in chronic arthritis, *Physiotherapy, 55*, 51-56.

Ruch, T C, Patton, H, Woodbury, J and Towe, A, 1965, *Neurophysiology*, Philadelphia: WB Saunders Co.

Scott, P, 1969, Clayton's electrotherapy and actinotherapy, *Balliere, Tindall and Cassell, London*.

Showman and Wedlick, 1964, The use of cold instead of heat for the relief of muscle spasm, *Aust J of Physio, 10*, 85.

Stangel, L, October 1975, The value of cryotherapy and thermotherapy in the relief of pain, *Physio, Canada, 135*.

Stockmeyer, S A, 1967, An interpretation of the approach of Rood to the treatment of neuromuscular dysfunction, *Am J of Phys Med, 46*, 900-956.

Till, D, 1969, Cold therapy, Congress Lecture, *Physiotherapy, 55*, 461.

Viel, E, 1959, Treatment of spasticity by exposure to cold, *Phys Ther Rev, 39*, 598-599.

Waylonis, G W, 1967, The physiologic effects of ice massage, *Arch Phys Med Rehab, 48*, 37-42.

Wise, D, 1972, Pain relief and increase of quadriceps contraction in menisectomy patients through application of cold, London, Ontario, *Center for Treatment of Sports Injuries*, University of Western Ontario.

Wise, D D, October 1973, Ice and the athlete, *Physiotherapy, 25*, No 4.

Wolf and Basmajian, J V, 1973, Intramuscular temperature changes deep to localised cutaneous cold stimulation, *P T, 53*, 1284.

5 Ultrasonic Therapy

Some Key Points in this Unit

Ultrasonics is the name given to the technology associated with mechanical vibrations of frequencies above those to which the ear can respond. The upper limit of audibility varies from person to person, but the average is 20 000 Hz. Ultrasonic frequencies range from 20 kHz to 10 GHz.

Longitudinal or compression waves are the to-and-fro oscillations of particles in a medium in the direction of the propagation of the wave, giving rise to alternate compressions and rarefactions. The waves can occur in solids, liquids and gases.

Shear or transverse waves generally occur in solids. The particles of the medium oscillate in a direction at right angles to the direction of propagation.

Insonation is the art of irradiating the tissues of the body with ultrasound energy.

Piezoelectric effect. When crystals are subjected to pressure or tension, they develop electric charges on opposite crystal surfaces. The conversion of high frequency alternating voltage into a mechanical vibration is accomplished by the reversal of the piezoelectric effect.

Acoustic impedance of a material is its characteristic resistance to the propagation of ultrasound. The acoustic impedance (Z) is directly proportional to the density of the material and the velocity of ultrasound in it.

Velocity of ultrasound is the rate at which the successive zones of compression travel through a medium. It depends on the compressibility and density of the tissue through which it passes.

Infrasonic wave is a longitudinal mechanical wave with a frequency below the audible range and is usually generated by large sources. Earthquakes are examples of infrasonic waves.

Attenuation of ultrasonic energy is the progressive loss of intensity. It is the opposite of amplification.

Phon — the unit of loudness. A sound is said to be x phons if it is x decibels louder than the quietest sound of 1 kHz which can be heard by the normal ear.

Decibel — the unit of sound intensity. An increase of 1 decibel is an increase of power by 26%.

Cavitation is the momentary development of cavities within a liquid during the passage through the liquid of the rarefaction (low pressure) phase of an ultrasonic wave.

Transducer is a device which changes energy from one form to another. Transducers are used when energy is available in one form, but required in some other.

For example, it is difficult to generate directly a continuous 1 MHz ultrasonic signal, but relatively simple to generate a continuous 1 MHz electrical signal and apply it to a piezoelectric crystal which converts the electrical energy into an ultrasonic form. The principle is employed in all currently available ultrasonic therapeutic generators.

The efficiency of a transducer is expressed as $\frac{\text{power out}}{\text{power in}} \times 100\%$, which, in the case of our therapeutic generator, equals $\frac{\text{ultrasonic power (watts) leaving the crystal}}{\text{electrical power (watts) entering the crystal}} \times 100\%$ and can vary from almost zero to above 90%.

5.1 Ultrasonic Therapy

TERMS USED IN ULTRASONICS

Ultrasound is a form of acoustic vibration propagated in the form of longitudinal compression waves at frequencies too high to be heard by the human ear.

All sound waves are longitudinal mechanical waves. Sound waves from 20 Hz to 20 000 Hz are within the *audible* range. Waves below the audible range are called *infrasonic* waves.

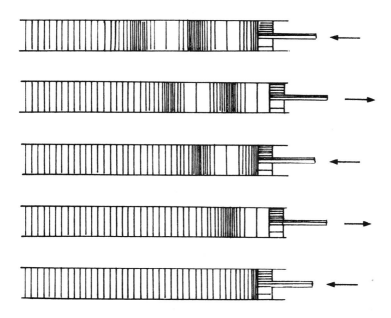

Sound waves being generated in a tube by an oscillating piston. The vertical lines indicate the variations in density of the compressible medium in the tube.

Longitudinal waves cause the articles of a medium to oscillate to and fro in the direction of the propagation of the wave, giving rise to alternate conditions of compression and rarefaction.

The *amplitude* of a longitudinal wave is the greatest distance which a particles moves from its rest position.

The *wavelength* of a longitudinal wave is the distance from the middle of one compression to the middle of the next. As ultrasound has a fixed speed for a particular medium, then it naturally follows that there will be a different number of compressions and rarefactions in a given distance, depending on the frequency of the oscillation. If the frequency is 1 MHz and the velocity is about 1500 m.s^{-1} in water and tissue, then the distance from one compression to another will be one-millionth of 1500 m, or 1.5 mm.

At higher frequencies the wavelength will be less.

The *frequency* of a longitudinal wave motion is the number of complete waves which pass a fixed point in unit time.

Wavelength frequency and velocity of a wave are linked:

velocity = frequency × wavelength.

Most human ears cannot detect frequencies beyond 20 kHz. It is known that some animals, including dogs, are able to hear higher frequencies. Bats can 'see' in the dark by using organs which can produce ultrasonic vibrations with frequencies as high as 150 kHz.

Medical frequencies of ultrasound. Most medical applications employ frequencies between 1 MHz and 15 MHz:

Physiotherapy equipment	—	0.75 MHz, 0.87 MHz, 1 MHz) (average)
		1.5 MHz, 3 MHz)
Diagnostic equipment	—	between 1 MHz and 10 MHz
Surgical equipment	—	between 1 MHz and 5 MHz
Ultrasonic equipment	—	4 MHz or 8 MHz.

Propagation and speed of ultrasound waves. The human body possesses a characteristic resistance against the propagation of ultrasound. Each tissue in the body has a characteristic impedance (Z). It is directly proportional to the velocity of propagation (V) and the density (P) of the tissue.

$$Z = PV.$$

The *velocity* of ultrasound is the rate at which successive zones of compression travel through a medium. It varies with different media.

Density of various media and the corresponding velocity of the ultrasound wave

	VELOCITY (V) m.s.$^{-1}$	DENSITY (P) g.cm^{-3}
bone	3360	1.8
liver	1590	1.06
muscle	1590	1.03
blood	1560	1.06
air at 20°C	340	0.0012
normal saline at 37°C	1535	1.01
distilled water at 37°C	1535	1.0

It is important to realise that the flow of ultrasonic energy can occur without a net movement of the medium: the particles simply oscillate about their mean positions, and, in this way, energy is transferred through the medium. The propagation velocity is controlled by the density and elasticity of the medium.

At intensities of 1 to 4 w.cm^{-2}, the following figures have been recorded:

Amplitude of displacement   — 1×10^{-6} to 6×10^{-6} cm

Particle velocity   —   10 to 26 cm.s^{-1}

Acceleration of particles   — 5×10^7 to 16×10^7 cm.s^{-2}

(This represents an acceleration which is 100 000 times that of gravity.)

Acoustic impedance. Tissues of the body have specific acoustic impedances which offer resistance to the ultrasonic energy passing through it. The characteristic impedance (Z) is the product of the density of the tissue and the velocity.

PRODUCTION OF ULTRASOUND

The brothers, Pierre and Jacques Curie, discovered that, when a quartz crystal is stressed, a potential difference is produced across its faces. This is called the piezoelectric effect.

In 1917 Langevin discovered that by vibrating a quartz crystal with a high frequency alternating current, ultrasound could be produced. All therapeutic ultrasound generators use the reverse piezoelectric effect. Quartz or ceramic materials are used by manufacturers today.

Piezoelectric effect. A crystal usually vibrates at a natural frequency which depends largely on its thickness. The actual amplitude of movement is small (of the order of 1 or 2 μm). Since the crystal will vibrate efficiently at only a single frequency, the generator must be tuned to it. The frequency of vibration remains constant for a given generator, but the intensity, in terms of amplitude, can be varied.

Certain crystals such as quartz, tourmaline, and Seignette's salt, produce electric currents when they are alternately compressed and relaxed in certain directions. Conversely the crystals will contract under the influence of an electric current, and expand when the current is switched off (reverse piezoelectric effect). By continuously varying the direction of the current, the crystal will be made to vibrate and the vibrations produce sound waves.

Most generators are constructed on the reverse piezoelectric principle. When the vibration frequency of the crystal corresponds to the frequency of the alternating current, the waves produced will be amplified by resonance. The object is to cut the crystal platelets carefully so the resonance is greatest at the desired frequency. The vibrations are then conducted to the transducer head, which transmits them to the body tissues.

The ultrasonic generator. The therapeutic ultrasonic valve generator produces a high frequency AC from about 0.75 MHz to 3 MHz. The resonant frequency of the current is at the same natural frequency as that of the crystal. The high frequency current is applied to the crystal. In front of the crystal lies the transducer head which is made to vibrate mechanically by the acoustic vibration energy of the crystal.

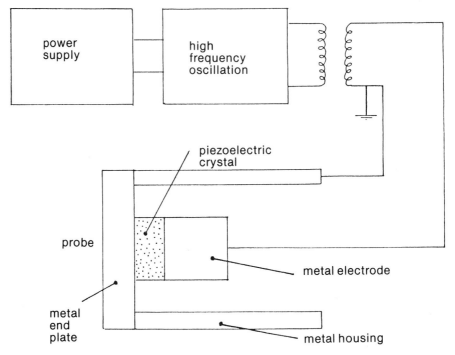

Schematic diagram of ultrasonic generator

The basic components of the generator are the power supply, the oscillating circuit producing the high frequency current, and the transducer circuit.

The *power supply* has full wave rectification and filtering in order to provide a steady output.

The *oscillating circuit* is similar to that of the valve generators producing short wave diathermy. The capacitance and the inductance of the oscillating circuit are selected to produce an alternating current of the same frequency as the mechanical resonance frequency of the crystal of the transducer. The 50 Hz alternating current must be converted to high frequency oscillations of up to 3 MHz, and the voltage is increased before application to the transducer crystal.

The high frequency generator may be connected directly to the crystal through a cable, or a transformer may be incorporated into the transducer treatment head to couple the crystal to the oscillator circuit, so that the impedances of the crystal and the output circuit are matched. Some generators have a variable capacitor with which to adjust the frequency. In other generators, tuning is eliminated by a frequency-stabilising device.

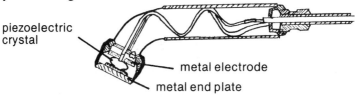

The head of the ultrasonic generator

The *transducer* or treatment head is a crystal inserted between two electrodes. The crystal or synthetic ceramic is cut according to the electrical axis of the crystal lattice. The crystal translates the electrical oscillations directly into mechanical vibrations which pass through a metal cap into the body through the coupling medium.

The intensity distribution of the ultrasonic field produced by the transducer head is measured along the axis of the beam. The maxima and the minima of the near field extend from the sound head. The last maximum is about 170 mm from the head, and marks the beginning of the far field (170 to 250 mm).

Many machines use barium titanate crystals which produce an uneven intensity distribution across the transducer head. Other machines use quartz crystals which produce an even intensity distribution which is preferable as it minimises adverse effects.

For therapeutic purposes, the applicator should have a radiating surface which is slightly smaller than the total applicator surface. This makes it easier to maintain full contact between the head and the treatment area, and at the same time make use of the total surface of the applicator.

When the machine is switched on, the high frequency energy applied to the crystal is increased to the required level. The average ultrasonic intensity is expressed in watts per square centimetre (w.cm^{-2}). It is obtained by measuring the total output of the applicator (power), and then dividing it by the size of the radiating surface of the applicator (area). Large applicators are preferable to small ones.

The angle of divergence of the beam is less if an applicator with a large diameter is used. It would also be difficult to reach deep tissues with a small beam. Therapeutic applicators are usually in the range of 70 to 130 mm. Intensities found useful in the therapeutic range are from 0.5 to 3 w.cm^{-2}. A machine with 30 watts total output and a transducer head of 10 cm^2 surface area has an average intensity of 3 w.cm^{-2}.

SOME PHYSICAL PHENOMENA OF ULTRASOUND
Ultrasound behaves similarly to rays of light and generally follows the laws of optics.

Reflection. When ultrasound passes from one medium to another it is important to know the acoustic impedance (Z) of each medium. If there is an *acoustic mismatch* between the two media, that is, if each medium has a different acoustic impedance, a certain amount of reflection will occur at the *interface* between the media. If the two media have the same characteristic acoustic impedance, there will be no reflection. The amount of reflected energy depends on the difference in the acoustic impedances of the media, and may be calculated by the formula

$$x = \frac{Z_1 - Z_2}{Z_1 + Z_2}$$

where Z_1 and Z_2 = characteristic impedances

and x = the intensity of reflection coefficient

The reflected power is always smaller than the incident power.

Impedance values

MEDIUM	IMPEDANCE (Z) $\times 10^5$ g.cm^{-2}.s^{-1}
bone	6.0
liver	1.68
fat	1.43
brain	1.56
blood	1.65
air	0.0004
normal saline	1.55
water	1.54
muscle	1.64
forearm	1.55
calf	1.55
face	1.65
upper arm	1.65

Bone-periosteum interface. As periosteum and bone tissue have different acoustic impedances, about 70% of the energy is reflected, and the balance (30%) is absorbed by the bone. The total load on the periosteum is equal to the total incident power plus the reflected power. This causes *shear waves* to occur around the periosteum.

The particles of both media oscillate at right angles to the direction of propagation and, as the wavelength is different in each medium, the particles move in different directions and cause a shear stress at the boundary. This is called a *shear stress wave*, and is rapidly absorbed at the periosteum. The periosteum is avascular, and no cooling effect occurs, so it quickly heats up and causes a periosteal pain. The patient will soon complain of the heating sensation, because the periosteum is temperature-sensitive, and thus it helps to safeguard the patient against burns.

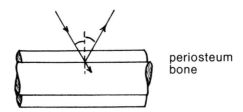

periosteum
bone

The principle of reflection

Tissue-air interface. Reflection also occurs at the tissue-air interface. Here air acts as a reflector, and the ultrasound beam is reflected back to the surface of the tissue area being treated. Excessive heating will occur, causing a heating pain in the skin. This can occur if ultrasound is given to a thin area such as the palm of the hand, where ultrasound will go through the tissues and then meet the air on the opposite side. Pain will be felt in the area of the skin opposite the transducer head.

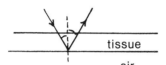

Reflection at the air-tissue interface

Transducer head-skin interface with an air pocket. If the metal of the ultrasound head and the tissue are not completely in contact with one another, and there is a small air pocket, reflection into the transducer head of the machine will occur, with no acoustic power going into the patient. The head will be heated rapidly and cause excessive heating of the skin. There is minimal transmission of ultrasound and danger of a burn.

Refraction. When the angle of incidence is 15°, refraction of a beam is 90° and will run parallel to the interface. Refraction is deviation. It means that the ultrasonic energy impinges the tissue at one angle and continues at a different angle (angle of refraction). Only for angles of incidence of less than 15° will any energy pass into the tissues. Refraction occurs particularly where tendon joins bone and leads to concentration of energy.

The angle of 15° is the *critical angle* concerning the index of refraction. For angles greater than 15° no refracted beam exists, the wave is fully reflected. For angles of incidence of less than 15° there is a reduction of energy going through the tissues. Hence it is important to hold the transducer head perpendicular to the tissues.

Transmission of ultrasound is the passage of ultrasound from the transducer head to the site of the lesion. It is better studied in terms of attenuation and absorption.

Attenuation is the progressive loss of acoustic power, as ultrasonic energy travels through a medium. The amount of attenuation varies from tissue to tissue.

It is worth noting that biological media show attenuation which is linear and inversely proportional to the frequency. If the frequency is changed from 1 MHz to 3 MHz, the attenuation in muscle changes from 2% to 6% per millimetre. For a frequency of 3 MHz, attenuation is 50% (half value) at 25 mm, while at 0.75 MHz half value is at 90 mm.

Absorption of ultrasound. It is generally accepted that absorption of ultrasound energy takes place at a molecular level. A series of investigations has established that proteins are the major absorbers of ultrasound among the molecular constituents of soft tissue.

The protein in *nerve* is sensitive to ultrasound. *Muscle* absorbs twice as much as *fat*. The haemoglobin of *blood* absorbs ultrasound. There is some absorption in the structural content of *cell membranes*. Basically, ultrasound is absorbed at the molecular level, and the absorption coefficients of the tissues are due primarily to the presence of macromolecular tissue contents. Absorption in *fluids* is determined mainly by viscosity and heat conduction. Absorption of ultrasound in *air* is 500 to 1000 times that in water. The absorption in *water* is very small (0.9993) and hence water is a good coupling medium for the transmission of ultrasound.

The *viscosity* of the medium opposes the particle motion, and so absorption of energy occurs. An important contribution to the absorption which occurs in biological materials is due to relaxation mechanisms. Energy can exist in a system in various forms such as molecular vibrational energy, lattice vibrational energy, and translation energy. All the different forms in which the energy is stored are coupled together. The equilibrium which exists between the various forms of energy is disturbed by the passage of an ultrasonic wave. As the equilibrium times are not instantaneous, energy-phase relationships which result in absorption may occur. The mechanism is known as relaxation. *The absorption increases with frequency*.

Frequency dependence of absorption

FREQUENCY	ABSORPTION COEFFICIENT		
MHz	muscle	fat	blood
1	0.12	0.04	0.18
2	0.24	0.10	0.40
3	0.36	0.16	0.58
4	0.48	0.30	0.80

The higher the frequency, the shorter the wavelength, and the greater the absorption, but there is a greatly reduced half value thickness.

Absorption of ultrasonic energy depends on the following:
acoustic impedance of the tissues;
propagation velocity of sound;
density of tissues;
frequency of ultrasound;
protein content;
fat and water content;
angle of incidence of acoustic energy;
mismatch of impedance;
viscosity of fluid;
reflection;
refraction;
diffraction;
shear waves.

Accoustic properties of media

MEDIUM	PROPAGATION VELOCITY $(m.s^{-1})$	CHARACTERISTIC IMPEDANCE $(g.cm^{-2}.s^{-1} \times 10^5)$	ABSORPTION COEFFICIENT $(dB.cm^{-1})$ at 1 MHz	DENSITY $(kg.m^{-3})$	ATTENUATION in 1 mm at 1 MHz
muscle	1585	1.64	0.12	1100	2.0%
bone	3360	6.0	13	1800	1.5%
fat	1450	1.43	0.04	940	0.5%
blood	1560	1.65	0.18	1060	0.1%
water	1480	1.54	0.0022	1000	0.001%
air	340	0.0004	12	1.2	2.0%
steel	5850	47.0	—	8000	

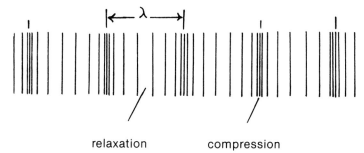

relaxation   compression

Micromassage is the alternate compression and relaxation of tissue by the pressure of sound waves and the mechanical reactions of the tissues.

Motion and amplitude. The forces of sound pressure will set up in tissues a stress pattern which will produce a reciprocating movement of the cells, in such a manner that there is dispersion and aggregation of the molecules occurring alternately as compression and relaxation. The pressure extremes, maximum and minimum, are separated by one half wavelength. For a frequency of 1 MHz the distance is 0.75 mm (750 μm). There is a positive maximum pressure and a negative minimum pressure. There are two million changes of direction of movement every second, hence a great difference of pressure occurs over a relatively small distance, and in a short period of time.

Oscillation of particles. There is also mechanically-caused oscillation of particles in the media.

Friction. The alternate compression and relaxation by the elastic ultrasound waves causes friction between cells. This causes a thermal component.

Cavitation is an important feature of high-intensity ultrasound and care must be taken that it does not occur with therapeutic administration. Cavities can be produced during the phase of relaxation or rarefaction. Threshold intensities required to produce cavitation are 1 to 2 w.cm^{-2} with a stationary head and above 4 w.cm^{-2} when a moving applicator is used.

Since there are dissolved gases always present in biological media, gas-filled cavities may be produced in the fluid media during the period of rarefaction, when high intensities of ultrasound are given to the tissues. During the phase of compression, the cavities may collapse, creating a high concentration of energy. Mechanical destruction will occur when the gas bubble is large enough to vibrate in resonance with the sound waves or when the cavities collapse.

THE ULTRASONIC FIELD

An ultrasound wave is propagated unidirectionally as a non-uniform beam of acoustic energy. The movement of the particles or molecules in the media occur parallel to the direction of wave propagation. The sound beams produced by therapeutic applicators are almost cylindrical in shape.

The beaming properties of the sound applicator depend on the presence of a medium that can be compressed, as propagation does not occur in a vacuum. They depend also on the wavelength and the diameter of the sound applicator. A

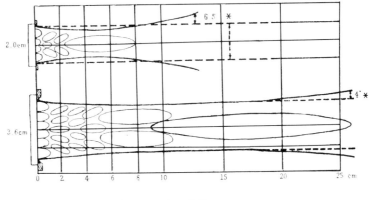

* = angle of divergence

The ultrasound beam (from Pohlman)

transducer operating at 0.9 MHz and having a radiating surface diameter of 20 mm produces a divergence of the beam of about 6.5°, while an applicator of 36 mm will produce an angle of divergence of approximately 4°. The beam spread is inversely proportional to both the diameter of the source and to the frequency.

Sound intensity across the beam. It is characteristic of the ultrasonic field that, in contrast to light, it is not homogeneous with respect to the distribution of power in front of the applicator. A distinctive pattern of maxima and minima spreads over a certain distance called the near or interference field. Beyond this non-homogeneous field, the distant field extends as a homogeneous sound field. If measurements are made of the sound intensity along the central axis of a beam produced by a therapeutic applicator, the intensity distribution shows maxima and minima near the applicator, and then a gradual decline beyond the last maximum. Waves originating from two parts of the transducer may arrive at a point out of phase, leading to a decrease in intensity, as the waves cancel one another.

Waves from the transducer may also meet at a point in phase, causing an increase in intensity of ultrasonic energy. In practice the interference patterns are a matter not only of spatial distribution but also of power content.

The whole power can be considered as bunched into a beam with most of it concentrated in a central pencil of ultrasound, the diameter of which is approximately one-third the dimension of the quartz disc. Therefore this factor and the uneven distribution pattern make it essential that the applicator be moved over the treatment area.

PULSED ULTRASOUND

An ultrasound beam can be administered as a continuous beam or produced in bursts that are pulsed. It is normally pulsed at a frequency of 500 Hz. The time between pulses is 10 ms. This means the ultrasound is pulsed in the ratio of 1:5, which means it is 'on' for only one-fifth of the insonating time. Thermal effects of ultrasound are reduced if the pulsed beam is used, but pressure and amplitude (the micromassage effect) remain unaltered. The shape of the pulse is rectangular.

Heat production is not completely eliminated with a pulse of 1:5. Most equipment has a pulse ratio of either 1:5 or 1:4. Some equipment also provides a 1:1 ratio.

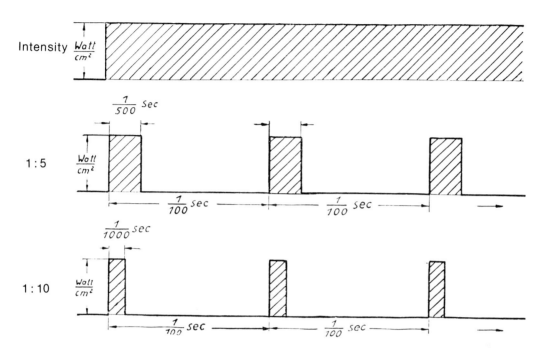

Diagrammatic representation of continuous, pulsed 1 : 5, and pulsed 1 :10 ultrasound.

If heat exacerbates pain, then the pulse ratio of 1:5 or 1:4 should be used. If high intensities are being given and the problem of heating of the sound head arises, the ratio of 1:1 can be used in place of continuous ultrasound. It is also useful when there is a lot of reflection from subcutaneous bone, as in epicondylitis, because it will minimise the heat from the shear waves, but still give the overall effect of heat and micromassage.

Using pulsed ultrasound for 10 minutes with a ratio of 1:5 means that the patient will only receive 2 minutes of ultrasound.

THE PHYSIOLOGICAL EFFECTS OF ULTRASONIC ENERGY

We have seen that high frequency electromagnetic radiations such as infrared and microwave cause mainly thermal effects in the tissues of the body. Electromagnetic radiations below 300 nm wavelength cause other effects besides heat. Waves such as ultraviolet, X-rays, and gamma rays are in this category. Ultrasonic waves are not electromagnetic waves but are mechanical acoustic waves. They range in frequency from 0.75 to 3.5 MHz for physiotherapeutic clinical use.

The main properties of ultrasound will be studied under the following categories in order to evaluate the physiological responses of ultrasound in the body: (*a*) micromassage, (*b*) thermal reactions, (*c*) chemical effects, and (*d*) electrical effects. It must be remembered that ultrasound may display several kinds of behavior simultaneously, and you need to know a number of variables such as frequency, density, accoustic impedance, velocity and intensity, reflection, refraction and diffraction, in order to compute the total biological effects of ultrasound on the body tissues. Also you have to look at the pathology of the lesion, and the patency of neural and circulatory mechanisms.

Micromassage (mechanical effects). When ultrasound waves are absorbed in the tissues (remembering that acoustic waves show mechanical properties of compressions and rarefactions of the tissues), there will be immense mechanical forces working in the tissues which cannot be compared with any other physical agent. The alternation of positive and negative pressures at the frequency of the machine causes the micromassage effect of ultrasound. The following biological effects are caused:

loosening of the microscopic cell structure;
friction, which will produce a thermal effect;
oscillation of particles in a fluid medium;
acceleration of the diffusion processes across the cell membrane;
intracellular massage;
breakdown of complex, biochemically active molecules;
depolymerisation of proteins, especially those which are found in nerve, muscle and collagen cement;
excitation of calcium bound to proteins;
reversible decrease of viscosity of intra- and extracellular colloidal substances;
transport of drugs;
specific effects on neural and circulatory mechanisms;
with high intensities it will cause gaseous cavitation as discussed earlier.

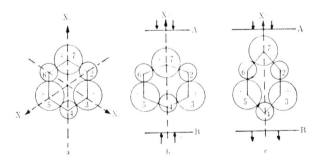

Compression and rarefaction of the quartz crystal (from Bergman)

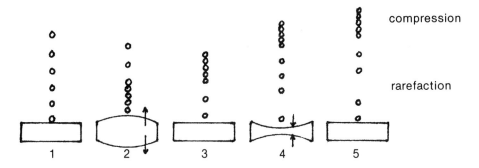

The interaction of the transducer head with its vibrating piezoelectric disc and the tissues of the body in contact with the head.
Phase 1 — the crystal's normal shape
Phase 2 — expansion of the disc pushes the particles closer together (positive phase of pressure cycle)
Phase 3 — the disc returns to normal
Phase 4 — the disc is thinner in the negative phase of the pressure cycle and the particles move apart
Phase 5 — the disc returns to normal

Thermal reactions. Any medium exposed to ultrasound will undergo heating proportional to the energy absorbed, the time insonated, and the specific frequency of the machine. A tissue volume of 50 mm depth heats up with a speed of 0.2°C per minute if an energy of 0.1 watts per minute is applied and there is no mismatch of impedance.

The friction caused by the micromassage effect of ultrasound causes production of heat in the tissues. As an intact blood supply is generally operating, there is a constant dissipation of any increase of temperature. The greatest advantage is that deep-seated areas can be effectively heated, as there is no loss of energy in the skin and subcutaneous fascia, as there is with short wave and microwave.

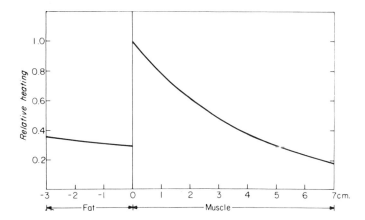

Patterns of relative heating produced by ultrasound in fat and muscle tissue. (From Schwan: Biophysics of Diathermy. In Licht, S.: Therapeutic Heat. New Haven, Conn., Elizabeth Licht, 1958.)

Owing to the mismatch of impedance at the bone-muscle interface, there is reflection, and some shear waves occur which then cause increased heating effects around a joint or bone. So, if any increase of heat is desired in a muscle or around a joint or bone, ultrasound can effectively produce it.

The maximum effective depth of penetration, and therefore temperature rise in that area, will depend on the frequency of the machine, the intensity, and the duration of treatment. It was found that in treating joints with only a thin layer of muscle, skin, and superficial fascia, lower intensity was needed for the increase of temperature, but if there was more than 80 mm of muscle, fat and fascia, then greater intensities for a longer period of time were needed to produce the desired temperature.

Temperature rise in muscle	2°C to 3°C
Temperature rise inside joints	7°C to 8°C
Temperature rise in the area around the joint	3°C to 5°C

Different thicknesses of subcutaneous fat at differing frequencies will alter the heat distribution. The efficiency of ultrasound with a frequency of 1 MHz is decreased by 50% with 20 mm of subcutaneous fat, and it is reduced by 77% with 30 mm of fat. With higher frequencies, a greater percentage is lost.

If ultrasound is applied to a liquid, considerable rise of temperature may take place in seconds. The following values were noted by Dognon and Biancani when ultrasound was given for 10 seconds in 2 ml of liquid:

water	2°
alcohol	3.5°
wax	44°
gelatine gel	1°
glycerol	10°
liquid paraffin	10°

Therapeutic dosages of ultrasound, and the dissipation of heat by the circulation reduce any danger of overheating with ultrasound, though care must be taken to consider the patency of the circulation and the nervous control of sensation before applying treatment.

The degree of heating of tissues depends on the frequency of the generator, the absorptivity of the tissues, the reflection by interfaces and the shear waves.

Chemical effects. Ultrasound can produce effects such as inversion of sugar, changes in crystallisation, hydrolysis, crystallisation of supersaturated solutions, oxidation, and depolymerisation of substances (for example, starch, rubber, and gum). Certain effects, mechanical, thermal and chemical, may involve each other.

In the clinical field nothing significant has been proved regarding the utilisation of any chemical effects. In general, chemical changes are accelerated by ultrasound. There has been noted a drop in blood sugar level, and this could be due to overdosage. Patients who habitually use ephedrin or adrenalin react less favorably with ultrasound, but this is connected with its reactions on the neural elements.

Electrical effects. Generally ultrasound will affect electrode processes and electrolytic solutions, and cause the disturbance of the thin layer of ions at the boundary between a solid and an electrolytic solution. Fukuda reports that large biological molecules, such as proteins and cellulose, exhibit the piezoelectric effect. When subjected to pressure, they exhibit electrical charges on their surface. It could well be that insonation with ultrasound causes the proteins to attract the electrophylic metabolites liberated during ischaemia and pain.

Effects on the circulation. *The main effects of hyperaemia — vasodilatation, and acceleration of lymphatic flow* — are due to the thermal effect of ultrasound. The combination of the thermal and micromassage effects produces the histamine-like substances which cause capillary hyperaemia. Recent experiments have shown that a rise in temperatures does not increase blood flow in muscles. It has been suggested that weak muscles generally have increased circulation, but are unable to use the substrates in the circulation. An increase in temperature would aid metabolism and help the muscle to use its substrates more effectively.

In conditions of the arthritic group, heat can aggravate the symptoms. The normal temperature of joints is 30°C, while the temperature of the inflamed joint is much higher. A rise of 5°C in the joint produces enzymatic lysis of human cartilage collagen by the rheumatoid synovial collagenase. The intra-articular temperature in rheumatoid arthritis is about 36°C and this accelerates cartilage destruction. It is important then to review the effect of raised temperature on specific pathological lesions before administering a modality that causes increased temperature.

According to Gordon, ultrasound does not affect the collagen content of large arteries and arterioles. The semi-permeable membrane of erythrocytes causes a concentration of potassium ions to the exclusion of sodium ions which accumulate in the plasma. Insonation with intensities of 1 to 2 w.cm^{-2} will inhibit the passage of potassium ions from the cell into the surrounding membrane. Absorption of ultrasound in normal blood is proportional to the frequency of the generator.

Blood is a hydrosol and must be regarded as having numerous interfaces. A suspension becomes more heated than a clear liquid, and when ultrasound is beamed through blood, where there are particles such as erythrocytes, leucocytes, and platelets suspended in a fluid, the particles will oscillate. The erythrocytes produce thrombus-like accumulations, between which the plasma remains clear. Normal circulation prevents the formation of ultrasonic thrombi, but if the circulation is impaired great care must be taken to prevent the formation of a thrombus. Generally, though, the thrombus disintegrates once the insonation is stopped, and is thus termed an *ultrasonic parathrombus*.

Ultrasound with intensities of 2 to 3 w.cm^{-2} increases blood velocity.

Effects on nerve tissue. The work of Andersen and Herrick have established that 'B' fibres are the most sensitive to ultrasound, followed by 'C' fibres, and last of all the 'A' fibres were the least sensitive, particularly the gamma group. As the classification of nerve fibres depends on the degree of myelination, there seems to be no correlation with the protein content of nerve fibre and absorption. It has been shown that ultrasound does reduce nerve conduction velocities. This is not due to its thermal effects but to its mechanical and electrochemical effects.

Results from studies have shown that specific intensities of ultrasound alter peripheral nerve propagation.

0.5 w.cm^{-2} — increase motor nerve conduction
$1 \text{ to } 2 \text{ w.cm}^{-2}$ — decrease the conduction velocity
3 w.cm^{-2} — increase nerve conduction velocities.

If ultrasound were to decrease nerve conduction velocities due to its thermal effects, then intensities of 1 to 2 w.cm^{-2} should cause a rise in nerve conduction velocity. With high intensities, the thermal effect may play a role in the reduction of nerve conduction velocities provided it is given for sufficient time to cause a rise in temperature over the nerve. Ultrasound in high dosages should not be given over nerve roots or over the spinal cord, since nerve cells are especially sensitive to sound. The work of Fry (1960) and Ballantyne and Lindstrom has established the following:

cell bodies are more susceptible to ultrasound than the cerebral cortex;

white matter is more sensitive than the cerebral cortex;

fibre tracts are more vulnerable than aggregates of cell nuclei or vascular structures;

the vascular system can be left anatomically functioning and intact in both grey and white matter when all neural components have been destroyed;

the white fibre tracts can be irreversibly changed without destruction of the nerve cell bodies;

reproducible and reversible changes can occur in the brain with appropriate doses;

it is possible to give a low enough dosage to the cell to interrupt function with subsequent complete recovery;

it is possible to selectively produce lesions of the brain, of any area and size, without causing damage to the adjacent structures.

Clinically, diagnostically and with surgery, using varying dosages and intensity, physiotherapists and doctors have utilised all the above effects.

Effects on the autonomic nervous system. It has been found that pulsed ultrasound in the ratio of 1:5 is most suitable to insonate sympathetic ganglia or sympathetic nerve fibres for the production of a change in neural activity. The central nervous system is more sensitive to the thermal effects than to the mechanical effects, so only pulsed ultrasound should be used. Ultrasound has a pronounced vasodepressor effect on nerve roots and thus insonation inhibits the sympathetic system. Patients who are taking ephedrin or adrenalin habitually react less favorably to insonation. Diabetes mellitus patients can be affected by a reduction in blood sugar, so these patients may feel sleepy or begin to go into a coma, and hence it is advisable to give them a drink of glucose immediately after treatment.

Effect on proteins. It is generally accepted that the absorption of ultrasound energy takes place at a molecular level. It has been well established that proteins are the major absorbers of ultrasonic energy among the molecular constituents of soft tissue. It has also been established that there was no significant difference in absorption by proteins wherever they were found in the tissue.

It has been shown by Schwann and other workers that less intensity is required to break the linkage between the amino acids which have combined to form proteins, or between the amino acids and their ions, such as calcium, sodium, or potassium, than is required to rearrange carbohydrates and fat molecules. Schwann has estimated that 80% of absorption by soft tissue is due to the protein it contains.

Effect on drugs. An ultrasonic beam will drive a substance which is dissolved or suspended in the coupling fluid through the skin into the underlying tissue. This is known as *phonophoresis*. The drug to be transported is generally suspended or dissolved at the ratio of 1:10 in a suitable coupling medium such as water, alcohol, glycerol, or liquid paraffin. If the drug is soluble in water or alcohol, then the viscosity can be increased by adding glycerol.

Phonophoresis differs from *iontophoresis* in several important ways. Iontophoresis has a penetration which is only skin deep, whereas phonophoresis can drive a molecule at least 50 mm in depth. With iontophoresis the substance is not transported in its entirety but is dissociated as a positive or negative ion, whereas with phonophoresis the whole molecule is driven in.

Ultrasound at 3 w.cm^{-2} will increase the permeability of the cell membranes by 200%. If the input is reduced by pulsating the beam, the permeability is reduced. The high acceleration will cause increased diffusion without allowing the diffusion of the protein molecules. Phonophoresis using 1% or 10% hydrocortisone cream for subcutaneous inflammations has been used by physiotherapists.

Drugs commonly used include hydrocortisone, lasonil and Vitamin E.

INDICATIONS

Adhesions. It is well known that, following trauma, the connective tissue element of fascia, skin, muscle, and tendon predisposes to adhesions. Connective tissue is loose, dense, or organised. It contains reticulin, collagen, and variable elastin fibres in a ground substance. The collagen fibril is an aggregation of tropocollagen rods in staggered array. Chemical bonding between the tropocollagen molecules leads to increased insolubility and tensile strength. However the process is reversible.

With the formation of adhesions following trauma, there is formation and maturation of collagen bonds, and collagen adhesions form at the site of injury within 36 hours. Ultrasound is thought to aid resorption of the adhesions by the depolymerisation of mucopolysaccharides, mucoproteins or glycoproteins, or by reducing the viscosity of hyaluronic acid in joints.

In joints the increase of adhesions and intracellular substances responds to ultrasound by being converted from the gel to the sol state. It is thought that resorption of adhesions is brought about by both the heating effect of ultrasound and its micromassage effect. The quick rise in temperature, which penetrates deeper, and lasts longer at an effective temperature, helps in the process.

Conditions suitably treated with ultrasound where adhesions are the major problem include:

joint contractures resulting from trauma to periarticular structures,
capsule, muscles, and tendons around joints;
tendon and muscle contractures following trauma;
joint and muscle contractures as symptoms of chronic osteoarthritis;
adhesions of structures around a joint, following insertion of metal implants;

inflammation of a bursa, such as subdeltoid bursitis and olecranon bursitis;
traumatic synovitis;
plantar fasciitis;
stenosing tenovaginitis;
cases of early Dupuytren's contractures.

Pain and muscle spasm. "Pain is the total set of responses an individual makes to a stimulus which causes or is about to cause tissue damage" (Sternbach). If the nervous system is intact, pain can be relieved by various mechanisms which prevent pain volleys from reaching the supraspinal structures. The interference can be achieved by the micromassage effect on the nerves, or by raising the temperature of the part. Ultrasound intensities at 1 to 2 w.cm^{-2} will reduce the nerve conduction velocities of the 'C' fibres carrying pain. 'C' fibres are readily affected by ultrasonic energy.

If pain is due to the accumulation of metabolites causing ischaemia and swelling in the region, ultrasound alters the permeability of cell membrane and aids in accelerating phagocytosis and the absorption of exudate. It also helps to attract the electrophylic pain metabolites and disperse them from the site of the lesion.

It is also thought to cause capillary hyperaemia by the release of histamine-like substances which are produced by the thermal effects of ultrasound. This will help remove the pain metabolites.

Pain caused by sympathetic dysfunction. For conditions such as shoulder-hand syndrome, Sudek's atrophy, reflex sympathetic dystrophy, or post-traumatic dystrophy, the peripheral and central pathways of pain are not well understood. Theories are based on the unproven presence of pain fibres in the sympathetic nervous system. Insonation with pulsed ultrasound on the sympathetic ganglion for the shoulder and reflex sympathetic dystrophies, or insonation of the stellate ganglion have proved effective. 1 w.cm^{-2}, pulsed, for 5 to 10 minutes is generally sufficient to relieve symptoms.

Post-herpetic neuralgia. Insonation of the affected nerve root with pulsed ultrasound for 5 minutes at 1.5 w.cm^{-2} has been found useful. It must be done daily.

Neuroma. Small neuromas which may be found at the end of stumps or where there has been neural damage are treated effectively with low-dosage pulsed ultrasound. 0.5 to 0.8 w.cm^{-2} for 5 to 8 minutes is given. 0.5 w.cm^{-2} for 3 minutes continuous could also be used. Phonophoresis with hydrocortisone has been found to be effective.

Traumatic prepatellar neuralgia. Ultrasound is useful where there is contusion of the neurovascular bundle in front, which, if left untreated, will become adherent to surrounding tissues. A 3 MHz frequency with a dosage of 0.5 to 1 w.cm^{-2} for 4 to 5 minutes is effective. Higher dosages will increase pain.

Calcified tendinitis. Ultrasound causes excitation of calcium bound to proteins. Patients who have calcified supraspinatus tendinitis have been treated successfully with ultrasound to promote resorption of the calcium. Ultrasound-driven hydrocortisone is also useful for the resorption of calcium.

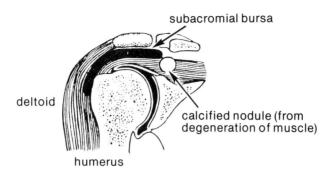

Calcified nodule in the supraspinatus muscle has caused, by friction, a swelling of the subacromial bursa.

Haematomas. In the first 48 hours, low dosage ultrasound to the surrounds of the haematoma with a 3 MHz frequency is useful to prevent the organisation of the exudate. This is best combined with *ice, compression, and elevation*. Later, if it is an intermuscular haematoma, the whole area is insonated, particularly the attachments of the muscle as this is where fluid tracks down and collects, causing pain and exudate adhesions. If it is an intramuscular haematoma, care must be taken to prevent calcification of the muscle, where it has torn its periosteal attachments. Low-dosage ultrasound should be given. For large muscle haematomas the 1 MHz machine could be used. Depending on the extent of the exudate the dosage can be increased.

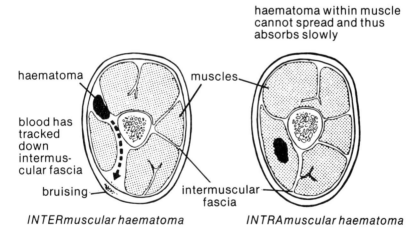

Swelling is often a complication of trauma. It can occur as a result of microtrauma from habitual postures insulting the area, or from a macrotrauma. Effusions of the knee joint, tenosynovitis of the wrist, bursitis of various regions, tendinitis in different muscles, gravitational oedema, and swelling in the tissue spaces following injury to the ankle joint are some of the traumatic swellings that present for physiotherapy treatment. Ultrasound with a dosage of 3 w.cm^{-2} can alter the semi-permeability of the cell membrane 200%. Overdosage can cause the escape of the protein plasmas, so care must be taken not to give large intensities.

Ultrasound also causes capillary dilatation which will then help to remove waste products. Lymphatic circulation is also accelerated by ultrasound. Dosages can be calculated depending on the acuteness or chronicity of lesion, the cause of the lesion, and the quality and quantity of exudate. The following examples will give some directive over selection of dosage.

Acute effusion of knee (traumatic). Treatment is started straight away with the leg in elevation, and ultrasound given to all aspects of the knee joint. Low dosage with a 3 MHz machine is given to prevent the exudate from organising into a tenacious exudate. The area should include 30 mm over the patella to include the suprapatellar bursa under the quadriceps muscle. If the swelling is gross and not organised, it is best to reduce the swelling with ice packs and compression, and then treat with ultrasound.

Chronic synovitis should be treated with the knee bent to 90° within the limits of pain, thus exposing the whole joint line. The knee should be treated anteriorly and posteriorly. Care should be taken of the neurovascular regions in the popliteal fascia, and the pad of fat through which the ultrasound has to penetrate. The insertional areas of the muscles should also be insonated. Dosage could be higher and the use of continuous ultrasound with a 1 MHz frequency is useful. If the joints are well padded, then a lower frequency of 0.75 MHz or 0.8 MHz can be used, where the penetration is deeper.

Fractures. There have been conflicting reports on the use of ultrasound at a fracture site, but ultrasound does not interfere with the healing process and the formation of callus, except perhaps in the very early stages when the blood clot proceeds to form granulations. Ultrasound may interfere with the procedure, particularly if high doses are given. Fractures of the calcaneum are treated successfully for the control of the swelling with ultrasound and ice in the early days. Low dosage with 1 MHz frequency for large soles and a 3 MHz frequency for thin soles is recommended.

Healing of wounds. The work of Dyson and Pond has shown that low-dosage ultrasound using 0.8 w.cm^{-2} pulsed ultrasound promotes the formation of granulation tissue in the healing of wounds in the absence of bacteria. Great care must be taken to use aseptic procedures, since slow healing wounds are easily infected and have a low resistance to infection.

Plantar warts (verruca vulgaris) generally form at points of pressure on the balls of the feet. Occasionally they are grouped and several contiguous warts fuse together and appear as one. The wart virus parasitises several epidermal cells and is probably transmitted by contact. They are generally seen in school children in ages from 12 to 16 years. Warts sometimes disappear for no known reason, particularly at puberty. With adults they seem to persist for longer periods. Reid has done a literary search on the methods used for the treatment of plantar warts with ultrasound, and has arrived at the conclusion that the use of ultrasound is indicated if the following clinical features are exhibited:

    discoloration and blackening of the wart;

    dimpling of the core;

    warts have been present less than one year;

multiple isolated warts;
younger patients.

A poor prognosis may be expected in mosaic warts, long-standing warts, or if there is no response after 12 treatments with no pain relief.

Treatment is given using 1 MHz apparatus with a continuous beam and an intensity of 0.75 to 1.5 w.cm^{-2}, as high as can be tolerated, for 15 minutes. The head should keep constant contact with the wart. Treatments are given once a week for 8 to 15 treatments. An occlusive dressing should be used in between treatments. The direct contact treatment seems to be more effective than the underwater treatment. The use of a paraffin wax ball as a couplant between the wart and the transducer head has been tried with strong doses of 2 to 3 w.cm^{-2} for 3 to 5 minutes. This is a painful method and must be tried on stubborn cases only (Patrick and Sumner).

Bacteria. Ultrasound in high doses is said to have a bactericidal effect, for example, 15 minutes with 3.5 w.cm^{-2} is a lethal dose. Low intensity ultrasound at 0.5 w.cm^{-2} for 2 minutes could destroy B. coli. As, generally speaking, high doses are needed to be lethal to the bacteria, it is not feasible for the therapist to utilise this effect.

Bone. High intensity ultrasound applications associated with pain can produce pathological fractures, sub-periosteal damage, or retard growth. However these effects are not seen with the modern therapeutic machines which have an applicator with a radiating surface of an average 10 cm^2, a total output of 30 w, giving an average output of 3 w.cm^{-2}. Ultrasound over epiphyseal plates is considered destructive by some.

Metal. Surgical metal implants constitute artificial interfaces. The acoustic impedance of stainless steel, vitallium, and titanium was found to be quite different from that of bone or other soft tissues. Work done by Lane and Brunner produced the following data regarding acoustic impedance in metal implants.

Metal and sound

SOLID	SOUND VELOCITY m.s^{-1}	THERMAL CONDUCTIVITY	ACOUSTIC IMPEDANCE g.cm^{-2}.s^{-1}
titanium	5723	105	2.575×10^6
stainless steel	5858	113	4.699×10^6
muscle	1558	0.0012	1.667×10^5
cortical bone	2900	0.0035	4.459×10^5

Thus there is a marked mismatch between the metal used in implants and the tissues. Marked reflection occurs, resulting in the development of patterns of standing waves. Local concentrations of energy may occur in the vicinity of the implant. This causes a large increase in ultrasonic intensity close to the metal. Metal implants have a high thermal conductivity. Thus heat energy is removed from the areas of increased intensity more rapidly than it is absorbed. Lehmann, Brunner and McMillan showed that there was no selective rise in temperature close to those areas heated by ultrasound. Ultrasonic energy is the only type of diathermy which can be used with metal implants in the treatment field.

The metals used for implants are vitallium (a non-ferrous alloy containing chromium, cobalt, and molybdenum), and stainless steel containing chromium, nickel, and molybdenum (18/8 Mo steel).

CONTRA-INDICATIONS

Brain and spinal cord. Ultrasound with a high therapeutic dose will produce irreversible changes in nerve cells and fibre tracts.

Pulsed ultrasound is safer than continuous ultrasound. If treating the back extensor muscles adjacent to the spine, it is advisable to treat one side, then the other, thus only crossing the spinal cord once.

Eyes. High doses could harm the optic nerve, and cavitation may occur in the fluid.

Reproductive organs and abdominal organs. The abdominal organs contain gas and thus there is a danger of reflection and a burn.

Pregnant uterus. There is controversy over the giving of ultrasound over a pregnant uterus, but patients with sacro-iliac strain or low back pain and sciatica can be insonated with ultrasound.

Acute infections or sepsis. Here ultrasound could spread the infection.

Tumors. Ultrasound even in low dosages is thought to stimulate the growth of tumors. Metastases can grow while having ultrasound.

Patients having deep X-ray therapy or radium isotopes have impaired sensation and are greatly sensitised to ultrasound.

Deep vein thrombosis or arterial disease. Patients with either of these complaints must not be insonated because of the danger of causing an embolus or a further thrombus.

Haemophilia. The danger of producing more bleeding is possible.

Tuberculosis of lungs or bone. Ultrasound aggravates the condition.

Anaesthetic areas. Ultrasound should be applied with caution over anaesthetised areas. High intensities should not be given.

DANGERS

Burns. The main causes of burns are:
   over-dosage;
   too slow a movement of the transducer head over the lesion;
   right angle application of transducer head over the lesion is not maintained and there is occurrence of shear waves which produce heat;
   insufficient couplant;
   too much liquid paraffin as a couplant;
   irregular bony surface which negates absolute contact with surface;
   entrapped air in the couplant;
   air bubbles against the head or patient's skin in underwater treatment;

reflection from air when low frequencies are insonated through thin tissue such as the palm of the hand; burning sensations occur on the opposite side;
high dosages over bones produce shear waves at the bone-periosteal interface causing periosteal pain from heat.

Shock

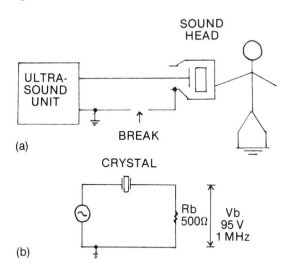

(a)

(b)

Hazard analysis
(a) Person touching metal sound head while complete break occurs in ground connection.
(b) Equivalent circuit of (a).
(from Cheng and Johnson, Physiotherapy Canada, 1976)

Deterioration of the cable connection to a movable angle transducer head could cause a shock. Improper use could cause the cable to be pinched between the metal head and the handle bar. This presents a potential shock hazard when somebody touches the sound head. The shock power could go up to 18 w, which is sufficient to give a burn. It is also possible in this case that the output of the machine could vary with the angle of the head.
Deterioration of the metal casing could also cause a shock.

Inaccurate and reduced power output from generators could be due to:
inaccurate tuning of the frequency of the crystal with the resonant frequency of the oscillator;
poor quality of the crystal;
wear and tear of electrical components;
wear and tear or damage to the crystal (the crystal generally has a long life).

PRECAUTIONS

Air-filled cavities. In the treatment of sinusitis, over lung tissue and pelvic organs, reflection could occur and care must be taken to ensure that the circulation is intact. It is advisable to use low dosages.
Sinusitis
Maxillary (1 MHz) 1 w.cm^{-2} continuous for 2 to 3 minutes $\Big\}$ or pulsed for 4 to 5
Frontal (3 MHz) 0.8 w.cm^{-2} continuous for 2 to 3 minutes $\Big\}$ minutes (1:5 ratio)

Pleurodynia (intercostal muscle contusions)
3 MHz – 1 w.cm^{-2} continuous for 4 minutes.

Water-filled cavities. Fluid media generally have the same acoustic impedance values as other soft tissues and hence there is no reflection, but care must be taken that the surrounding area has a good circulation. The fluid medium in the eye is less viscous and has few cells, and thus there is a danger of cavitation occurring. (Cavitation occurs more readily in fluids of low viscosity and low cellular content (Lehmann).)

Reproductive organs. Even though the current knowledge of effects on reproductive tissues concludes that ultrasound is contra-indicated, fibrous scars, for example, on the testicles can be treated with a 3 MHz machine. Sacro-iliac strains, too, can be treated during late pregnancy, again by using the 3 MHz frequency machines.

COUPLING MEDIA

Ultrasound differs from electromagnetic radiations such as microwave, infrared, and ultraviolet, in that energy is propagated as longitudinal waves, and at this frequency a coupling agent is required between the body and the vibrating source. There has to be intimate contact between the transducer head of the machine and the body surface to allow maximum transfer of energy from the head to the tissues. Even minute amounts of air can disrupt the flow of energy. Therefore in clinical practice the space between the transducer and the patient is filled with a thin layer of a coupling fluid which will allow the transmission of sonic energy.

Coupling media are selected for their high sound transmissivity. Transmissivity is the fraction of ultrasonic energy which is transmitted through a medium. Water has an absorption quotient of only 0.0022 and hence is a good transmitter. Patrick and Sumner state that the most suitable liquid couplant is the one which has a characteristic impedance halfway between that of metal (steel or aluminium) and human tissue. Thus matched, it will reduce transfer losses and minimise reflection. Coupling media should have negligible absorptivity powers, and be viscous so that they stay on the skin during treatment.

Water absorbs very little ultrasound, but is of insufficient viscosity to stay on the skin. It is used when there are prominent bony areas in the site of lesion. An underwater technique uses degassed (boiled) water.

Oils and liquid paraffin are fairly viscous, but their impedance does not match that of the tissues, and when used they are inclined to overheat locally. There has been recent controversy on the amount of energy transmitted when the commonly used agent liquid paraffin is used. Reid and Cummings claim that liquid paraffin transmits only 19.06% (S.D. ± 1.0%), but Warren and others state that there is very little difference between the media, and variables such as the amount of oil and pressure make the difference.

Glycerol is viscous and has a good affinity to skin. It is water-soluble. Reid and Cummings state it is an acceptable substitute and has a fair transmissivity (a mean of 67.5%). Again Warren feels that there is little difference; in fact glycerol tends to be more variable than liquid paraffin.

Aquasonic gel is a thixotropic agent, that is a solid medium which liquefies under insonation. Reid and Cummings showed a transmissivity of 72.6%, while Warren showed almost 90% transmissivity. Warren tried other similar thixotropic agents, such as Soni-gel, Ultraphonic, and Medco, and found that Soni-gel was the most efficient of all coupling media.

ECG couplant is a salt-based paste which, according to Reid, has a decreasing efficiency since it transmits only 26.6% of the ultrasound.

Hydrocortisone cream (Cortril) is used sometimes as an ointment or cream. It generally traps air on a microscopic scale, and hence has reduced transmissivity, according to Warren. The transmissivity varies from 26% with Cortril, 47% with pharmaceutically prepared hydrocortisone, and 65% with the commercial hydrocortisone cream.

Lanolin-based creams are opaque to ultrasound and will cause the head to heat up considerably in a few minutes.

Distilled water, which has had all gas bubbles removed, is, according to Reid and Cummings, less efficient than aquasonic gel. It has a transmissivity of 59.38%. Generally about 25% is added to the calculated dose when an underwater treatment is given.

Physiotherapists should, if possible, use the commercially prepared *thixotropic couplant media* such as Aquasonic gel, or Soni-gel, for the best effects. *Boiled degassed water* will ensure that the transmissivity is at its maximum. Only a *thin film of couplant* should be used, because too much couplant reduces transmissivity. Again care must be taken to apply *an even, but not too light or too heavy a pressure of the transducer head* on the tissues during treatment. Uneven pressure reduces transmissivity.

Transmissivity of media with transducer voltage control (Warren)

MEDIA	TRANSMISSIVITY (approximately)
degassed H_2O (reference standard)	100%
Soni-gel	100%
Aquasonic gel	90%
Ultraphonic	95%
mineral oil	90%
glycerol	75%

DOSAGE

The effectiveness and safety of ultrasonic treatments will depend on the availability and reliability of suitable equipment. The following factors influence the effectiveness of ultrasound dosage.

The frequency of the machine. Ultrasonic equipment today provides the physiotherapist with frequencies from 0.75 MHz to 3 MHz. The selection of these frequencies is based on the adequacy of depth of penetration into specific tissues that are generally treated in the clinical situation.

The effective penetration of specific frequencies (approximate values)
(Gordon, Goldman and Heuter)

FREQUENCY MHz	HALF VALUE PENETRATION mm
0.75	100
0.85	90
1	65
1.5	55
3	30

It is also accepted that at lower frequencies the non-thermal effects are predominant. It has been noted that at a frequency of 3.5 MHz there are minimal thermal effects, but much vibration. Occasionally patients may complain of a painful audible sound during treatment which is not heard by anybody when using low frequencies such as 0.9 MHz machines.

The quantity of ultrasound absorbed is also frequency-dependent. The higher the frequency, the shorter the wavelength and the greater the absorption (the tables of frequency and absorption have been discussed earlier in this unit). The skin load is an important factor. If greater intensities are needed for a deep-seated lesion which is covered with fat, fascia and muscle, the superficial skin area may not be able to tolerate the intensity, and the use of a lower-frequency machine is necessary to achieve effective penetration.

The size of the transducer head
Most transducer heads have a radiating surface of from 5 to 13 cm^2. Smaller applicators are unsuitable because of the greater divergence of the beam, and dilution of its intensity in the deeper tissues.

The total effective radiating area. The whole power of the transducer head is bunched into a beam with most of the power concentrated in a central pencil of ultrasound, the diameter of which is approximately one-third the dimension of the piezoelectric disc (Gordon and Sumner). The near field (Fresnel Zone) is non-uniform, and has interference patterns, but the far field (Fraunhofer Zone) is more uniform. This necessitates moving the head during treatment.

Gross acoustic power transfer. It is important that we should distinguish between the terms *dose* (that which is monitored by the power meter or dial) and *absorption dose* (the energy absorbed from an ultrasonic field by the medium). We measure the total power delivered by the transducer to the tissues to which it is coupled. Most meters have a range of 30 watts. The intensity can be increased from 0.1 to 3 w.cm^{-2}, either in discrete steps on a power control measuring acoustic power, or on a meter measuring electrical signals.

Ranges in dosage
Intensity — 0.1 to 3 w.cm^{-2}
Duration — 3 to 10 minutes (continuous)⎱ for areas up to 50 cm^2
5 to 15 minutes (pulsed)   ⎰
If the area is larger, for example 16 cm × 8 cm, then the dose must be given for twice the selected time.
If the area is 70 cm^2, then the same dose is given for 1½ times the selected time.

The time of insonation. The maximum limits of safety in ultrasound dosage are:

Continuous   —   10 minutes
Pulsed   —   15 minutes.

The time selected depends primarily on the size of the area to be treated. Acute conditions should be treated for a shorter time to reduce the thermal effects which increase with the length of insonation.

Existing pathophysiology. The presenting problems of the lesion should be examined. Priority should be given to the patient's problems. For example: should the pain or the cause of the pain be tackled first? Or should we tackle pain and the cause of pain together in an endeavor to reduce the period of recovery? The priority of the problems should be related to the effects of ultrasound on the pathophysiology of the tissues and organs.

Couplants. In view of the controversy that exists about their efficiency, the following values should be borne in mind when selecting couplants.

For all bony and uneven areas where there is a possibility of reflection of waves, underwater treatment with degassed water should be used. There is no loss of power during the passage of ultrasound through water, and no attenuation. Half value intensities are calculated from the skin. If maximal heating effects are required, 5 to 10% increase of dosage can be made to allow for the cooling effect of the water (Kossoff).

It has been shown that thixotropic agents such as Aquasonic gel, Soni-gel and Ultraphonic are superior to mineral oils, glycerol and ECG couplants. The transmissivity differences lie between 10% and 15% (Warren). However Kossoff states that there is little difference in the agents in regard to transmissivity. The most important factor is to *minimise the quantity of couplant*, since too much couplant, particularly paraffin oil, causes heating. 10% of the dosage could be deducted when using a good thixotropic agent such as Soni-gel. Reid, too, differs in his findings on the transmissivity of couplants.

Pulsed versus continuous ultrasound. *Pulsed currents* in the ratio of 1:10 are used if no heating effects are needed with lower power.

The ratio of 1:5 or 1:4 is used when minimal heating effects are needed. The ratio of 1:1 is used if heating effects are required, but the insonation is producing too much heat from teno-periosteal and bone-periosteal interfaces.

Pulsed ultrasound is used when heat exacerbates pain, or when reduction of nerve conduction velocities is required in nerve fibres, nerve roots or ganglia. Pulsed ultrasound with low dosages is also used for the regeneration of tissues, as in the healing of wounds, and to aid resolution of acute non-infective inflammation.

Continuous ultrasound is used when vigorous thermal and non-thermal effects are needed.

Calculation of dosage. The following dosage ranges can be used as a guideline for treatment. The dosages are for an area up to 70 cm^2.

For relief of pain

1 to 2 w.cm^{-2} continuous to nerve fibres, for 3 to 5 minutes.

0.5 to 1 w.cm^{-2} continuous to nerve roots and ganglia, for 3 to 4 minutes, or pulsed for 6 to 8 minutes.

For adhesion reduction

1.5 to 3 w.cm^{-2} continuous for 4 to 6 minutes. A vigorous effect is needed here for the resorption of adhesions by the depolymerisation of mucopolysaccharides and tropocollagen cement bonds.

For absorption of exudate

(a)   *Acute:* 1 to 2 w.cm^{-2} for 4 to 5 minutes.

(b)   *Chronic:* 1.5 to 2 w.cm^{-2} for 4 to 6 minutes. Care must be taken not to give 3 w.cm^{-2} for long periods of time as this will cause escape of plasma proteins.

Ultrasound causes a streaming of fluid across the cell membrane and alters the viscosity of colloids.

For wound repair

Pulsed ultrasound at 0.5 to 0.8 w.cm^{-2} for 3 to 4 minutes.

For haematomas

(a)   *Acute:* 0.5 to 0.8 w.cm^{-2} to the surrounds (3 MHz).

(b)   *Chronic:* 1.5 to 2 w.cm^{-2} to the haematoma.

Plantar warts

0.75 to 1.75 w.cm^{-2} for 15 minutes continuous, once a week.

Progression of dosage. There is no need to progress dosage. If high intensities are to be used, then progress with intensity and time can be made, but must be stabilised within 2 or 3 treatments. Again the existing pathophysiology must be reviewed daily so that the dosage is adjusted to the pathology. There should be some immediate relief of symptoms. If there is no relief within 4 treatments even after adjusting the dose, then ultrasound should be stopped. Always assess before and after treatment.

Duration and frequency. Ultrasound treatment should be given daily. Ultrasound should not exceed 2 courses of 10 ultrasound treatments, unless the pathology requires it, and the patient is improving. The maximum time per area is 10 minutes for continuous ultrasound, or 15 minutes for pulsed ultrasound.

The following tables may be helpful in determining ultrasound dosage, but some variations may be required to maximise specific physiological effects.

Questions to ask
- What is the nature of the lesion?
- What are the accompanying pathophysiological changes?
- Is the lesion acute, subacute or chronic?
- Is the lesion superficial or deep?
- Is the lesion localized or diffuse?
- Do you want the micromassage effects?
- Do you want the thermal effects?
- Do you want both micromassage and thermal effects?
- What type of tissue are you trying to treat?

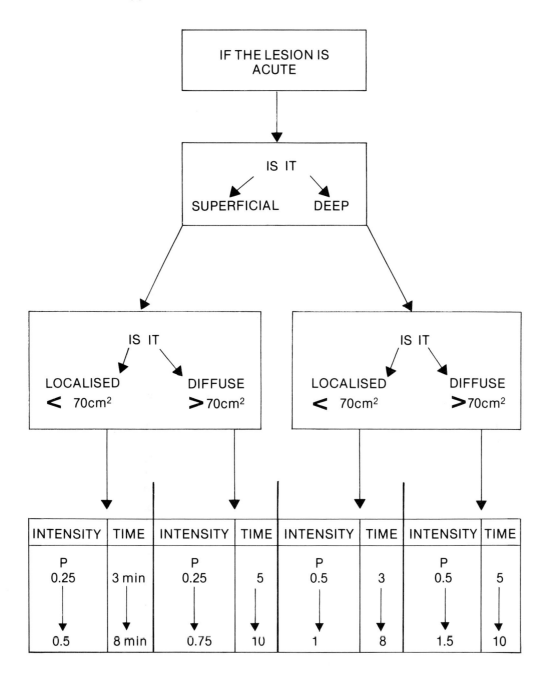

P = pulsed ultrasound
Intensity in watts cm²,
↓ = approximate range (i.e. up to this figure)

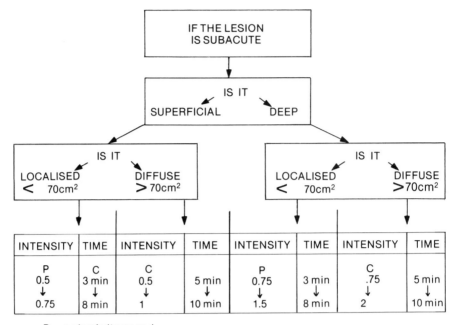

INTENSITY	TIME	INTENSITY	TIME	INTENSITY	TIME	INTENSITY	TIME
P 0.5 ↓ 0.75	C 3 min ↓ 8 min	C 0.5 ↓ 1	5 min ↓ 10 min	P 0.75 ↓ 1.5	3 min ↓ 8 min	C .75 ↓ 2	5 min ↓ 10 min

P = pulsed ultrasound
C = continuous ultrasound
intensity in watts cm²
↓ = approximate range (i.e. up to this figure)

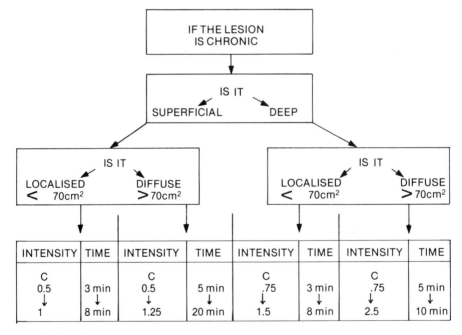

INTENSITY	TIME	INTENSITY	TIME	INTENSITY	TIME	INTENSITY	TIME
C 0.5 ↓ 1	3 min ↓ 8 min	C 0.5 ↓ 1.25	5 min ↓ 20 min	C .75 ↓ 1.5	3 min ↓ 8 min	C .75 ↓ 2.5	5 min ↓ 10 min

C = continuous ultrasound
Intensity = watts per cm²
↓ = approximate range (i.e. up to this figure)

METHODS OF APPLICATION

The moving sound head technique

In order to get a more uniform heating effect in the near field zone and utilise the central area of the far field, and also to enlarge the treatment area, a stroking technique is used. The near field has maximum and minimum intensity spots in the interference field and thus there is a very uneven heating field in the near zone.

The movement can cover an area from the size of the ultrasound head to about 50 to 70 cm^2, depending on the size of the transducer head. It is essential to move the beam to obtain an even heating effect on the lesion. The transducer head is moved slowly at the rate of approximately 25 mm.s^{-1} with circular or parallel strokes. One stroke must overlap about 50% of the previous stroke. The applicator head must be held parallel to the tissues of the body. Great concentration is needed to maintain an even, firm pressure consistently.

The pressure must simulate a gentle firm massaging action and must not be too heavy or too light. If the head is tilted, even 10° to 15°, the ultrasound is reflected and no intensity is transmitted to the patient. Some of it will go back to the head, causing the head to heat up. There are two methods of moving the head: one is in a circular manner, and the other is parallel strokes done transversely, longitudinally or diagonally. Transverse strokes are done over muscle fibres as they obtain better absorption. *Never stroke parallel to a main artery as it can cause a parathrombus.*

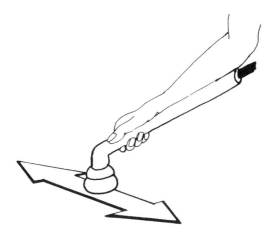

Parallel stroking with the sound head

Stationary technique

This can be used when small localised areas are being treated with small dosages of under 0.8 w.cm^{-2} continuous, or 1 w.cm^{-2} pulsed. There is uneven heating.

It is important to ensure that there is no danger of shear waves occurring from the bone-periosteum interface that would cause periosteal pain to the patient. Uneven surfaces must not be insonated with a stationary technique unless done under water with a reflector.

Underwater techniques
The limb or part of it is treated in a large bowl or bath. It is submerged in water with the treatment area well beneath the surface of the water. The treatment head is also well submerged. The therapist's hand should not be in the water. Make sure that, if tap water is used, no air bubbles adhere to head and skin. Boiled water generally prevents this occurrence, but it is not practical in a busy department.

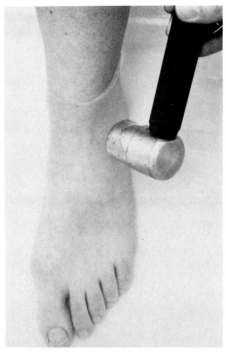

Underwater technique

The distance between the head and the treatment area is up to 50 mm. The usual distance is 10 to 20 mm. Great care must be taken that the beam is accurately positioned on the exact treatment area.

Underwater treatment with a stand reflector makes it possible to 'turn' the beam. The use of a stand reflector with a treatment head located at the bottom of the water bath can be used to produce sonic treatment at the surface. The reflector should be so angled that the beam of ultrasound will strike it and be reflected on to the target. This reflection technique is difficult to apply accurately. Care must also be taken to ensure that no air bubbles collect on the reflector. Treatment heads are made with the effective area at right angles to the longitudinal axis of the transducer.

If complete immersion is not possible, a sub-aquatic treatment can be maintained by using a reflector which is situated at the bottom of the bath. The beam on the reflector produces a fountain of water rising above the surface. The part needing treatment is brought against the fountain. This can be used in teno-periosteal lesions around the elbow.

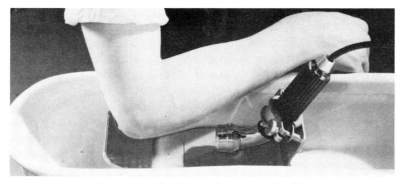

Underwater technique using a stand reflector

Water applicator (bag technique)
For the treatment of small areas with uneven surfaces and open areas, such as hydroadenitis or fistulas which cannot be treated with the fountain technique, the use of a water applicator is helpful. The applicator is a plastic bag which is sealed off under water once it has been filled, care being taken that there are no air bubbles in the bag. Rubber gets too hot easily and perishes, so a strong, heat-resistant plastic bag must be used. The transducer head is slowly moved over the bag, which is held in contact with the part. This technique is also useful for the treatment of areas which are very bony and irregular, but are not suitable for immersion, for example, the knee or the shoulder.

TECHNIQUE OF ULTRASOUND THERAPY

IN CONTACT APPLICATION

Equipment required
ultrasound unit
sheets for draping the patient
sheet of plastic
towels
cotton wool
contact medium (couplant): aquasonic gel, liquid paraffin oil, or glycerol
substance for removal of the contact medium: soap and water, or methylated spirits
soap and water, or methylated spirits
   Position the patient comfortably with the area to be treated adequately exposed, supported and relaxed.
   Explain to the patient the rationale for treatment, ultrasonic energy and the sensation to be experienced.
   Examine the area to be treated. Note any cuts, skin lesions or inflammation (danger of spreading infection).
   Accurately *locate* the anatomical site of the pathology and the radiation of any pain.
   Assess the symptoms or pathology to be treated.
   Check that there are no contraindications to treatment with ultrasound.
   Skin test the patient to ensure intact thermal and pain sensation.

In cold weather preliminary warming of the part, the sound head and the oil may be necessary to eliminate the reduction of the desired pathophysiological effects because of the lowered temperature on the affected area.

Ensure that there are no lanolin-type creams on the affected part, as these are opaque to ultrasound and cause the sound head to heat up considerably.

Test that the machine is producing ultrasound by covering the sound head with a thick coating of the couplant selected for treatment. Select pulsed or continuous ultrasound according to what will be used in the treatment of the patient. Turn the intensity *rapidly* to maximum, and *rapidly* back to zero to minimise the length of time the machine is on, as the ultrasound will be reflected by the air back through the couplant and into the sound head, potentially causing damage. Check that the couplant bubbles with increasing intensity as the ultrasound intensity is increased, and that the needle on the meter (if present) rises and falls smoothly. This also serves to demonstrate to the patient that something is being produced by the machine, even though nothing may be felt.

Place a piece of protective plastic and a towel under the part to be treated, the towel being next to the patient's skin.

Using the sound head, apply the couplant to the skin in sufficient quantity to provide an air-free contact. For perfect transmission of power from the treatment head to the body, the head must be applied perpendicularly to the skin surface (the emitting surface will be parallel to the tissues being insonated). *Do not use too much couplant.*

Warn the patient that there should be no increase in the presenting symptoms and no periosteal pain. Only minimal perceptible warmth should be felt under the sound head, which could be caused by friction forces. Any concentration of heat under the sound head or any hot spots must be reported immediately. The patient must be told not to move or touch any of the equipment.

Tell the patient that there is a possibility of a burn occurring if these precautions are ignored.

The therapist should be seated with the forearm supported and relaxed, and with the machine conveniently placed for manipulating the controls.

Check that all controls are at the zero position.

Plug into the mains power supply and switch on.

Select 'Pulsed' or 'Continuous' ultrasound as required.

Set the timer.

Maintaining absolute contact with firm pressure, keep the sound head moving and stroke the affected part while turning the intensity control to the desired intensity. Stroking must be comparatively short — 50 mm up to 120 mm in length, each stroke overlapping 50% of the previous one.

Great concentration is needed not to tilt the head, as even an angle of 10° to 15° will reflect the sound waves and the treatment will be totally ineffective.
Stroking can be done in a parallel or circular manner. Parallel strokes are preferable as it is easier to control deflection.
The rate of stroking is about 25 mm.s^{-1} or 2 to 3 s for 1 revolution if done in a circular manner.

Movement of the sound head must be *slow, smooth* and *rhythmical* with even pressure.

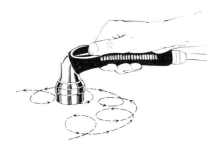

Illustration of circular motion employed in the application of ultrasound

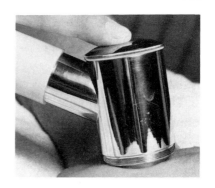

max. 120 mm

Parallel stroking technique

Dosage is selected according to the pathophysiology of the lesion, the desired effects, the site of the lesion and the depth of tissues to be insonated.

If large areas are being treated at one time, cool the transducer head in water after 10 minutes. If the head heats up in the first 5 minutes check:

(a) intensity;

(b) tilting of the head;

(c) couplant;

(d) transducer mechanism.

In most machines the ultrasound is automatically switched off by the timer at the conclusion of treatment. Return all controls to zero. Switch off at the mains and unplug the unit.

Clean the part to remove the contact medium.

Clean the sound head with methylated spirits or ether.

Assess the patient's symptoms for any relief and instruct the patient to note any further effect of the treatment so that he can report this at his next visit.

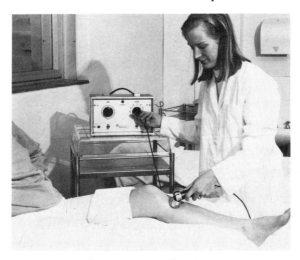

In contact application

Sub-aquatic Application

Equipment required
ultrasound unit
plastic
towels
suitably sized water container (bowl, basin, baby's bath)

Position the patient, explain the treatment, assess the area, check contraindications and skin test for thermal and pain sensation as described in the in contact technique.

Test the machine by immersing the sound head in the water so that it points at an angle to the surface of the water. This prevents reflection of the ultrasound back into the sound head. Ensure that there are no air bubbles on the sound head. Select pulsed or continuous ultrasound according to what will be used in the treatment of the patient. Turn the intensity to maximum and back to zero, watching the ripples produced on the surface of the water. The rippling should increase in magnitude as the intensity is increased. Check that the needle on the meter (if present) rises and falls smoothly. This also serves to demonstrate to the patient that something is being produced by the machine even though nothing may be felt.

The limb, or part of it, is submerged in the bowl, basin or bath, so that the area to be treated is well beneath the surface of the water. The working surface of the treatment head is also submerged. The distance between the working surface and the skin can be from 10 to 50 mm (usually 10 mm or 20 mm).

Maintain distance to keep the head parallel to the part.

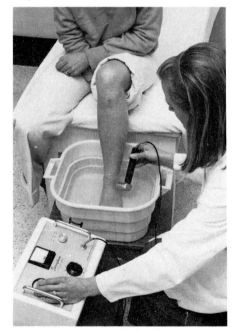

Subaquatic Technique

Care should be taken to ensure that there are no air bubbles adhering to the patient's skin or the treatment head during treatment as this causes reflection of the sound waves. Remove the bubbles by turning the sound head away from the part and wiping them off. If the bubbles are numerous, switch the machine off, remove the sound head and limb from the bath, wipe off the bubbles and resume treatment.

Do not put your hand under water.

Switch on the machine, selecting the dosage as described in the in contact technique.

The sound head is moved in a circular or parallel stroking technique, as described in the in contact technique. Great care must be taken to maintain the distance of the sound head from the part and to ensure that the ultrasound beam is perpendicular to the tissues. This is easier if the part can be positioned with the lesion to be treated facing the side of the bath, so that the sound head can be seen to be parallel and at a constant distance from the part.

Conclude the treatment as described in the in contact technique.

USE OF ULTRASOUND WITH OTHER MODALITIES

Acute traumatic conditions

Pain, swelling and tenderness. The regime of ice packs to reduce swelling, followed by low dosage ultrasound, has been found effective. If the swelling is not too gross, interferential therapy followed by ultrasound is useful. Crushed hands and acute tendinitis are cases where this regime has been effective. For muscle belly injuries, short wave or microwave followed by ultrasound is also effective in the sub-acute stages.

Chronic traumatic conditions

Pain, swelling and tenderness. Post-traumatic, gross insidious swelling can be managed by the use of interferential therapy and ultrasound. If the area is large, then alternate hot packs and ice packs for 30 to 40 minutes followed by ultrasound and mobilisations are useful. The mobilisations and exercises can be done before the ultrasound.

Chronic pain and swelling. If the pain has been a long-standing problem, interferential dosage for pain and ultrasound dosage for absorption of exudate make a good combination.

Chronic swelling. The use of the Masman pump after insonation with ultrasound has been found to be effective. Ultrasound and faradism combined by using the sonadyne machine which simultaneously gives both treatments, has been used in North America and Europe. Results have been effective in selected cases. When giving ultrasound after the application of ice treatments, care must be taken to monitor the dosage within thermal limits of safety. Dosages at 1.5 $w.cm^{-2}$ and above must be carefully administered.

5.2   Efficiency of Ultrasound Equipment

(Included with the permission of the author, Stuart Tyler, Electronics Engineer, Watson Victor Ltd.)

Crystal efficiency

The ultrasound transducer head converts a continuous x MHz frequency electrical signal by means of the piezoelectric crystal into a continuous x MHz ultrasonic signal. Piezoelectric crystals used in the domestic record player are required to maintain high efficiency (as far as is possible) over the complete range of audible frequencies in order to reproduce faithfully those sounds which have been recorded.

At the high powers used in therapeutic generators, such a 'wide' frequency response is very difficult to obtain, and since it would have very little therapeutic value, the designers of therapeutic equipment use crystals which are efficient at (or near) only one frequency — called the *resonant frequency*. The crystal is driven by an electrical signal of exactly that same frequency in order to obtain maximum efficiency of transduction.

As with TV sets, radios and all other pieces of electronic equipment, the ultrasonic generator may, from time to time, require servicing. That parameter most likely to need regular attention is the *electrical frequency being generated*. If the electrical signal becomes 'out of tune' (that is, drifts away from the crystal's resonant frequency), the efficiency of the transducer will drop markedly. This means that, for the same electrical power fed into the crystal, the output (ultrasonic) power is much reduced. The danger here is that the operator may have little or no indication of this deterioration without some independent instrument which responds directly to acoustic power.

Note: When electrical power is being fed into a crystal transducer, and ultrasonic power is not being taken out, there is a resultant accumulation of energy, which presents itself in the form of heat. An operator may be able to gain some indication of a transducer's efficiency by the coolness with which it operates.

Meters on therapeutic machines. In order to gain 'sales mileage', some manufacturers of ultrasonic equipment fit a meter to indicate either output power or output intensity. This can be misleading as usually such devices respond only to the electrical voltage applied to the crystal regardless of how poorly that voltage is tuned to the resonant frequency of the crystal. It is reasonable to assume that, if the signal drifts away from the crystal's resonant frequency, this voltage which drives the meter could increase (thereby causing an increase in indicated output) while the acoustic power (or intensity) generated, in fact, actually drops. A reliable form of indication can be obtained only by an instrument which is actually driven with the acoustic power being measured. Unfortunately, such devices are not readily available, and cannot be constructed without considerable difficulty.

Testing acoustic power. When acoustic (or ultrasonic) radiation impinges on an interface separating media with different acoustic properties, a steady force is exerted on the interface in the direction of the energy flow. The time-averaged force per unit area of the interface being insonated by the beam is known as the Langevin Radiation Pressure, and it is dependent on the relative amounts of energy transmitted, reflected and/or absorbed.

This principle may be employed to deflect a thin metal vane which, in turn, can

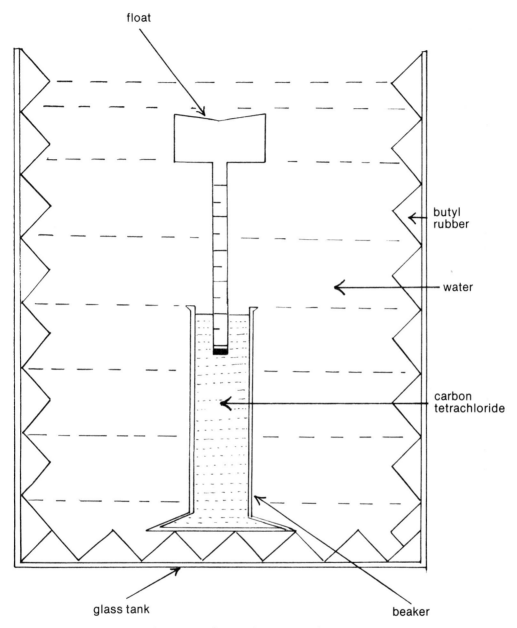

Apparatus for testing accoustic power

deflect a pointer against a scale which gives a direct indication of ultrasonic intensity. Such a device is available from E.M.S., America, but will give only an approximate indication of output power.

The most reliable and accurate technique yet developed employs this same principle (Langevin Radiation Pressure) to deflect a submerged float downward into a heavy liquid. The system requires a tank of degassed, distilled water, lined with sound-absorbing material (for example, butyl rubber), to completely surround an inner container of some slightly denser, immiscible fluid (such as carbon tetrachloride). The weight of the float is adjusted so that it just sinks in the water, and obtains equilibrium when its stem is partially immersed in the denser liquid. Radiation pressure causes the float to immerse further into the denser liquid, and the stem may be calibrated to read directly the acoustic power. The power (w) divided by the area of the generating source (cm^2) yields the ultrasonic intensity (w/cm^2).

One feature which makes this system superior to all others is that it can be calibrated directly by placing known masses on the float and measuring the deflection which results. A known mass has a known force due to gravity (its weight). By knowing force and velocity, we can calibrate in terms of power.

$$P = FV$$

5.3   Ultrasound for Diagnosis

The use of diagnostic ultrasound in medicine is assuming ever-increasing importance since its development in the early 1950s. For the past thirty years ultrasonics has been used therapeutically by physiotherapists, but in the last twenty years it has been developed for diagnosis and surgery. The importance of ultrasonics in medicine arises because its properties are fundamentally different and safer than those of other diagnostic agents. Thus the information that can be obtained by the use of ultrasound in diagnosis is unique in some situations. Kossoff states that the ability to provide accurate cross-sectional views of soft tissue is the distinguishing feature of diagnostic ultrasound.

Medical diagnostic equipment uses frequencies in the range of 1 to 5 MHz. At these frequencies it is possible to obtain a beam of sound from the source and direct it at the tissues of the body, where the sound wave is transmitted through the media at a constant velocity and is partly reflected at interfaces. This reflected wave is called an *echo* and can be recorded and measured. Reflections occur at the surface between the two tissues if the speed of sound in the two tissues is different. The greater the difference, the larger the reflection. If a series of reflections or echoes is charted, a sectional picture of the tissues can be obtained. This is the basis of diagnostic ultrasound.

Ultrasound is complementary to other diagnostic aids. The diagnostic value of X-rays depends on the different absorption coefficients of tissues containing varying proportions of elements of differing atomic number. Ultrasound is based on the filtering densities, propagation velocities and absorption rates of different kinds of tissues.

PRINCIPLES

The sound waves are directed to the tissues through the skin. The incident sound beam is reflected at the interface of two media in the tissues and returns to the transducer probe, which acts as both transmitter and receiver. The reflected wave is an echo. From the transducer probe, the mechanical vibrations of the echo are converted into electrical voltage oscillations and passed by way of an amplifier to a cathode ray tube to make them visible.

ADVANTAGES OF ULTRASOUND DIAGNOSIS

The examination technique is simple and causes no discomfort or suffering to the patient.

The importance of ultrasound is that the risk of damaging tissues under investigation is negligible, because it produces no ionising radiations. It produces no significant biological changes in the tissues because of the short duration of the ultrasonic probe.

Accurate localisation of areas in the human body can be undertaken. For example, in the case of intracranial disease the midline of the brain can be localised by obtaining the distance between the temple and the third ventricle. In eye diseases the length of the optic axis, the thickness of the lens, or the depth of the anterior chamber of the eye can be assessed.

Ultrasound is capable of detecting abnormalities in living soft tissues. This is a definite advantage over the use of X-rays in diagnosis.

DISADVANTAGES

The interpretation of the ultrasound image becomes difficult at times when the images presented on the screen are not very clear, and the 'noise' which interferes with the diagnosis also presents a problem. The accuracy of the result depends on the skill with which the data are interpreted. New methods of data presentation with three-dimensional display or the use of cine-ultrasound techniques, such as are used in cardiology, may be of help in accurate diagnosis.

The micromassage effect of ultrasound by acceleration (g) of the intracellular structures of $10^5 g$, with peak power of 14 w.cm^{-2} at 1 MHz, has been proved to produce no injury to tissue. Nevertheless therapy machines using higher energies than diagnostic equipment should not be used on the central nervous system, the foetus, or the reproductive organs.

TECHNIQUES USED IN DIAGNOSIS

There are five methods used in diagnosis. A-mode technique is a one-dimensional study of biological tissues. B-mode technique is used for cross-sectional scanning. M-mode is a time-motion study of moving objects. This is valuable in cardiology. The Doppler technique compares the frequencies of the ultrasonic emission with the frequencies of the received signals. C-mode, or constant depth technique, provides a view of the image that is at right angles to that which is obtained with the B-mode.

A-mode technique
The probe usually acts as a receiver and transmitter, and thus sound waves reflected at interfaces of tumors or other pathological disturbances are returned to the probe.

The probe converts the mechanical vibrations into electrical voltage oscillations which are passed on by way of an amplifier to a cathode ray tube, where they are made visible as vertical deflections from the horizontal baseline. The height of the deflection represents the strength of the echo and the distance along the baseline represents the depth from which the echo arises. A knowledge of anatomy is necessary for the accurate interpretation of the scans, so that the nature of the various interfaces which gives rise to the echoes may be identified. A-mode techniques are valuable in echo-encephalography and echo-opthalmology.

The units used are simple to operate and portable, and results can be rapidly evaluated.

Clinical application of A-mode

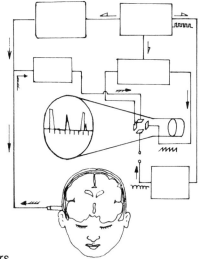

Diagnosis of cranial tumours

Echo-encephalography is the evaluation of intracranial haemorrhage after trauma, and for the diagnosis of space-consuming tumors in the brain.

B-mode technique
In this technique a probe is moved manually or automatically to obtain a sectional image. Short pulses of ultrasonic energy are emitted by the transducer and are reflected at discontinuities in acoustic impedance. The energy that is reflected to the transducer is converted back into an electrical impulse and displayed as an increase in the brightness of a trace of an oscilloscope. The direction of the trace represents the direction of the propagation of the energy. A cross-sectional view or echogram can be obtained.

The range of information obtained in an A-mode is presented in the form of an intensity modulated B-mode, in which each echo is registered as a bright spot at the appropriate point on the time base. By continuously photographing the display while the probe is moved around the patient, a cross-sectional picture in the plane of the scan is built up on the film. The probe is oscillated as it moves around.

Ultrasonic imaging equipment available works either with a probe which is moved over the surface of the body, the image being built up by way of an image score tube or by a scanning technique which makes it possible to display sectional images of organs in a rapid sequence of the display tube. Thus the observer can distinguish not merely stationary situations but also kinetic processes directly and immediately.

Clinical application of B-mode

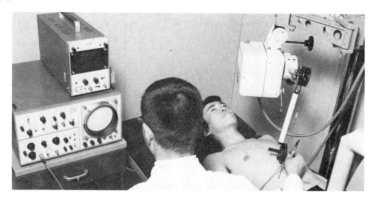

Diagnosis of abdominal lesions

Abdominal tumors can be explored without causing trauma. B-mode techniques are useful for identifying cysts or parenchymatous tumors in the abdomen, which cannot be identified by palpation, X-ray examination or by scintillograms. Using ultrasound, most masses throughout the body can be measured. By increasing the gain of the ultrasonic equipment it is possible to differentiate between fluid-filled or solid masses. Fluid-filled masses produce no echoes, whereas solid masses will produce multiple echoes. Masses containing both fluid (cystic) and solid components, such as necrotic tumors or abscesses, will show patterns combining features of both types of masses.

Using the ultrasonic technique, masses have been measured in all parts of the body with greater than 95% accuracy. One of the most important uses has been for differentiating solid from cystic pelvic masses. Ovarian cysts or tumors, cysts in the pancreas or kidneys can be identified. Polycystic liver disease, secondary liver cancer, liver abscess or liver cirrhosis can be identified with B-mode scans of the liver. With these scan pictures the size, internal structure and base of the growth can be examined.

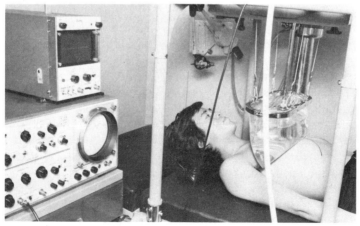

Diagnosis of thoracic lesions

In the field of *obstetrics* the rapid B-mode technique is useful for measuring the biparietal diameter of the foetal skull, determining the position of the child, the differential diagnosis of a twin pregnancy, a hydramnion, a hydatidiform mole or tumor.

Ultrasonic Doppler effect. The Doppler effect can provide data on the motion of structures and blood. The Doppler effect is the change in frequency that occurs when the transmitter and the receiver are in relative motion, or the propagating medium is in relative motion to either of them.

Application to circulatory conditions. Clinical assessment of extensive deep-vein thrombosis has been shown frequently to be inaccurate. Ultrasonic findings correlate well with those of phlebographic, radio-isotopic and post-mortem studies.

The use of ultrasound for the diagnosis of venous disease was first suggested by Strandness, Schultz, Sumner and Rushmer (1967) following the development of the transcutaneous Doppler flowmeter by Rushmer, Baker and Stegall (1966). With their apparatus operating at 5 MHz it was possible to detect venous flow from the calf to the groin. A change of apparatus and transmission frequency to 2 MHz (Evans and Cockett, 1969) has permitted detection of venous flow from the calf to the inferior vena cava. This form of examination promised to be simple, quick, repeatable and without hazard or discomfort to the patient.

Principles of the Doppler method. A continuous wave oscillator excites a piezoelectric crystal at frequencies up to 10 MHz. The crystal vibrates to produce 'sound waves' at the oscillator frequency. The waves are reflected at interfaces and the reflected waves are detected by a second piezoelectric crystal. The waves reflected from a moving target have a slightly different frequency from that of the transmitted waves. This *Doppler shifted frequency* can be modulated, amplified and displayed in the appropriate way.

It is usual to have two transducers in one housing with the angle between them fixed at a value dependent on the anticipated depth of the target. If the signal is fed to a loudspeaker, a change in pitch indicates a change in the velocity of the target (for example, in blood flow). For quantitative measurements, changes in frequency are either measured by a zero crossing rate-meter or by a sound spectrum analyser, which gives more information than the zero crossing rate-meter. A single implanted crystal can be used alternately as transmitter and receiver.

The Doppler method has the advantage of being non-invasive, but it produces problems in the techniques used for blood flow measurement. The Doppler blood flow velocity meters transmit pulses of ultrasound through the intact skin by a hand-held transducer head, which picks up the signals reflected from the blood corpuscles within the vessel on which the beam is focused. A shift in frequency between the transmitted and reflected signals occurs, which is proportional to the particle velocity.

In the conventional instrument the frequency difference is detected as an audible tone, the pitch of which depends on the velocity of the moving particles. If there are streams of particles moving at different velocities within the vessel, because of the varying radial position of the corpuscles within the vessel, a mixture of Doppler shift frequencies are obtained. Conventional instruments do not detect the various components and a search is being made for an understanding of the flow characteristics within arteries and veins (Yeo and Needham).

Technique for the detection of thrombosis. The transcutaneous Doppler flow velocity detector can be used to examine individual arteries selectively and directly. The instrument is portable and is simple to use. Pulses not palpable because of obesity or oedema are immediately detected, and a permanent record can be made simultaneously on an electrocardiogram machine.

"The ultrasonic flow velocity detector is placed at an angle of 45° to the artery and then detects and amplifies the frequency shift that occurs when ultrasound passes through moving blood. An audible signal, rising in pitch with increasing blood velocity, is produced. The angle and alignment of the probe are important, and the loudest obtainable signal should be maintained throughout the recording period.

"Normal arterial flow produces a signal with first and second sounds. Converted to wave form, the pattern has two components, corresponding to systole and diastole. The signals are easily distinguished from the more continuous flow signal from veins, and with experience the sounds of collateral and stenotic flow can readily be identified. For example, flow through a stenotic segment usually produces a high-pitched sound, while signals distal to an occlusion have a low-pitched first sound and no second sound." (Evans)

Patients are examined sitting in bed, flexed at the hips to 45° or more, with the knees straight and the feet supported to prevent pressure on the legs and allow good filling of the calf veins. With olive oil as a coupling medium, the transducer is applied to the skin overlying the vein to be examined. The transducer is placed over the superficial femoral veins 100 mm below the inguinal ligament, over the common femoral veins, over the external iliac veins, and over the inferior vena cava. Veins are usually located by detecting flow through the adjacent artery and then moving the transducer accordingly.

Use is made of the augmentation wave (A-wave) to obtain easily detectable signals. If the velocity of venous flow is suddenly increased by squeezing, more sound is reflected back at a changed frequency, producing an easily audible roar from the amplifier. With the transducer over the common femoral vein, the leg is squeezed successively over the upper thigh, mid-thigh, and lower thigh at the level of the adductor canal and calf.

Normal flow is indicated by the presence of a roar while obstruction is shown by the absence of sound. Similar observations are made with the transducer over the superficial femoral veins, external iliac veins, and inferior vena cava. The site of obstruction and upper extent of a thrombus in many cases can be indicated in this way.

Complete examination is obviously essential, for abnormalities will usually be detected only between the site of squeezing and the transducer. *Where there is a collateral circulation, thrombus may be missed, especially when multiple channels are present. Where vein occlusion is only partial, acceleration in venous flow can occur. A small non-occlusive thrombus may thus be overlooked.*

However, as thrombi enlarge to the point of occlusion, obstruction will be demonstrated.

Little is known at present about the rate at which thrombus is formed, or whether it varies between individuals. Research in this field suggests that in many cases thrombosis starts during an operation and subsequently extends. Extension would seem to be gradual as death most frequently occurs from massive pulmonary embolism around the tenth post-operative day. In the light of present knowledge it would appear, therefore, that twice-weekly screening by experienced personnel, using a good analyser that detects turbulence and considers dynamic flow characteristics, is adequate to detect potentially dangerous thrombi.

5.4   Summary of Ultrasonic Therapy

Ultrasonics is the name given to the science or technology associated with frequencies above 20 000 Hz which is the general upper limit of audibility. Ultrasound waves are longitudinal mechanical waves causing alternate compressions and rarefactions of the media they pass through, and oscillating the particles of the media in the direction of the propagation of the wave.

Ultrasonic therapeutic equipment utilises frequencies from 0.75 MHz to 3 MHz, with penetration of from 60 mm to 200 mm. The primary reaction to the ultrasound beam of therapeutic intensities from 1 to 4 w.cm^{-2} is directly related to particle movement as a result of wave propagation. The acceleration rates to which the particles are subjected are 5 to 16×10^7 cm.s^{-2}, which is 100 000 times that of gravity.

The ultrasound energy produces both thermal and non-thermal effects on the tissues of the body. *Ultrasound adds more energy per unit of time than exposure of the patient to any other form of heat, such as infrared, short wave diathermy or microwave.* More energy per unit of time can be added with no danger to the patient, because of its deeper penetration and selective absorption in the tissues of the body.

The physiological effects of ultrasound depend on the amount of absorption that occurs. Absorption is dependent on two factors: protein and fluid content. Tissues with high protein content and low fluid content are the best absorbers of ultrasound. Absorption is also frequency-dependent. The higher frequencies have a greater absorption in the tissues, but have shorter penetration distances. Ultrasound energy is also attenuated in the tissues as it travels. This alters with the frequency.

The phenomena that occur when ultrasound energy penetrates into the living tissues are *absorption, reflection, refraction and transmission.* Reflection and refraction occur where there is a mismatch of acoustic impedance of tissues, as at the bone-periosteum interface, thus causing increased heating around joints and bones.

The possible mechanisms of the physiological responses of the thermal and non-thermal effects of clinical ultrasonic energy are:

(*a*)   depolymerisation of proteins, especially those which are found in nerve, muscle and tropocollagen cement;

(*b*)   decrease or increase of nerve conduction velocities depending on the dosage;

(c)   reversible decrease of viscosity of intra- and extracellular colloidal sub-
      stances by altering the permeability of the cell membrane;
(d)   excitation of calcium bound to proteins;
(e)   gaseous cavitation with absorption of large quantities of ultrasonic energy.
Parameters which can alter the clinical effects of ultrasound are as follows:
      efficiency of the transmission of energy from the transducer to the patient;
      the frequency of the ultrasonic apparatus;
      the size of the transducer head;
      the protein content of the tissues;
      the duration of the exposure in terms of pulsed, continuous or stationary
      techniques;
      the quantity of bone and its proximity to the skin;
      the depth of the lesion and density of tissues;
      the quantity of peripheral nerve in the area of the lesion;
      the amount of fluid and its relative velocity in the area to be treated;
      air in the pathway of the ultrasonic energy.

References

Bierman, W, 1954, Ultrasound in the treatment of scars, *Arch Phys Med and Rehab, 35*, 209-214.

Blitz, J (3rd Ed), The fundamentals of ultrasonics, *Butterworth*.

Buchan, J F, September 1970, The use of ultrasonics in physical medicine, *Practitioner, 205(227)*, 319–26.

Buchan, J F, January 1972, Heat therapy and ultrasonics, *Practitioner, 208(243)*, 125–31.

Clarke, G R and Stenner, L, 1976, Use of therapeutic ultrasound therapy, *Physiotherapy, 62*, No 8.

Dyson, M and Pond, J B, 1970, The effect of pulsed ultrasound on tissue regeneration, *Physiotherapy, 56*, 136–142.

Dyson, M and Pond, J B, 1973, The effects of ultrasound on circulation, *Physiotherapy, 59*, 284–287.

Dyson, M, Pond, J B, Joseph, J and Warwick, R, 1968, The stimulation of tissue regeneration by means of ultrasound, *Clin Sci, 35*, 273–285.

Dyson, M and Taylor, K J W, 1972, Possible hazards of diagnostic ultrasound, *Brit J Hosp Med, 8*, 5, 571–577.

Faris, P, 1969, Ultrasound: The dosage question, *J Can Physio Assoc, 21:3*, 155–159.

Farmer, W C, 1968, Effects of intensity of ultrasound on the conduction velocity of motor axons, *Phys Ther Rev, 48*, 1233–1237.

Friedland, Frietz, 1957, Present status of ultrasound in medicine, *JAMA, 163*, No 10.

Garg, A G and Taylor, A R, 1967, Effects of ultrasound with special reference to the nervous system, *Biomedical Engineering*.

Gordon, Jean, 1974, Effect of ultrasound on the elasticity of arteries, *W.C.P.T. Congress — Montreal (Lecture)*.

Grieder, A, Vinton, P W, Cinotti, W R and Kangur, T T, January 1971, An evaluation of ultrasonic therapy for temporomandibular joint dysfunction, *Oral Surg, 31(1)*, 25–31.

Griffin, J et al, Patients treated with ultrasonic driven hydrocortisone and with ultrasound alone, *Physical Therapy, 47*, No 7.

Griffin, J E, January 1966, Physiological effects of ultrasonic energy as it is used clinically, *J Amer Phys Ther Assoc, 46*, 18–26.

Griffin, J E, Echternach, J L and Bowmaker, K L, 1970, Results of frequency differences in ultrasonic therapy, *Phys Ther Rev, 50*, 481–495.

Griffin, J E, 1980, Transmissiveness of ultrasound through tap water, glycerine and mineral oil, *Physical Therapy*, 60, 8, 1010–1016.

Halle, J S et al, 1981, Ultrasound's effect on the conduction latency of the superficial radial nerve in man, *Physical Therapy*, 61, 3, 345–349.

Hueter and Bolt, 1955, Sonics, *John Wiley & Sons Inc*.

Kaiser, H S, July 1970, A new method of applying ultrasonic therapy, *J Am Podiatry Assoc, 60(7)*, 280–2.

Kleinkort, A J and Wood, F, 1975, Phonophoresis with 1 per cent versus 10 per cent hydrocortisone, *Physical Therapy*.

Kossoff, 1962, Calibration of ultrasonic therapeutic equipment, *Acustica, 12*.

Kossoff, G, 1976, Techniques for measurement of attenuation and velocity, *Nat Bur Stand Spec Pub*, No 453, Sydney.

Kossoff, G, Research papers in ultrasonic diagnostic and surgical techniques and measurement of ultrasonic power and dosimetry, *Comm Ac Lab, Sydney*.

Krusen, F H, Kottke, F J and Ellwood, P M, 1971, Handbook of physical medicine and rehabilitation, *Philadelphia: W. B. Saunders*, 314–315.

Lehmann, J F, Dehateur, B J and Silverman, D R, 1966, Selective heating effects of ultrasound in human beings, *Arch Phys Med, 46*, 331–339.

Lehmann, J F and Guy, A W, 1972, Ultrasound therapy: Proceedings of a workshop on interaction of ultrasound and biological tissues, *U.S. Dept. of Health Ed and Wel, Maryland*.

Lehmann, J F et al, 1959, Comparative study of the efficiency of short wave, microwave and ultrasonic diathermy in heating the hip joint, *Arch Phys Med and Rehab*, December.

Lehmann, J F et al, 1974, Therapeutic heat and cold, *Clin Orthop and Rel Res*, No 99.

Licht, S, 1965, Therapeutic heat and cold, *Maryland: Waverley Press*.

Madsen, P W and Gertsen, J W, 1961, Effects of ultrasound on the conduction velocity of peripheral nerves, *Arch Phys Med, 42*, 645.

Markham, D E and Wood, M R, Ultrasound for Dupuytren's contracture, *Physiotherapy*, 66, 2, 55–58.

Miller, J T, 1967, The principles of ultrasonics, *Biomedical Engineering*, October.

Patrick, M K, 1966, Ultrasound in physiotherapy, *Ultrasonics, 1*, 10–14.

Quin, C E, 1969, Observations on the effects of X-ray therapy and ultrasonic therapy in cases of frozen shoulder, *Ann of Phys Med, 110*, 64–69.

Reid, D C, Redford, J B and King, P, 1972, The influence of ultrasound and high frequency radio waves on the rate of absorption of experimental hematomas in training: Scientific basis and application, Ed. Taylor, A W, *Illinois: Charles C. Thomas Company*.

Reid, D C, 1977, The use of couplants in ultrasound, *Physiotherapy*, September.

Robinson, Garrett, Kossoff, 1970, Safety margins in diagnostic ultrasonics, *Comm Ac Lab*.

Russell, J G B, 1973, Radiology in obstetrics and ante-natal paediatrics, *London: Butterworth & Co*.

Stangel, L, 1975, The value of cryotherapy and thermotherapy in the relief of pain, *Physio Can, 27*, No 3.

Stewart, H F et al, 1980, Considerations in ultrasound therapy and equipment performance, *Physical Therapy*, 60, 4, 424–428.

Sumner, W and Patrick, M K, 1964, Ultrasonic therapy, *Elsevier Publishing Co., Amsterdam*.

Tymkio, R, William, F O and Goldberg, B, Practical uses of diagnostic ultrasound, *Rad Tech, 43*, No 5.

Valtonen, E J, 1968, A historical method for measuring the influence of ultrasonic energy on living tissue under experimental conditions, *Acta Rheum Scand, 14*, 35–42.

Vaughen, J L and Bender, L F, 1959, Effects of ultrasound on growing bone, *Arch. Phys. Med. and Rehab.*, 158–160.

Wells, P T, 1970, Physical principles of diagnostic ultrasound, *Academic Press*.

Wright, E T and Haase, K H, 1971, Keloids and ultrasound, *Arch Phys Med, 52*, 280–283.

Yeo, S T, Hobbs, J T and Irvine, W T, 1968, Pulse examination by an ultrasonic method, *Brit Med J* (30th Nov.), 555–557.

Yeo, S T, Hobbs, J T and Irvine, W T, 1969, Ankle systolic pressure measurement in arterial disease affecting the lower extremities, *Brit J Surg, 56*, 676–679.

6   Phototherapy

6.1   **Ultraviolet Rays for Treatment**
6.2   **Ultraviolet Rays for Diagnosis**
6.3   **Summary of Ultraviolet Therapy**
       References

Some Key Points in this Unit

Ultraviolet rays are electromagnetic rays lying between visible light and X-rays in the electromagnetic spectrum.

UVA are the longer ultraviolet rays which have wavelengths of from 290 to 390 nanometres.

UVB are the shorter ultraviolet rays which have wavelengths of from 180 to 290 nanometres.

Erythema is reddening of the skin.

Desquamation is the casting off of dead cells from the surface of the skin.

6.1   Ultraviolet Rays for Treatment

Ultraviolet rays are electromagnetic waves with frequencies of from 0.8×10^{15} to 20×10^{15} Hz, lying between visible light and X-rays in the electromagnetic spectrum. The wavelengths of ultraviolet rays used in therapy are from 180 to 390 nanometres. Ultraviolet rays are further categorised by their wavelengths into

UVA (long rays) — 290 to 390 nm
UVB (short rays) — 180 to 290 nm.

The natural source of ultraviolet rays is the sun. However, for therapeutic purposes, ultraviolet rays are generally produced by mercury vapor lamps.

They consist of a quartz burner tube evacuated of air and containing traces of argon gas and mercury under reduced pressure. An electrode is inserted at each end of the burner tube. Current is applied to the electrodes, the mercury vaporises, and the passage of the electrons through the vapor establishes the ultraviolet arc. All ultraviolet lamps also produce visible light and infrared rays.

Due to the production of infrared rays, the quartz burner will heat to temperatures varying from 60°C to several hundred degrees Celsius. It is therefore necessary to incorporate a cooling device into the lamp, particularly if the lamp is to be used close to, or in contact with the patient. Devices commonly used include air cooling (using air circulation which may or may not be assisted by a fan), and water cooling (using a water jacket surrounding the burner with continually circulating water).

A wide range of apparatus is available for the therapeutic application of ultraviolet rays. They can be grouped as follows:

(a) *Air-cooled lamps* — for example, the Hanovia Alpine Sun Lamp, the Hanau Hohensonne, and the Birtcher. The wavelengths of the rays produced are concentrated primarily at the 253 nm level, called UVB (short wavelengths), although some rays down to the 184 nm level are also produced. These lamps are generally recommended for the treatment of generalised skin conditions such as acne and psoriasis. The Birtcher is designed for the treatment of more localised lesions such as pressure areas or ulcers.

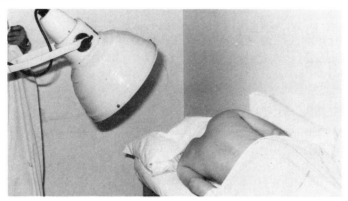

An air cooled ultraviolet lamp — the Hanovia Alpine Sun Lamp

(b) *Water-cooled lamps* — for example, the Kromayer lamp. The wavelengths of the rays produced are concentrated at the 366 nm level, but a wide range of both UVA and UVB rays are produced. The lamps are designed for the treatment of localised lesions such as pressure areas and ulcers, and, with the attachment of appropriate applicators, for the treatment of shelves and sinuses in open areas.

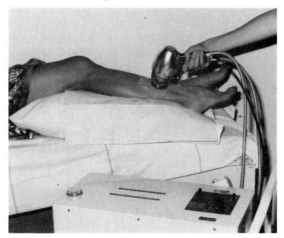

*A water cooled lamp —
the Kromayer Lamp*

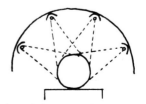

*An ultraviolet tunnel containing
four fluorescent tubes*

(c) *Fluorescent tubes* — for example, the Theraktin lamp consists of a number of fluorescent tubes incorporated into a semicircular tunnel. The wavelengths produced are virtually all between 290 and 350 nm, that is, entirely UVA (long wavelengths). The lamps are recommended for the treatment of conditions such as psoriasis affecting large body areas.

Physical behavior of ultraviolet rays. As ultraviolet rays are electromagetic radiations, they will be governed by the same phenomena and laws as microwave diathermy and infrared rays. Reflection, refraction, penetration, absorption, and the law of inverse squares have been discussed in Unit 3.

PHYSIOLOGICAL EFFECTS OF ULTRAVIOLET RAYS

Ultraviolet rays penetrate the skin to a maximum depth of 2 mm so that all ultraviolet rays will be absorbed by the cells in the epidermis and the superficial dermis. The effects produced by the absorption of the ultraviolet rays are primarily local, although some general effects do occur if large areas are treated with high doses.

LOCAL EFFECTS

Erythema is reddening of the skin and is the first observable effect of ultraviolet irradiation. It will not be visible for at least one hour, and will reach its maximum in about 24 hours. The erythema is the result of an inflammatory reaction stimulated by the ultraviolet rays. The ultraviolet rays cause irritation and degenerative changes in the epidermis, and the prickle cell layer of the skin with a resultant release of a histamine-like substance. This stimulates the triple response of dilatation of capillaries and arterioles, and exudation of fluid into the tissues. The erythema is produced primarily by rays with wavelengths of from 240 to 300 nm, and to a lesser extent by rays with wavelengths of from 330 to 420 nm.

Pigmentation, or tanning, of the skin follows the erythema. The amount of pigmentation produced varies with the intensity of the erythema, and with low-intensity erythema may be visible only after repeated exposure to ultraviolet rays. The pigmentation is due to the increased deposition of the pigment melanin, formed in the basal cell layer of the skin by the melanoblasts, and which then migrates to the more superficial layers of the epidermis. It is thought that ultraviolet rays accelerate the production of melanin by stimulating the production of the enzyme tyrosinase in the melanoblasts.

Desquamation, or peeling, is the casting off of the cells which have been destroyed by the ultraviolet rays. The extent of the desquamation is proportional to the intensity of the erythema. With mild degrees of erythema, fine desquamation may be seen only after repeated exposure to ultraviolet rays.

Growth of epithelial cells is increased as part of the repair process which follows the erythema. The cells in the basal cell layer proliferate to replace the cells in the epidermis which were damaged or destroyed by the ultraviolet rays. Distinct thickening of the epidermis occurs as a result.

Antibiotic effects, or destructive effects of ultraviolet radiation include the destruction of viruses, bacteria, and other small organisms on the skin surface. This effect is produced primarily by rays in the UVB range (short rays).

GENERAL EFFECTS

Formation of Vitamin D is accelerated by ultraviolet radiation. Vitamin D is required to assist in the absorption of calcium and phosphorus from the intestine into the blood stream.

The esophylactic effect, whereby the resistance of the body to infection is increased is enhanced, particularly if general irradiation of UVA is given. This is thought to be the result of stimulation of the reticulo-endothelial system, the cells of which ingest bacteria and produce antibodies against bacteria and toxins.

Variations in responses to ultraviolet rays. There is a wide range of individual variation in responses to ultraviolet rays. The variations have been attributed to variations in skin types, degree of pigmentation, and are also said to be influenced by the age of the subject. It is well recognised that the reaction to ultraviolet also varies from one area to another on the same person. Wet skin, for example, apparently absorbs ultraviolet rays to a greater extent than dry skin.

Natural protection against ultraviolet rays. It is recognised that, with repeated exposure to ultraviolet rays, the sensitivity of the skin to ultraviolet rays generally decreases. The thickening of the epidermis, and in particular the stratum corneum, following ultraviolet radiation is the major factor responsible for the development of this protection.

Previous theories that the increased pigmentation contributed to the development of protection against ultraviolet radiation have been abandoned. The pigment is deposited in layers of the skin deeper than those in which the erythema primarily occurs.

THERAPEUTIC EFFECTS

The effects generally required for therapeutic purposes are primarily the local effects. Although the general effects of increase in Vitamin D formation and the esophylactic effect are beneficial to the patient, it is extremely rare for ultraviolet rays to be used primarily to achieve these effects.

The erythema is useful in conditions where an increase in the circulation of the skin is required. It is beneficial in situations where infection is present, such as in acne or infected wounds, and in situations where the skin condition is poor, such as in pressure areas or around ulcers. The marked inflammatory reaction associated with a marked erythema may also be used for its counter-irritant effect in the relief of pain. However this effect is rarely used today.

Pigmentation is not generally required as a therapeutic effect of ultraviolet radiation.

Desquamation is useful in conditions where the pores and hair follicles have become blocked, such as in acne.

Growth of epithelial cells is a major effect used in the treatment of open areas such as pressure areas, ulcers, and slow healing surgical incisions. It is also desirable in the treatment of dermatological conditions such as acne.

Antibiotic effects are the second major effect required in the treatment of infective conditions such as acne, pressure areas and ulcers.

DOSAGES OF ULTRAVIOLET RAYS

Levels of ultraviolet erythema

Ultraviolet dosages are graded into levels of the erythema reaction according to the intensity of the reaction. It is important to remember that the characteristics of the different levels described here are based on *the reaction observed on normal skin.*

A *minimal erythema dose* (MED) is the length of ultraviolet exposure required to produce a mild erythema, which appears within 6 to 8 hours, and which is still just visible after 24 hours.

A *first degree erythema dose* (E_1) is the length of ultraviolet exposure required to produce a mild erythema, which appears within 6 to 8 hours, and which has just disappeared in 24 hours. Pigmentation is seen only after repeated exposures. Very fine desquamation will also only occur after repeated exposures.

A *second degree erythema dose* (E_2) is the length of ultraviolet exposure required to produce an erythema which appears within 4 to 6 hours, and which disappears within 48 hours. It resembles a mild sunburn reaction and a little discomfort may be felt. It is followed by definite pigmentation, and powdery desquamation usually occurs within 1 to 2 weeks.

A *third degree erythema dose* (E_3) is the length of ultraviolet exposure required to produce a marked erythema which appears within 2 to 4 hours, and which lasts for 72 to 96 hours. It resembles a severe sunburn, and is associated with oedema and tenderness. Subsequent pigmentation and desquamation are marked, with the skin peeling in sheets or flakes.

A *fourth degree erythema dose* (E_4) is the length of ultraviolet exposure required to produce an intense erythema which appears within 2 to 4 hours, and which may last for a week or more. Oedema and exudation of fluid into the tissue layers results in blister formation. Multiples of an E_4 may be given to areas which have been denuded of skin.

Calculation of dosage. The basis for any calculation of ultraviolet dosage is the E_1, which is determined for each individual patient by performing a skin test. From this point all other doses of ultraviolet rays can be calculated. The two significant units of measurement are:

(*a*)   the length of time (usually measured in seconds);
(*b*)   the distance from the source of ultraviolet to the patient (usually measured in millimetres).

Four levels of dosage-intensity are commonly used — E_1, E_2, E_3 and E_4. After the E_1 has been determined from the skin test, the E_2, E_3 and E_4 are calculated using the formulas:

$$(a) \quad E_2 = 2\tfrac{1}{2} \times E_1$$
$$(b) \quad E_3 = 5 \times E_1$$
$$(c) \quad E_4 = 10 \times E_1$$

Examples:
(*a*)   If the E_1 of the patient is 25 s at a distance of 100 mm, calculate the E_3 at 100 mm.

$$E_1 = 25 \text{ s at } 100 \text{ mm}$$
$$E_3 = 5 \times E_1$$
$$\therefore E_3 = 5 \times 25$$
$$= 125 \text{ s at } 100 \text{ mm}$$

(b)   If the E_1 of the patient is 1 s in contact, calculate the E_4 in contact (I/C).

$$E_1 = 1 \text{s I/C}$$
$$E_4 = 10 \times E_1$$
$$\therefore E_4 = 10 \times 1$$
$$= 10 \text{ s I/C}$$

Progression of dosage of ultraviolet rays. Because ultraviolet, when applied to *normal skin*, causes reactions which thicken the superficial layers, each dose must be progressed in a specific way to reach the same effective level of ultraviolet at each treatment. Doses are progressed as follows:

E_1 is progressed by 25% of the preceding dose
E_2 is progressed by 50% of the preceding dose
E_3 is progressed by 75% of the preceding dose

It is unusual to apply doses of the intensity of an E_4 to areas of normal skin. A dose of this intensity is usually used for the treatment of conditions such as ulcers where slough is present. Whilst normal skin develops a resistance to successive doses of UV, non-skin areas do not, and it is thus possible to treat an area not covered by skin with the same dose on successive days to achieve the same result.

Example: If the E_1 is 30 s at 450 mm, find the second progression (P_2E_1).

$$E_1 = 30 \text{ s at } 450 \text{ mm}$$
$$P_1E_1 = E_1 + 25\%E_1 = 30 + \frac{30}{4} = 30 + 7.5$$
$$= 37.5 \text{ s}$$
$$P_2E_1 = P_1E_1 + 25\% \ P_1E_1$$
$$= 37.5 + \frac{37.5}{4} = 37.5 + 9.4 = 46.9$$
$$\therefore P_2E_1 = 47 \text{ s at } 450 \text{ mm}$$

Alteration of intensity with distance. The law of inverse squares states that, as the distance between the source and the patient increases, the intensity decreases in proportion to the square of the distance, and this is represented in the equation:

$$\text{new time (nt)} = \frac{\text{old time} \times (\text{new distance})^2}{(\text{old distance})^2}$$
$$\text{that is nt} = \frac{\text{ot} \times (\text{nd})^2}{(\text{od})^2}$$

Using the Kromayer, the source of ultraviolet is a U-shaped burner situated behind a water jacket, and the burner lies 25 mm from the outer window of the treatment head. Thus the patient will always be at least 25 mm from the source of ultraviolet. Because this distance is a constant, it is not included in the description of the dose (for example, the expression I/C indicates contact of the outer window with the patient, and a distance therefore of 25 mm between the patient and the source of ultraviolet), *but it must be included in all calculations*.

Example: Using the Kromayer, if the E_1 of the patient is 1 s I/C, find the E_1 at 100 mm.

$$nt = \frac{ot \times nd^2}{od^2}$$

$nt = x$
$ot = 1$ s
$nd = 100 + 25$ (constant) $= 125$
$od = 25$ (constant)

$$x = \frac{1 \times 125^2}{25^2} = \frac{1 \times 25}{1}$$

$$= 25 \text{ s}$$

$\therefore$ if the E_1 I/C is 1 s, the E_1 at 100 mm is 25 s

Using air-cooled lamps, the distance is measured from the burner of the lamp to the patient.

Example: Using the air-cooled lamp, if the E_1 at 900 mm is 60 s, find the E_1 at 450 mm.

$$nt = \frac{ot \times nd^2}{od^2}$$

$nt = x$
$ot = 60$ s
$nd = 450$ mm
$od = 900$ mm

$$x = \frac{60 \times 450^2}{900^2} = \frac{60}{2 \times 2} = \frac{60}{4}$$

$$= 15 \text{ s}$$

$\therefore$ if the E_1 at 900 mm is 60 s, the E_1 at 450 mm is 15 s

It will often be necessary to combine the above types of calculations.

Example: Using the Kromayer, if the E_1 I/C is 1 s, find the E_3 at 100 mm.

Step 1 $E_1 = 1$ s I/c
                       $E_3 = 5 \times E_1 = 5$ s I/C

Step 2
$$nt = \frac{ot \times nd^2}{od^2}$$

where $nt = x$
         $ot = 5$
         $nd = 125$
         $od = 25$

$$nt = \frac{5 \times 125^2}{25^2} = 125 \text{ s at 100 mm}$$

$\therefore$ E_3 at 100 mm $= 125$ s

Example: The dose given yesterday was the second progression of an E_1 at 900 mm, where the E_1 is 60 s at 900 mm. What dose was given, and what time will be necessary for treating today if the dose is progressed and the distance changed to 450 mm?

Step 1 $\qquad E_1 = 60$ s at 900 mm

$\qquad\qquad P_1E_1 = E_1 + 25\%E_1 = 60 + 15$

$\qquad\qquad = 75$ s at 900 mm

Step 2 $\qquad P_2E_1 = P_1E_1 + 25\%P_1E_1$

$$= 75 + \frac{75}{4} = 75 + 18.75$$

$\qquad\qquad = 93.75$ s at 900 mm

$\qquad\qquad$ The actual dose given would be 93 s.

Step 3 $\qquad P_3E_1 = P_2E_1 + 25\%P_2E_1$

$$= 93.75 + \frac{93.75}{4} = 93.75 + 23.44 = 117.19$$

$\qquad\qquad = 117.2$ s at 900 mm

Step 4 $\qquad$ To find P_3E_1 at 450 mm, use the equation

$$nt = \frac{ot \times nd^2}{od^2}$$

$$x = \frac{117.2 \times 450^2}{900^2} = \frac{117.2}{2 \times 2} = \frac{117.2}{4}$$

$\qquad\qquad = 29.3$ s

$\qquad\qquad \therefore$ the dose to be given (P_3E_1 at 450 mm) is 29 s

Calculation of doses to be given using an applicator. When using an applicator attachment to the Kromayer lamp, the dose must be adjusted to compensate for the loss in intensity of the ultraviolet as it passes through the applicator. The dose required for the sinus or shelf to be treated must be calculated first as an in-contact dose. The applicator dose is then calculated as follows:

$\qquad$ Applicator dose = in-contact dose $\times$ coefficient of the applicator

The manufacturer of the applicator should test each applicator to determine the loss of intensity which occurs and should thus calculate the coefficient necessary to compensate for this loss of intensity.

For practical purposes the coefficient of the applicator is usually taken as the length of the applicator measured in millimetres, divided by 25.

Example: Calculate a $4E_4$ using a 120 mm applicator if the E_1 of the patient is 1 s in contact.

$$E_1 = 1 \text{ s I/C}$$

$$E_4 = 10 \times E_1 = 10 \text{ s I/C}$$

$$4E_4 = 4 \times E_4 = 40 \text{ s I/C}$$

$\qquad\qquad$ Using 120 mm applicator

$$4E_4 = 4E_4 \times \text{coefficient}$$

$$= \frac{4E_4 \times 120}{25} = \frac{40 \times 120}{25}$$

$$= 192 \text{ s}$$

SELECTION OF DOSAGE LEVEL

The dosage level is selected according to the effects required for the treatment of the presenting condition. However it is not recommended that large areas be exposed to high doses of ultraviolet rays. The following guidelines should be followed:

(*a*)   An E_1 or MED may be given to the total body area.
(*b*)   An E_2 may only be given to up to 20% of the total body area.
(*c*)   An E_3 may only be given to up to 250 cm² of normal skin.
(*d*)   An E_4 may only be given to an area of up to 25 cm² of normal skin, but is usually only given to non-skin areas where the size of the area is not important.

Frequency of treatment. The frequency of treatment depends upon the level of erythema produced. *Successive doses of ultraviolet must never be given to normal skin while the erythema produced by the preceding dose is still visible.* The following guidelines should be followed when treating normal skin:

(*a*)   An E_1 or a MED may be given daily.
(*b*)   An E_2 should be given every second day.
(*c*)   An E_3 should be given every third or fourth day (twice weekly).
(*d*)   An E_4 may only be given once a week, or even once a fortnight, provided the effects of the previous dose have subsided.

However, when *treating non-skin areas* such as pressure areas or ulcers, *all doses may be given daily* as there is no erythema reaction produced.

Effect of desquamation on dosage. When desquamation occurs, the natural protection developed against the ultraviolet rays is lost to a varying extent, depending on the amount of desquamation. In order to prevent damage to the newly exposed skin, the successive dose should be reduced. As a general rule, after desquamation the dose is reduced to the original erythema level and progressed again at each successive treatment. For example, a patient who had been receiving a P_3E_3 would be reduced to an E_3; or a patient who had been receiving a P_6E_1 would be reduced to an E_1.

INDICATIONS

Ultraviolet rays are used in the treatment of some dermatological conditions, and infected and non-infected skin lesions.

Acne. Treatment of acne, using ultraviolet rays, is aimed at producing desquamation to open the blocked pores and hair follicles, erythema to improve the condition of the skin, stimulation of growth of healthy epithelium, and antibiotic effects to destroy the infecting organisms. Acne is usually found affecting the face, front of the chest, neck, and the upper part of the back and shoulders.

The ideal dose for the production of the effects required would be an E_3. This may be given safely to small areas on the back and shoulders, but would not be tolerated on the face, chest, or neck by most patients, as these areas tend to be more sensitive to ultraviolet. Therefore an E_2 dose would be given to the face, chest and neck. For cosmetic reasons, some patients may not tolerate doses higher than an E_1 to the face. An air-cooled lamp is generally used.

Psoriasis. Ultraviolet radiation is often given as part of a regime of treatment for psoriasis. The aims of treatment with ultraviolet rays are to decrease the DNA synthesis in the cells of the skin, with a resultant decrease in the proliferation of the skin cells which causes the silvery plaques so characteristic of the disease, and to improve the skin condition. Two regimes of treatment are commonly used today.

Leeds Regime consists of the patient having a coal tar bath, gently rubbing the skin to loosen and remove the psoriatic plaques. The patient is then treated with ultraviolet rays, using an E_1 dose progressed daily. As coal tar sensitises the skin to the effects of ultraviolet rays, it must be applied prior to the skin test so that its effect on each patient is known before treatment is commenced. If only localised areas of the body are affected by the psoriasis, or if the condition is resistant to treatment, an E_2 dose may be given every second day, progressing the dose at each treatment. After irradiation with ultraviolet rays, dithranol cream is applied to the psoriatic plaques. A large air-cooled lamp is generally used.

Photochemotherapy is a recently developed regime gaining popularity in the treatment of psoriasis. It is based on the combination of ultraviolet therapy using waves of the UVA range (long rays), together with the systemic administration of a photosensitising drug, 8-methoxypsoralen, and is commonly known as the *PUVA regime*. The dosage of 8-methoxypsoralen is determined by the patient's body weight.

A skin test is performed 2 hours after the patient has taken the drug, to determine the minimal phototoxicity dose (MPD), which is measured in $J.cm^{-2}$ and can be measured accurately using a meter. The MPD produces an area which is barely pink 72 hours after exposure to ultraviolet rays. The patient is then treated 2 to 4 times weekly, each treatment being given 2 hours after taking 8-methoxypsoralen. The ultraviolet dosage is progressed at each treatment according to the patient's skin type. Patients who always burn in the sun are progressed by $0.5 J.cm^{-2}$, while those who rarely or never burn are progressed by $1 J.cm^{-2}$.

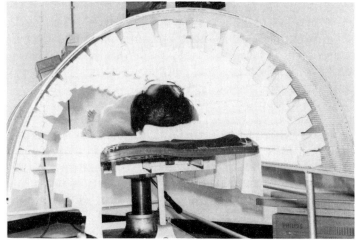

A patient receiving treatment for psoriasis using a fluorescent tunnel as part of the PUVA regime

The lamp used is generally a tunnel containing fluorescent tubes which emit UVA primarily in the range between 350 and 365 nm. The lamp is tested for intensity each month, and the treatment time adjusted to produce a constant intensity of treatment.

Incipient pressure areas. Ultraviolet rays may be used to prevent the skin over an incipient pressure area from breaking down and producing an open, infected wound. The aims of treatment with ultraviolet rays are to improve the skin condition, to stimulate the growth of epithelial cells, and to destroy surface bacteria.

An E_1 dose, progressed daily, is generally given using the Kromayer lamp. In areas such as the heels or elbows, where the skin is thicker, an E_2 may be preferred.

Non-infected open wounds. Ultraviolet rays may be used to promote the healing of non-infected open wounds such as surgical incisions, pressure areas, or venous or arterial ulcers. The aims of treatment with ultraviolet rays are to stimulate growth of the granulation tissue, to promote healing by stimulating growth of the epithelium, and to prevent infection by the destruction of any surface organisms.

The granulation tissue should not receive any more than an unprogressed E_1, or overgranulation may occur. The surrounding skin is generally treated with an E_1 progressed daily, although areas such as the heels and ankles may respond better to a progressed E_2 given every two days. The Kromayer lamp is generally used.

Infected open wounds. Ultraviolet rays may be used in the treatment of infected surgical incisions, pressure areas, and arterial and venous ulcers. The aims of treatment with ultraviolet rays are to destroy and remove the slough (infected material), stimulate growth of healthy granulation tissue, and promote healing by stimulating growth of the epithelium.

The skin surrounding the area should be irradiated with an E_1 dose, progressed daily. Any healthy granulation tissue should not receive any more than an unprogressed E_1, or over-granulation may occur.

If the slough is only a fine film, giving the granulation tissue a yellowish appearance, an E_3 dose should be sufficient. All surrounding skin and granulation tissue must be screened so that it does not receive this destructive dose. The dose may be given daily and is not progressed, as it is not being applied to normal skin.

When a definite layer of yellow or green slough is present, an E_4 or a multiple E_4 (up to 20 E_4) dose may be given, depending on the thickness of the slough and its resistance to treatment. All tissue surrounding the slough must be screened to protect it from this highly destructive dose. The dose may be given daily and is not progressed, as it is not being applied to normal skin.

Some open areas are covered initially by a thick, dark brown or black, leathery scab. This is known as black slough and will not be penetrated by even the highest doses of ultraviolet. To remove this black slough, an E_4 or a multiple E_4 is given to 5 mm of the healthy skin surrounding the slough. This dose is repeated daily until the edges of the slough start to lift away from the skin. The black slough can then be gently cut away with a scalpel blade, leaving the open area, generally with green or yellow slough underneath, exposed for treatment. Excising the black slough is generally not painful as there are no sensory nerves in the slough, so no anaesthesia is necessary.

Shelves and sinuses should be treated with an applicator of an appropriate shape, as the effects of the ultraviolet will not otherwise penetrate to these areas. The Kromayer lamp is generally used.

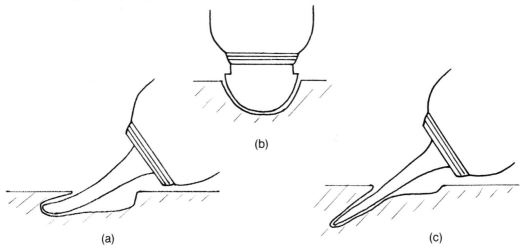

Applicators for the irradiation of (a) shelves; (b) deeply eroded wounds; and (c) sinuses.

Counter-irritation. Ultraviolet may be used for its counter-irritant effect in the relief of pain. A small area of skin is given an E_4 dose, so that the discomfort produced masks the pain caused by deeper structures. After administering the dose, the area must be covered with a dressing to prevent infection as the blisters form and rupture. The Kromayer lamp is generally used.

CONTRA-INDICATIONS

Dermatological conditions. Certain conditions, such as acute eczema, lupus erythematosis, and herpes simplex, may be exacerbated by ultraviolet radiation.

Hypersensitivity to sunlight. Patients who are known to react adversely to even minimal exposure to sunlight should not be treated with ultraviolet rays.

Febrile disorders. Ultraviolet rays should not be applied to large body areas if the patient has a raised temperature, as a further increase in temperature may result.

Deep X-ray therapy. If the area to be treated with ultraviolet rays has received deep X-ray therapy within the preceding three months, it may be hypersensitive to the effects of the ultraviolet rays.

Infrared therapy. If infrared therapy has been given recently to the area to be treated, and the erythema produced is still present, there will be increased absorption of the ultraviolet rays, with a resultant increase in their effects.

Photoallergy. If the patient is known to develop a rash after exposure to sunlight, treatment with ultraviolet rays should be avoided.

Tuberculosis or tumours in the area to be treated may be exacerbated by the effects of the ultraviolet rays.

APPLICATIONS USING AIR-COOLED LAMPS

(*a*) **Skin test procedure.** Before any doses can be calculated, the E_1 of the patient must be determined, using the following procedure. The test doses are determined using a combination of factors: the E_1 of the lamp (that is an E_1 taken from an average population), the patient's normal reaction to sunlight, and whether or not the patient is taking any sensitising drugs.

If the patient burns after only a brief exposure to sunlight, use the E_1 of the lamp as the highest test dose.

If the patient has an average response to sunlight, that is, burns on average exposure but then tans, use the E_1 of the lamp as the middle test dose.

If the patient rarely burns, or burns only after long exposure to sunlight, and tans easily, use the E_1 of the lamp as the lowest test dose.

If the patient is taking sensitising drugs, use a set of test doses lower than would be normal for that patient.

The remaining test doses are selected so as to give intervals of one-third of the E_1 of the lamp. For example, if the E_1 of the lamp is 18 seconds, and the patient burns after only a brief exposure to sunlight, the test doses would be 6, 12, and 18 seconds. Or, if the E_1 of the lamp is 60 seconds and the patient rarely burns but tans easily, the test doses would be 60, 80, and 100 seconds.

Equipment required
ultraviolet lamp
sheets for screening
grey or black paper or plastic with three shapes cut out
scissors
sticking plaster
tape measure
cotton wool
2 pairs of goggles
stopwatch

The patient should be in a position of optimum comfort with the part to be tested exposed so that the lamp will not be placed directly over the patient.

Explain to the patient what you are about to do and why.

Tell the patient not to look to the lamp, or remove the goggles you have given him, because of the possibility of damage to the eyes (conjunctivitis).

Tell the patient not to move as there is a risk of overdose or inaccuracy in the test.

Tell the patient to call out if he feels distressed.

Assuming that there are no contra-indications to ultraviolet, proceed as follows:

Ascertain the E_1 of the lamp, which will be marked on the lamp, and the patient's normal sensitivity to sunlight. Check whether the patient is taking any sensitising drugs.

With the lamp positioned towards the floor, switch it on. If the lamp does not strike immediately, press the starter booster button. Leave the lamp away from the patient to stabilise. The head of the lamp should not be covered or in close contact with the floor or furniture as there is a risk of burning.

Prepare the skin test area in exactly the same way as the area to be treated will be prepared. For example, patients with psoriasis should have had a coal tar bath, or have taken their 8-methoxypsoralen as appropriate. Patients with acne may need to wash with a medicated soap.

Screen the patient with a double layer of sheeting, so that all exposed areas are protected. Ensure that the patient can still breathe when draping the head.

Cut three different shapes out of the paper or plastic and apply these to a suitable flat area of exposure to sunlight similar to the area to be treated. Hold them in place with sticking plaster. Never skin-test on the face.

Cover the patches with a small drape, marking the center of the test area with a crease.

Position the lamp and measure the distance from the burner accurately, ensuring that the rays will be perpendicular to the part (the rim of the lamp should be parallel to the part).

Check that the patient is still fully draped.

Do *not* touch the burner and do not position the lamp directly over the patient as there is a risk of the lamp falling on the patient, or the burner exploding or falling out.

Remove the small drape from all three areas and expose them for the shortest test dose required. Cover one area. The second area has already received a dose. Continue exposure for the extra time needed to complete the second test dose required. Cover this area as well as the first, and continue to irradiate the remaining area until the largest test dose has been completed. Then cover the entire area. The test doses must be timed accurately, using a watch with a second hand.

Example:

AREA 1	AREA 2	AREA 3
$\diamondsuit$	$\bigcirc$	$\square$
12 seconds	18 seconds	24 seconds

Expose all areas for 12 seconds. Cover Area 1.
Expose Areas 2 and 3 for 6 more seconds. Cover Areas 1 and 2.
Expose Area 3 for 6 more seconds. Cover Areas 1, 2 and 3.
Switch off the lamp and remove it.
Undrape the patient immediately.

Instruct the patient, a relative, or the nursing staff to inspect the area which was irradiated 6 to 8 hours after exposure (give the patient specific times) and mark on the diagram you have given them any areas which are showing pink or red. Make arrangements to see the patient again 24 hours later.

Always record:
date;
time;
anatomical location of exposure;
the lamp used and its E_1;
the distance of the lamp from the patient;
time of each exposure;
physiotherapist's signature.

Example: 19th November, 1977 at 2.00 pm. UV skin test on the inside of the left forearm using the OPD air-cooled lamp at 240 mm. E_1 of lamp = 18 s at 240 mm.

HAND ◇   ◯   □ ELBOW

12 seconds   18 seconds   24 seconds

J. JONES.

Determination of the E_1

The patient should be seen 24 hours after the skin test. The E_1 is determined as that area which appeared erythematous at 6 to 8 hours and which has just disappeared at 24 hours.

(b)   Treatment procedure

Equipment required
ultraviolet lamp
sheets for screening
tape measure
goggles
stopwatch

The patient should be positioned comfortably so that the area to be treated is exposed and the lamp need not be placed directly over the patient.

Explain to the patient what you are about to do and why.

Tell the patient not to look at the lamp, or remove the goggles because of the risk of conjunctivitis.

Tell the patient not to move as there is a risk of inaccuracy or overdose.

Tell the patient to call out if he feels distressed.

Check that the patient has not commenced taking, or altered the dose of any sensitising drugs. If so, the skin test should be repeated.

Assess the area to be treated and determine the dosage level to be given. Calculate the dosage accurately.

With the lamp positioned towards the floor, switch it on. Do not cover the lamp or position it close to the floor or any furniture as there is a risk of burning.

Check that the patient has washed, had a coal tar bath, or taken his 8-methoxypsoralen as appropriate.

Screen all areas not to be irradiated with a double layer of sheeting, leaving the area to be treated exposed. *Use immovable bony landmarks to delineate the area so that it can be reproduced exactly* at the next treatment to prevent an overdose. Do *not* hold the screening in place with sticking plaster. Give the patient goggles, or cover the eyes with vaseline and cotton wool, and cover the head.

Cover the area to be treated.

Check that the patient is fully screened.

Align the lamp, so that it is parallel to the part to be treated, but not positioned directly over the patient. Measure the distance accurately from the burner to the part.

Remove the drape from the area to be treated to expose it for the dosage time.

The dose must be timed accurately, using a watch with a second hand, and the area recovered immediately with the drape.

Move the lamp away from the patient and position it towards the floor while preparing to treat another area, or switch it off if the treatment is completed.

Arrange for the patient's next treatment according to the dosage level given. Always record:

date;

time;

anatomical location of exposure, including the bony landmarks used for delineation of the area;

the lamp used and the patient's E_1;

the dosage given;

the distance from the patient;

physiotherapist's signature.

Example: 20th November, 1977 at 2.00 pm. UV treatment was given for acne of the back and shoulders. The patient's $E_1 = 18$ s at 240 mm using the OPD air-cooled lamp. Dosage given: $E_3 = 90$ s at 240 mm.

Area treated —

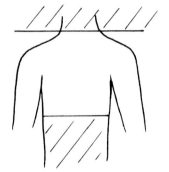

head screened to C7 spinous process

back screened to T8 spinous process, arms exposed

S. JONES.

Irradiation of large areas. If the area to be treated is too large to be irradiated adequately in one exposure, it should be treated in sections. For example, to treat a patient with total body psoriasis if a tunnel is not available, treat the back in two halves delineating the area at the posterior superior iliac spines, and the front in two halves delineating the area at the anterior superior iliac spines. All four areas may be irradiated at one treatment session. If the sides of the body require specific irradiation as well as the front and back, the sides should be treated on alternate treatment sessions to the front and back, to avoid overlapping the doses.

APPLICATIONS USING THE KROMAYER LAMP

(*a*)   **Skin test procedure.** Before any doses can be calculated, the E_1 of the patient must be determined using the following procedure. The test doses are determined using a combination of factors: the E_1 of the lamp (that is the E_1 taken from an average population), the patient's normal reaction to sunlight, and whether or not the patient is taking any sensitising drugs.

If the patient burns after only a brief exposure to sunlight, use the E_1 of the lamp as the highest test dose.

If the patient has an average response to sunlight, that is, burns on average exposure but then tans, use the E_1 of the lamp as the middle test dose.

If the patient rarely burns, or burns only after long exposure to sunlight, and tans easily, use the E_1 of the lamp as the lowest test dose.

If the patient is taking sensitising drugs, use a set of test doses lower than would be normal for that patient.

The remaining test doses are selected so as to give intervals of one-third of the E_1 of the lamp. For example, if the E_1 of the lamp is 2 seconds and the patient has an average response to sunlight, the test doses would be 1, 2 and 3 seconds.

The E_1 of the Kromayer is often 1 second, so that for patients who burn easily, or who have an average response to sunlight, test doses of less than 1 second should be selected. This, however, is impractical as these doses would be impossible to time accurately. In this situation, test doses of 1, 2 and 3 seconds are given and the E_1 is estimated from the reaction obtained. If an area becomes markedly red and has some oedema present, that is an E_3 reaction; divide that test dose by 5 to determine the E_1 of the patient. If an area becomes red and tender without oedema, that is an E_2 reaction; divide that test dose by 2.5 to determine the E_1 of the patient.

Equipment required
Kromayer lamp
grey or black paper or plastic
scissors
sticking plaster
stopwatch

Position the patient comfortably with the area to be tested exposed.

Explain to the patient the purpose of the test and tell him not to move so that the test will proceed smoothly and accurately. Warn the patient not to look at the lamp because of the risk of conjunctivitis.

Assuming that there are no contra-indications to ultraviolet, proceed as follows:

Ascertain the E_1 of the lamp and the patient's normal sensitivity to sunlight. Check whether the patient is taking any sensitising drugs.

Turn the pump on, then turn the burner on. If the lamp does not strike immediately, press the starter booster button. When the lamp has struck, leave it on for 5 minutes to stabilise.

Select an area of skin which has had similar previous exposure to sunlight to the area to be treated. The grey or black paper or plastic, with three different shapes cut out, should be secured with sticking plaster to the area chosen.

The skin test with the Kromayer is done in contact. For example, if the E_1 of the lamp is 1 second in contact, the test doses selected may be:

AREA 1   AREA 2   AREA 3

1 second   2 seconds   3 seconds

Take the cap off the Kromayer quickly and place on Area 1 for 1 second, timing with the stopwatch, then quickly replace the cap. Then take the cap off again, and place on Area 2 for 2 seconds. Do likewise for Area 3 for 3 seconds.

Turn the burner off, then wait till the head of the Kromayer is cool before turning the pump off (at least 3 minutes).

Instruct the patient, a relative, or the nursing staff to inspect the area which was irradiated, 6 to 8 hours after exposure (give specific times) and mark on a diagram any areas which are showing red or pink.

Always record:

date;

time;

times and distance of exposure;

anatomical location of exposure;

lamp used and its E_1;

physiotherapist's signature.

Example: 19th December, 1977 at 2.00 pm. Ultraviolet skin test on inside of (L) forearm using the ward Kromayer in contact. E_1 of lamp = 1s I/C.

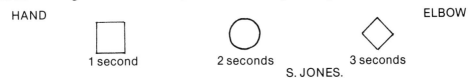

HAND   ELBOW

1 second   2 seconds   3 seconds

S. JONES.

Determination of the E_1. The patient should be seen 24 hours after the exposure. The E_1 is determined as that area which appeared erythematous at 6 to 8 hours and which had just disappeared at 24 hours.

(*b*) **Treatment procedure.** As most treatments given with the Kromayer lamp will be to open wounds, an aseptic technique must always be used. It is preferable to have two therapists, one performing the aseptic technique, the other applying the ultraviolet radiation.

Equipment required

Kromayer lamp

sterile dressing pack, swabs, and other dressings as required

sterile screening material, such as vaseline gauze or jelonet, which are usually available in 100 mm squares

stopwatch

ruler

sticking plaster

Position the patient comfortably with the area to be treated exposed.

Explain the purpose of the treatment and warn the patient not to look at the lamp because of the risk of conjunctivitis. Tell the patient not to move, or doses will be inaccurate.

Check that the patient has not commenced taking, or altered the dose of any sensitising drugs. If so, the skin test should be repeated.

Turn the pump on, then turn the burner on. If the lamp does not strike immediately, press the starter booster button. When the lamp has struck, leave it on for 5 minutes to stabilise.

Using an aseptic technique, clean the area thoroughly. Assess the area to be treated and determine the dosage levels to be given. Calculate the dosages accurately.

Attach a ruler to the head of the lamp with sticking plaster to measure the distance at which the doses to the skin and granulation tissue are to be given. Ensure that the ruler is attached at an angle so that it will not cast a shadow over the area irradiated. These doses are generally given at 100 mm, or sometimes at 50 mm, in order to irradiate as much of the skin surrounding the open area as possible. It is not necessary to screen any of the surrounding areas when using the Kromayer. The dose for the granulation tissue is given to the whole area first, timing accurately with a watch with a second hand (usually an unprogressed E_1). Then the granulation tissue is screened from all further doses using sterile vaseline.

If the skin dose is higher than the granulation dose (for example, a progressed E_1), the balance of the skin dose is then given to the area. Remove the ruler from the head of the lamp.

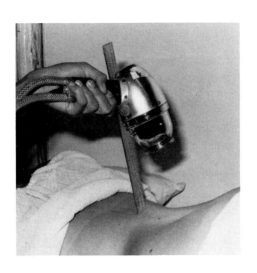
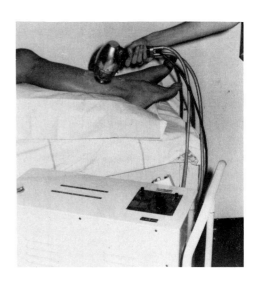

Administration of a skin dose using the Kromayer Lamp at 100 mm

Administration of a slough dose using the Kromayer Lamp in contact

Using an aseptic technique, screen the skin and granulation tissue with sterile vaseline gauze or jelonet to protect them from all further doses.

Give the destructive doses to the slough, with the head of the Kromayer gently in contact with the area to maximise the effects of the short rays. If there are several different slough doses to be given, the lowest dose is given first, and the area screened before the balance of the next dose is given. Before replacing the cap over the lamp window, wipe the window with a swab soaked in methylated spirits to remove all vaseline.

Example: (third treatment of the area)

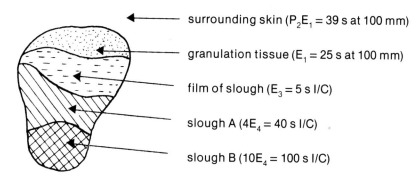

surrounding skin ($P_2E_1 = 39$ s at 100 mm)

granulation tissue ($E_1 = 25$ s at 100 mm)

film of slough ($E_3 = 5$ s I/C)

slough A ($4E_4 = 40$ s I/C)

slough B ($10E_4 = 100$ s I/C)

Step 1 — Give the entire area 25s at 100 mm (granulation dose).

Step 2 — Screen the granulation with sterile vaseline and give the area a further 14 s at 100 mm to complete the skin dose.

Step 3 — Screen the surrounding skin and granulation tissue with sterile jelonet and give the whole open area a further 4 s in contact to complete the E_3 to the film of slough. (It has already received an E_1 = 1 s in contact.)

Step 4 — Screen the film of slough and give a further 35 s in contact to the remainder of the open area to complete the dose for slough A.

Step 5 — Screen slough A and give a further 60 s to the remainder of the open area to complete the dose for slough B.

When all doses have been given, remove the screening and gently wipe off the excess vaseline before applying a sterile dressing.

Switch off the burner and leave the pump running to cool the head of the Kromayer (at least 3 minutes).

Arrange for the patient's next treatment, usually the following day.

Always record:

date;

time;

anatomical location of exposure;

the lamp used and the patient's E_1;

the doses given — a diagram is useful;

physiotherapist's signature.

Records of the progress of the area may be kept by taking a tracing of the area, using sterile cellophane, at intervals during the course of treatment.

Irradiation of large areas. If the area is too large to be treated with one application of the dose, it should be treated in suitably sized sections. Areas to be treated as separate sections must be covered with a sterile gauze swab, not vaseline gauze or jelonet, as these would leave a residue of vaseline which would screen out future doses. Care must be taken not to overlap doses to adjacent sections.

Irradiation using applicators. When the use of an applicator is required, the remainder of the area is treated in the normal manner. The sterile applicator is attached to the head of the Kromayer by an adapter, which also incorporates a shutter so that emission of ultraviolet can be easily controlled. The applicator is introduced gently into the shelf or sinus with the shutter closed to prevent emission of ultraviolet. When the applicator is positioned, the shutter is opened to irradiate the shelf or sinus for the desired dosage time, then closed before the applicator is removed gently.

DANGERS

Shock. As with any electrical apparatus there is the danger to both the patient and the therapist of sustaining a shock. The machine should be earthed and the mains power cord insulation intact.

Damage to the eyes. Irradiation of the eyes with ultraviolet rays produces conjunctivitis. Iritis may also be produced, and keratitis and opacity formation in the cornea has been found after higher levels of exposure. Massive doses of ultraviolet may result in lens opacity (cataract).

The eyes of both the patient and therapist must be protected. Goggles made of Chance Crooks A glass absorb all ultraviolet wavelengths and offer maximum protection. If the face is to be irradiated, as in the treatment of acne, the eyes should be covered by cotton wool balls held in place by a smear of vaseline.

The risk to the eyes is minimal when using the Kromayer lamp, and it is sufficient protection for both patient and therapist to avoid looking directly at the burner or the rays emitted.

Overdosage. There is a risk of producing an ultraviolet burn, characteristically an E_4 reaction, if an overdose is given. This may occur if care is not taken to prevent the overlap of doses or the exposure of previously untreated areas to progressed doses, by not using bony landmarks to delineate the area of exposure.

Accuracy in dosage calculation and progression is essential to prevent an overdose, and must be based on the patient's E_1, as determined by a skin test. When destructive doses (E_3 or E_4) are to be given, all other areas must be carefully screened.

Should an overdose of ultraviolet rays be given, its effects may be reduced if it is realised before the erythema has been produced. Infrared radiation is given over the area for 20 minutes in every hour for 6 to 8 hours, so that the increase in the circulation may dissipate the effects of the ultraviolet rays. Administration of infrared radiation should be followed by the application of hydrocortisone cream to reduce the inflammatory reaction.

Sensitising drugs. A number of drugs, and some foods in a few patients, are known to sensitise patients to the effects of ultraviolet rays. If the patient changes the dose of the drug taken, or commences or ceases a course of the drug, his reaction to the ultraviolet rays will alter, and the treatment will be either ineffective or may result in an overdose.

When skin-testing the patient prior to treatment, the effects of the sensitiser must be taken into consideration in selecting the test doses, and will be reflected in the E_1 determined for the patient. If the dose of the drug is then changed, or a course of sensitising drugs commenced during treatment with ultraviolet rays, the skin test should be repeated, so that accurate adjustments to the dosage of ultraviolet may be made.

Sensitising drugs include the following:

Thiazide diuretics	Aprinox (bendrofluazide)
	Chlotride (chlorothiazide)
	Doburil (cyclothiazide)
	Enduron (methcyclothiazide)
	Navidrex (cyclopenthiazide)
Sulphonamides	Gantrisin (sulphafurazole)
(anti-bacterial)	Lederkyn (sulphamethoxypyridazine)
	Furadantin (nitrofurantoin)
	Salazopyrin (sulphasalazine)
	Thalazole (phthalylsulphathiazole)
Tetracyclines	Achromycin
(antibiotics)	Aureomycin
	Mysteclin
	Reverin
	Terramycin
Anti-fungal agents	Fulcin (griseofulvin)
Phenothiazine tranquillisers	Largactil (chlorpromazine)
	Melleril (thioridazine)
	Stelazine (trifluoperazine)
Barbiturates	Amytal (amylobarbitone)
	Barbico (barbitone)
	Gardenal (phenobarbitone)
	Nembutal (pentobarbitone)
	Soneryl (butobarbitone)
Hypnotic drugs	Sulphonal
	Trional
	Veronal
Miscellaneous	Aspirin and its derivatives
	Alcohol
	Throid extract
	Insulin
	Coal tar
	Eithranol
	Gold injections
	Mercurochrome
	Eosin

Note that as **8-methoxypsoralen** is also a sensitising drug, its long-term use in conjunction with ultraviolet rays for the treatment and maintenance of patients with psoriasis requires that specific precautions be taken.

To prevent conjunctivitis and possible cataract formation, patients are instructed to wear good sunglasses for at least 5 hours after taking the drug, and the eyes are protected with both cotton wool and goggles during irradiation. In addition the patient should have an annual eye examination.

A full blood count and biochemical screen should be performed regularly to assess any actinic damage which may occur.

6.2   Ultraviolet Rays for Diagnosis

Patch testing for photoallergies. Some patients are found to be photoallergic, that is, allergic to a combination of ultraviolet rays and a particular drug or chemical. The condition generally manifests itself as a rash in the areas where the skin is exposed to sunlight, or to both sunlight and the chemical.

The drugs or chemicals suspected are determined by questioning the patient about drug therapy, and the soaps, powders and other cosmetics applied to the skin, since a component of one of these may be the cause of the allergy.

The diagnosis is confirmed by the use of a photopatch test procedure. A typical photopatch test would involve the irradiation of localised patches, to which the suspected substances have been applied, with ultraviolet rays. Often two sets of patches are irradiated, one with UVA and the other with UVB, to determine the wavelengths responsible, so that an appropriate filter cream may be prescribed.

If a drug is suspected, the patch test must be performed after ingestion of the drug. A control test is usually also performed without ingestion of the drug.

To ensure that the reaction is not due purely to the effects of ultraviolet rays, a control patch is included in all patch tests, which receives ultraviolet radiation only. In true photoallergy, there should not be any rash development in the control patch.

6.3   Summary of Ultraviolet Therapy

In Unit 6, the effects and uses of ultraviolet rays in the treatment of a variety of commonly encountered conditions have been described. The principles of dosage selection and calculation described must be followed accurately in order to ensure safe and effective treatment of these conditions. Although the dangers associated with treatment using ultraviolet rays are few, they are serious, and require that the recommended precautions are strictly adhered to.

References

Cotterill, J A, 1980, Acne vulgaris and its management, *Physiotherapy*, 66, 2, 41–42.

Enta, T and Dolphin, B, 1973, Therapeutic and diagnostic uses of ultraviolet light, *Physiother Can, 25*, 3, 159–160.

Epstein, Stephen, 1964, The photopatch test, *Ann of All, 22*, 1, 1–11.

Epstein, Stephen, 1966, Simplified photopatch testing, *Arch of Derm, 93*, 216–220.

Fugill, G C, 1980, Pressure sores, *Physiotherapy*, 66, 2, 46–47.

Fusco, R J et al, 1980, PUVA therapy for psoriasis, *Physiotherapy*, 66, 2, 39–40.

Glasgow, R M and Baldwin, J P, 1969, Reactions from phototesting procedures, *Cutis, 5*, 565–570.

Kalivas, James, 1969, A guide to the problem of photosensitivity, *JAMA, 209*, 1706–1709.

Klaber, M R, 1980, Ultraviolet light for psoriasis, *Physiotherapy*, 66, 2, 36–38.

Licht, Sidney (Ed.), 1967, Therapeutic electricity and ultraviolet radiation, *Baltimore: Waverley Press*.

MacKenna, R M B, 1953, Some of the uses of ultraviolet rays in dermatology, *Brit J Phys Med*, July, 1953.

Montgomery, P C, 1973, The compounding effects of infrared and ultraviolet irradiation upon normal human skin, *Phys Ther, 53*, 5, 489–495.

Schurr, Donald G and Zuehlke, Richard L, 1981, Photochemotherapy treatment for psoriasis, *Physical Therapy*, 61, 1, 33–36.

Scott, Pauline M, 1975, Clayton's electrotherapy and actinotherapy, *London: Balliere and Tindall*.

Ward, A R, 1976, Electricity fields and waves in therapy, *Science Press*.

Wolff, K et al, 1977, Phototesting and dosimetry for photochemotherapy, *Brit J Derm, 96*, 1, 1–10.

7 Direct Current

Some Key Points in this Unit

An **electron** is a fundamental particle of matter possessing a negative charge and a small mass.

Electricity is a form of energy which can be made to exhibit magnetic, chemical, mechanical, thermal, and electrostatic effects, and when at rest or in motion exerts a force on other electricity.

Electric current is a net movement of electrons through any material when a potential difference exists between the ends of the conducting pathways. Its unit of measurement is the ampere.

One ampere (1A) is the flow of 6.24×10^{18} electrons per second.

An electromotive force must be applied to produce a flow of electrons. The electric pressure required to send a current of one ampere through a resistance of one ohm is one **volt**.

A **voltmeter** is a meter designed and calibrated to measure potential difference.

An **Ammeter** is a meter designed and calibrated to measure current.

Direct current is a current that flows in one direction only. When used medically it is called 'galvanic' current. Most power supply is alternating current, in which the direction of flow of electrons changes by, say, 50 cycles per second.

An **electrode** is the part of the electric conductor by which the current is being applied.

Watts (w) are the units of electrical power. It is the power used when a current of 1 ampere at an EMF of 1 volt flows for one second.

$$\text{watts} = \text{volts} \times \text{amperes}$$

Transformers are devices to step up or reduce AC voltages. In medical apparatus a transformer steps down the mains voltage of 240 volts to an appropriate safe lower value.

Rectification is the conversion of alternating current to direct current, by either a diode valve or a metal semi-conductor rectifier.

Transducers are devices which are used in electrical circuits to turn energy such as sound, light or motion into current flow, and by converting the modified electrical signal into a form which can be detected by the senses.

A **cathode** is the negative pole or electrode of any electrical device.

An **anode** is the positive pole of an electrical device.

An **electrolyte** is a substance which contains ions, that is, charged particles.

Anion is an ion carrying a negative charge, and so is attracted to the anode of an electrolytic cell.

Cation is an ion carrying a positive charge, and so is attracted to the cathode.

Iontophoresis is the transfer of ions through the skin by the use of a constant direct current.

7.1 Direct Current

Direct current (synonyms: galvanism; constant current) is a unidirectional flow of electrons through a conductor. The rate of flow of electrons is known as the intensity of the current, and is conveniently measured in *milliamperes*. One milliampere is the flow of 6.24×10^{21} electrons per second.

Constant direct current treatments are rarely used today, but an understanding of the basic physics and physiological effects of direct current applications is essential to enable us to appreciate the effects of low and medium frequency currents on the body.

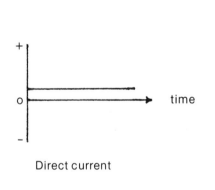

Direct current

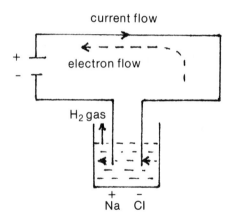

Passage of current through a solution

Electrolysis. In order to understand the physiological effects of direct current on the body, one must look at the chemical effects produced when a direct current is passed through an electrolyte. Saline solution (a solution of sodium chloride) is an electrolyte, meaning that it can conduct an electric current. It contains positive sodium ions, Na^+, negative chloride ions, Cl^-, and water molecules, H_2O. The electrode which is connected to the negative terminal of the DC supply becomes negatively charged and attracts the positive ions (cations) in the electrolyte. It is called the *cathode*. The other electrode, connected to the positive terminal becomes positively charged and attracts negative ions (anions), and is called the *anode*.

Electrons flow from the negative terminal to the positive terminal through the external circuit. Conventionally, the direction of current flow is said to be opposite to electron flow. Current leaves the positive terminal and flows through the circuit to the negative terminal.

In the electrolyte there is a migration of positive ions and polar water molecules to the cathode. The water molecules pick up electrons from the cathode, forming hydrogen atoms and thence hydrogen gas, and leaving hydroxide ions in solution.

$$2H_2O + 2e^- \longrightarrow H_2 + 2OH^-$$

Thus the solution near the cathode becomes alkaline. The positive sodium ions remain in solution.

At the anode, the chloride ions release electrons and become neutral atoms which form chlorine gas.

$$2Cl^- \longrightarrow Cl_2 + 2e^-$$

Some of the chlorine reacts with the water to form a mixture of hydrochloric and hypochlorous acids.

$$Cl_2 + H_2O \longrightarrow HCl + HClO$$

So the solution near the anode becomes acidic.

Physiological Effects

If we pass a direct current through the body, the area of tissue under the cathode will show an alkaline reaction, while at the anode there will be a weak acidic reaction. The alkaline reaction under the cathode produces a marked red coloration of the skin, due to capillary hyperaemia. There is less red coloration under the anode. Thus *a danger of chemical burn exists*, particularly under the area of the cathode.

When a constant direct current is applied to the body, the entire region between the electrodes is involved, in accordance with the electrical conductivity of the tissues. The conduction of the current depends on the water content of the tissues. Muscle has a good blood supply, so it will conduct current, while fat is a poor conductor. Current takes the path of least resistance. Skin has a high resistance of over a million ohms when it is dry, but only 20 000 ohms when it is wet. It varies from person to person, and from hour to hour.

When the skin is artificially heated and made to perspire, its resistance drops. The upper limit drops to 200 000 ohms, except in elderly persons with sclerotic blood vessels, where resistance is higher. Passage of a current through dry skin can produce a chemical burn; so, if a warm moist towel is applied to the part to be treated prior to current being passed, it will lower the skin resistance and also reduce the risk of a chemical burn.

Hyperaemia. The most marked circulatory changes take place in the skin and superficial tissues just under the electrodes. If sufficient intensity of current is given, to a maximum of 0.8 mA.cm^{-2}, there will be a marked counter-irritant effect produced by the capillary hyperaemia of the dermis. This will relieve pain in the treated area.

Sedation. At the anode, if a low dosage is given for a longer period of time, such as 0.3 mA.cm^{-2} for 30 minutes, then an analgesic effect is felt in the area just under the anode. The direct current is thought to reduce nerve conduction velocity.

7.2   Iontophoresis

Iontophoresis is the transfer of the ions of drugs into the body through the skin by the use of a constant direct current. The principle is based on the fact that ions will migrate to the electrode of opposite charge under the influence of an electromotive force. Since the ions migrate to the oppositely charged electrode, the positive ions must be introduced from the positive electrode and the negative ions from the negative electrode.

The hyperaemia which is produced following iontophoresis disappears after a few hours, but renders the blood vessels more sensitive to changes from thermal or mechanical stimuli, and hence vasodilatation occurs more easily in the treated area. Drugs are often more effectively transferred into the affected area than by topical application in the form of creams, liniments or lotions.

Strength of solution. It is important to make a dilute solution of the drug, since a high concentration reduces its conductance into the tissues. Generally a 0.1 molar (0.1 M) strength is sufficient. Specific ions have their own velocity in tissue. Also some ions, such as copper, zinc, and silver, precipitate more rapidly than others by forming insoluble proteinates.

Another factor to be remembered in evaluating the method is *the velocity of the existing blood flow* in the area to be treated. Blood flow will dilute the concentration of the drug.

Common drugs in usage today include renotin, for adhesions of ligaments and tendons; zinc sulfate, for vasomotor rhinitis (hay fever); glycopyrronium bromide, for excessive sweating; and acetic acid, for calcium deposits.

Some uses of drugs

CONDITION	DRUG	POLARITY
fungus infections	copper sulfate	copper+
scleroderma	mecholyl	choline+
varicose ulcers	mecholyl (to periphery)	choline+
indolent ulcers	zinc sulfate	zinc+
keloids	potassium iodide	iodide-
recent scars	sodium chloride	chloride-
calcium deposits	acetic acid	acetate-
chronic arthritis	mecholyl	choline+
traumatic lesions of ligaments and tendons	renotin	renotin+
hyperhidrosis (sweating)	glycopyrrolate	bromide+
vasomotor rhinitis	zinc sulfate	zinc+

Ion transfer. The principles of ion transfer are:
(*a*)   dissolving the medicinal substances in water breaks them into ions (ionisation).

(b)   like charges repel:
      positive ions are introduced into the skin or mucous membrane at the
      positive electrode, or anode;
      negative ions are introduced into the skin or mucous membrane at the
      negative electrode, or cathode.
(c)   deeper penetration is produced than would result from mere topical ap-
      plication of the medicinal substance.

APPARATUS FOR DIRECT CURRENT AND IONTOPHORESIS TREATMENTS

All modern low frequency generators provide both direct current and alternating
current circuits for connection to the patient. The DC is obtained from the mains
power supply after it has been rectified by suitable rectifiers, inductors, and
capacitors in the circuit. The term low voltage generator is used for a stimulator
that supplies both AC and DC and has the means to modulate them.

The direct current controls in low frequency apparatus. The basic requirements
for the application of DC in an apparatus are clearly indicated positive and
negative terminals. *Red* denotes the positive terminal, or the *anode*. *Black* indicates the negative terminal, or the *cathode*. The power output and the
milliammeter must be clearly indicated. Generally there will be two current
ranges. For example, the unit may have ranges from 0 to 12 mA and from 0 to 30
Ma. The dial indicating the range should be clearly marked. Siemen's Neurotron
626 has a choice of three ranges: 0 to 5 mA, 0 to 20 mA, and 0 to 80 mA.

There should also be a polarity reversal switch, which enables you to change
the polarity of the terminal. Also look for a clear ON/OFF switch connecting the
machine to the mains.

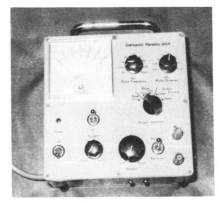

The galvanic-faradic unit

Some machines have the option of superimposing a faradic type current over
the DC. This will have a separate circuit. It is important to select the circuit that
produces a direct current only.

Accessories

The electrodes are made from aluminium foil or metal. Care must be taken that
the electrodes are smooth and have rounded edges. Circular electrodes are useful

in avoiding sharp edges and are easier to apply over joints. Rubberised carbon electrodes are often used in modern machines.

The pads may be made from any smooth absorbent material such as lint, gauze pads, sponge, or household absorbent cleaning cloth. The important factor is that when compressed the thickness of the pad should be 10 mm. Lint generally requires 16 layers, and household absorbent material requires 6 to 8 layers. The pad should be uniform in thickness.

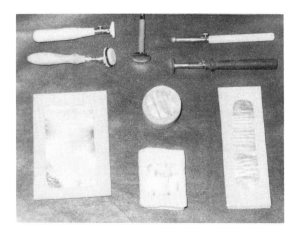

Electrodes and pads for direct current applications

Conducting leads with a variety of end fittings are provided with the apparatus. It is important to ensure that the fittings to the lead wires are firm and not broken.

INDICATIONS FOR DIRECT CURRENT AND IONTOPHORESIS

Relief of pain. *Cathodal galvanism* can be used to relieve cases of chronic pain caused by adhesions, swelling or pressure on nerves. The counter-irritant effect of cathodal galvanism produces a marked vasodilatation which, by helping to remove the pain factors, is responsible for the relief of pain. Also it is thought that the counter-irritation acts on the large sensory fibres to inhibit pain at the spinal level through pre-synaptic inhibitory mechanisms. However, in order to achieve this effect a maximum dosage must be given. It is useful for pain caused by ischaemia, such as in vascular or sympathetic disorders. Patients with painful amputation stumps, shoulder-hand syndromes and Sudek's atrophy are examples.

Anodal galvanism is thought to relieve pain by removing the increased concentration of H^+ and K^+ ions which accumulate in ischaemia or inflammation. The small hydrogen ions are easily repelled by the positive pole of the anode. In order to obtain benefit from anodal galvanism, a low dosage for a maximum length of time must be given.

Adhesions. Renotin, which is a derivative of histamine, can be used in iontophoresis. Renotin sets up a marked counter-irritation by producing the triple response to histamine — a feeling of increased heat, a marked vasodilatation, and a wheal. This affects the fibrous tissue of the adhesions and helps to resolve them. In cases of ligamentous and tendinous adhesions, renotin ionisation may be used. Care must be taken to give the correct dosage and treat the affected area accurately.

Chronic congestion of mucous membrane. Transfer of zinc sulfate into congested nasal membranes has proved beneficial for patients suffering with vasomotor rhinitis (hay fever). Fairly good results have been obtained.

Calcium deposits. Acetic acid transfer into calcium deposits has proved effective. Acetic acid is a drug which has been little used by therapists and perhaps should be encouraged. It relieves pain by reducing the size of the calcium deposit.

Idiopathic hyperhidrosis. Glycopyrronium bromide administered by iontophoresis has been recommended for the treatment of excessive sweating. It has been used successfully in some of the larger hospitals in Australia, where it was introduced by dermatologists a few years ago. The results have been variable, but it has been found that the drug works in many cases, provided the patients do not show any reaction to it. A reaction is uncommon, but care must be taken to look for side effects.

CONTRA-INDICATIONS

Open skin. As current tends to concentrate at these points, large broken areas must be avoided. Small areas can be insulated by the use of vaseline.

Infection. There is a danger of spreading infection if DC is given to an infected area.

Bony areas. Direct contact techniques with a pad are contra-indicated over bony areas, as they produce a burn. The uneven surfaces will prove to be an impediment when trying to gain even contact with the electrode pad.

Loss of sensation. It is important to evaluate the sensory function of the area to be treated, since loss of sensation can lead to a burn if an overdose is given inadvertently.

Dry scaly skin. If a patient exhibits a dry scaly skin, it is important to remove all scales and ensure that the skin is capable of being moistened. A wet pad placed on a dry scaly skin is no guarantee of reducing the skin resistance.

Skin lesions. Eczema, fungus, psoriasis, and other such conditions will be irritated by DC and made worse.

DANGERS

Shock can be caused by the following factors:
  inadequate earthing of the apparatus casing;
  faulty ammeters;
  faulty power points;
  wet floors and faulty earthing of apparatus;
  patients who touch a faulty machine while having current administered in a small bath;
  accidentally knocking off the mains switch when there is a high output of current going to the patient;

reversing the polarity during treatment;

increasing or decreasing the current too quickly.

Burns. Chemical burns can occur. Alkaline chemical burns occur at the cathode, and, if a strong saline solution is used, there will be an acidic burn at the anode.

They can be caused by the following factors:

contact of metal with the skin;

overdosage;

skin lesions;

concentration of current caused by:

(a)   the presence of undissolved salt in solution;

(b)   an uneven pad;

(c)   creases or raw edges on the pad;

(d)   pads unevenly moist;

(e)   skin abrasions, acne, blackheads, and any raised skin edges;

metal in the part, such as safety pins, hooks, or bare lead wire;

poor contact of the pad in the area allowing the electrode to slip.

DOSAGE

(a)   **Anodal galvanism** (low dosage for a long duration)

Intensity. 0.15 to 0.25 mA.cm^{-2} of the active (smaller) lint pad; that is, the area of skin receiving treatment.

Duration. 15 minutes for the first treatment, progressed by 5 minutes to 30 minutes.

(b)   **Cathodal galvanism** (higher dosage for a shorter duration)

Intensity. 0.5 to 0.8 mA.cm^{-2} of the active (smaller) lint pad; that is, the area of skin receiving treatment.

Duration. 10 minutes for the first treatment, progressed by 5 minutes to 20 minutes.

Both the intensity and the duration are primarily determined by the patient's tolerance.

Frequency. Treat on alternate days. Anodal galvanism may be given daily for a few days.

TECHNIQUES FOR APPLYING DIRECT CURRENT

Methods of application are either (a) in contact, or (b) through water.

IN CONTACT METHOD

Equipment required

a source of direct current

two leads of sufficient length with firm terminals or unfrayed bare ends

plastic sheet

towels

soap

insulating cream (vaseline, petroleum jelly, lanolin)

spatula

two small bowls of warm water

two moist pad electrodes 10 mm thick (16 layers of lint, 6 layers Wettex, sponge, or Chux towels 10 mm thick when compressed); the active pad electrode must be the exact size of the area to be treated, and the indifferent (dispersive) pad electrode as large as possible to reduce the current density to a minimum (2.5 times larger than the active is a fair guide)

two flat metal electrodes with rounded corners (10 mm smaller than the pads all round)

two pieces of plastic which must be just large enough to cover the surface of the lint pad and the depth of its thickness

two crepe bandages (or rubber bandages, in which case there is no need to cover the moist pads with plastic)

Position the patient comfortably with the part to be treated fully supported, easily accessible, and resting on the sheet of plastic which has been covered with a towel.

Describe to the patient:

(a)   the rationale for treatment;

(b)   the sensation to be experienced — as the current is turned on, a prickling sensation is felt which gradually passes off and is replaced by a feeling of warmth.

Accurately locate and measure the anatomical site of the pathology.

Examine the area to be treated. Note any cuts, skin lesions, or inflammation. Check that there is no metal on the skin or in the area between the two electrodes where the current will flow, as this will produce an electrolytic burn.

Over the skin areas where both the electrodes will be placed, test the patient's ability to differentiate sharp and blunt sensations, to ensure that the patient will be able to tell when prickling occurs, and also to detect immediately any increase in current.

With soap and water, wash the patient's skin to remove any grease where the electrodes are to be placed. Rinse with clean water.

Place a warm, moist pad over these areas to decrease skin resistance.

Warn the patient

(a)   not to move and not to touch any of the apparatus;

(b)   to report immediately if the prickling becomes too intense, or if it becomes more intense in one spot than over the rest of the area, or if a burning sensation is experienced either over the whole surface or in one spot, because there is a danger of a chemical burn occurring.

The therapist should be seated in front of the patient with the machine conveniently placed to manipulate the controls and read the meter accurately.

Check that all the controls are at the zero position.

Plug into the mains power supply and switch on.

Select settings for direct current.

Connect the leads *firmly* to the machine.

Test the machine — meter and polarity. After immersing the distal bare ends of the leads in water, turn the intensity control up, and check that the needle of the milliammeter moves smoothly through its full range. Check polarity by observing the many tiny bubbles of hydrogen formed rapidly at the cathode (and the fewer large bubbles of oxygen which appear slowly at the anode). It is standard practice for the cathode terminal to be black, and for the anode to be red.

Return the intensity control to zero.

Test the polarity reversal switch, if present, by checking that the hydrogen bubbles appear at the other electrode when polarity is reversed.

Soak the pads in warm water. The pads must be uniformly wet, otherwise most of the current will pass through the wetter parts, causing a high current concentration in the underlying skin which will produce a burn. Folded material pads must therefore be unfolded to be soaked.

Connect the leads *firmly* to the metal electrodes.

If applicable, fold the pads smoothly without wrinkles so that the smooth side of the material is against the patient's skin.

Calculate the dose on the area of the active (smaller) pad.

Cover the metal electrodes with the pads, and test the application on yourself by placing the dampened forearm and hand across the two pads, describing to the patient the sensation you feel.

Remove the hot soak, and if there are any breaks in the patient's skin insulate them with a small amount of vaseline, using the spatula. Skin lesions provide a pathway of low resistance, and thus the concentration of current would cause a burn.

Moisten the skin where both the electrodes will be placed. Cover the pads and electrodes with waterproof material and bandage on firmly with even pressure. Do not bandage the lead wire or electrode metal against the skin.

Turn the current up slowly and ask the patient to let you know immediately the prickling occurs. At first the current enters through the ducts of the sweat glands and the hair follicles, which are of lower resistance than the cornified layer, causing a prickling sensation. As the skin saturates and becomes a better conductor, the current flows evenly through the whole surface and the patient experiences a feeling of warmth.

The prickling is reduced and the treatment made more comfortable for the patient by the use of the hot soak and the moistening of the skin under the electrodes.

Wait for the prickling sensation to die down, then turn the current up again slowly.

Repeat until the prescribed dose, or the maximum tolerance level of the patient, is reached. This may take up to 5 minutes. Treatment is timed from here.

The physiotherapist must check constantly

(*a*)   the sensation being experienced by the patient;

(*b*)   the meter — if the current increases suddenly after stabilisation, it may be due to any of the following:

   (i) the skin has absorbed moisture and become a better conductor;

   (ii) there is a breakdown of the skin;

   (iii) there is a short circuit.

If the current decreases towards the end of treatment, it may mean that the pads are drying out, causing increased resistance.

Turn the current down slowly and return all controls to zero. Switch off the mains power supply, and remove the plug. Remove the pads and inspect the area. The skin under the anode will be pink, and under the cathode red. Any whealing indicates an overdose. In some patients the skin is more sensitive to direct current and a galvanic rash will be produced. If persistent, treat this as a contra-indication.

Wash the skin well to remove any chemicals and wash the pads well for the same reason.

Record the size of the pads, their position, the intensity tolerated, the duration of application, the effect on the skin and the effect on the condition being treated.

SUBAQUATIC METHOD

Equipment required
a source of direct current
two leads of sufficient length with firm terminals or unfrayed bare ends
plastic sheet
towels
soap
insulating cream (vaseline, petroleum jelly, lanolin)
spatula
two small bowls of warm water
a suitable sized water container (bowl, basin, or baby's bath)
trolley or small table
two metal electrodes (size does not matter)

A monopolar bath can often conveniently be used in the application of direct current, for example where the area to be treated is of uneven contour (active electrode), or where a large dispersive is required.

Position the patient, explain the treatment, assess and measure the area to be treated, test pain sensation, wash the skin and apply a hot soak as described in the in contact method.

Warn the patient as for the in contact treatment, but in particular *not to pull the limb out of the water*, as this will produce an uncomfortable galvanic shock. Also the patient must not touch the metal electrode in the bath as contact with metal will produce a chemical burn.

Test the machine as described previously.

One electrode is placed in the bath of warm water and the circuit completed by a second monopolar bath, or by a pad and electrode.

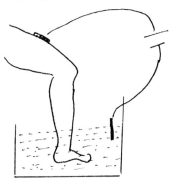

Subaquatic technique for direct current applications

In the bath some of the current passes through the water and some through the patient's tissues, but above the water line all the current passes through the patient's tissues and the current tends to concentrate at the surface of the water causing undue discomfort. This is avoided by applying insulating cream (vaseline) to the area of skin at the water line.

Turn the current up and down *very slowly*, as the skin resistance is reduced after several minutes' immersion.

Dosage can only be based on the patient's tolerance, but still maintaining the principle of low dosage of long duration with anodal and higher dosage for a shorter duration with cathodal galvanism.

Check carefully the patient's sensation and the meter as described in the in contact method. Conclude the treatment in the manner previously described.

IONTOPHORESIS TECHNIQUES

1. THE TREATMENT OF IDIOPATHIC HYPERHIDROSIS BY GLYCOPYRRONIUM BROMIDE IONTOPHORESIS

Risks with glycopyrronium bromide iontophoresis
Chemical burn, due to increased concentration at a particular part, especially at cuts and skin lesions.
Prevention: Insulate with vaseline.
Galvanic shock
Prevention: Turn the intensity up and down slowly.
Warn the patient not to move the hand or foot during treatment.

Side effects
Dryness of the mouth, which may vary in intensity from mild to severe.
Abdominal discomfort — uncommon and rarely troublesome.
Blurred vision — uncommon and rarely troublesome.
Urinary retention — rare.
These effects rarely last more than 24 hours and never more than 48 hours.

Contraindications
Patients with closed-angle glaucoma (cataract).
Patients with prostatic enlargement (especially elderly patients), coronary insufficiency or cardiac failure.
Patients with paralytic ileus (and constipation problems).
Patients on concomitant drug therapy, including antihistamines, phenothiazine tranquillisers and tricycle antidepressants.
Patients with a history of allergy to bromide or other halide salts.

Equipment required
a source of direct current
two leads and two metal electrodes
two large lint pads (16 thicknesses or, when compressed, 10 mm thick)
a plastic bowl big enough to fit a hand into
glycopyrrolate solution consisting of glycopyrronium bromide and distilled water in the following ratio: 0.1 g of glycopyrronium bromide : 100 ml of distilled water
vaseline

Technique for treatment of a hand

In treatments using glycopyrrolate solution for iontophoresis, the anode becomes the active electrode. This is essential if penetration of the drug into the skin is to be produced, since the glycopyrrolate ion is positive. The cathode therefore becomes the dispersive electrode.

In order to achieve concentration of the current under the anode, the dispersive skin area should be at least 2.5 times the area covered by the anode.

Warn the patient of possible side effects.

Set the machine as for any direct current application. Connect the leads and electrodes.

Cover any cuts or open areas on the skin with vaseline.

Place the *active* electrode — ANODE (red) — into a small bowl with the pad of lint on top. Pour in enough glycopyrrolate to saturate the lint.

The patient rests the hand on the lint pad so that the palmar surface is covered by the solution.

Place a large electrode, 2.5 times the area of the active electrode, on the upper arm or thigh.

Turn the intensity up slowly. For the first treatment the intensity should not exceed 10 mA. If side effects are not serious or troublesome, the intensity is gradually increased on subsequent treatments to the level of the patient's tolerance (15 to 20 mA)

Maintain for 10 minutes for the first treatment, and for up to 15 minutes for subsequent treatments when the patient's reaction to side effects is known.

Turn down slowly and repeat the procedure for the other hand.

For treatment to a foot, a larger plastic bowl may be needed. The foot is rested on a lint pad saturated with glycopyrrolate, and the hand and forearm on the same side as the foot being treated becomes the area for the dispersive electrode. Current tolerance in the foot will probably be reached at an intensity of 20 to 25 mA.

Frequency of treatment

Treat the patient twice a week for 6 treatments. The patient may need follow-up treatments from 2 months up to 12 months. It is usual to accept patients 12 months after treatment without a second referral. If the treatment is unsuccessful after 6 applications, send the patient back to the doctor.

2. ACETIC ACID IONISATION FOR THE TREATMENT OF CALCIUM DEPOSITS

Acetic acid iontophoresis has been effectively used in North America by Psaki and Carol in 1955, and by Joseph Kahn more recently. The acetic acid reacts with and dissolves calcium deposits.

Technique

Make a 2 to 5% solution of acetic acid. Make a pad about 10 cm^2 in area and soak the pad in the acetic acid. Connect the pad and electrode to the cathode terminal and bandage it firmly over the affected joint. Ensure that the middle of the pad is over the calcium deposit. Make a slightly larger indifferent pad and connect it to the anode. Position the pad and electrode on the same limb. Increase the current slowly. The dosage is 5 mA for 20 to 30 minutes, given three times a week for two weeks and thence once a week until the symptoms subside.

Kahn advocates giving surged sinusoidal current immediately after the iontophoresis, using the same electrode positions and a surged sinusoidal current at a frequency of 100 Hz and surged at 8 to 10 surges per minute, for 5 minutes. This is followed by infrared for 10 minutes, followed by massage and exercises.

The treatment relieves pain long before the X-ray shows disappearance of the deposits.

Precaution
Clean the area after treatment with an astringent lotion to reduce any irritation.

3.   ZINC SULFATE ION TRANSFER FOR THE TREATMENT OF ALLERGIC VASOMOTOR RHINITIS

Vasomotor rhinitis is hay fever, or allergic rhinitis with paroxysmal sneezing. The use of zinc sulfate for the treatment of chronic rhinitis has been discontinued in many centers because of the introduction of effective antihistamine drugs and desensitisation techniques. Nevertheless a few physiotherapists who work in ENT departments still use it successfully.

Contraindications
Asthma
Post-nasal drips
Respiratory infections
Sinusitis
Sneezing fits

Technique
Zinc sulfate solution can be made by dissolving $ZnSO_4,7H_2O$ crystals in lubricating jelly until a 2% solution is obtained (use Johnson & Johnson KY lubricating jelly). The gel can be easily introduced into the nasal cavity with minimal discomfort.

The patient is treated in the sitting position, with the negative electrode bandaged over the forearm.

The gel is inserted into the nasal cavity by means of a syringe with a rubber catheter. Position the patient with the head tilted forward and downward to prevent the gel going on the palate.

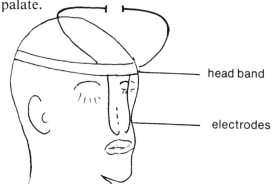

Technique for zinc sulfate iontophoresis for allergic vasomotor rhinitis

As an alternative a 1% solution of zinc sulfate is made. Ribbon gauze is soaked in this solution, gently wrapped around the electrode and inserted into the nasal cavity. The cavity is packed gently and firmly with ribbon gauze. Prior to insertion of the electrode and solution, the nasal fossae are sprayed with 4 parts of 10% cocaine to 0.1% adrenalin. The spray will anaesthetise the mucous membrane and also acts as a vasoconstrictor to cause shrinkage of the congested mucous membrane. This enables the nasal cavity to contain more gel.

The anode must be positioned centrally without allowing the central tip to touch the mucous membrane, or this will cause a burn. If wrapped well with ribbon gauze then this is prevented. The current is introduced gradually at an intensity of 3 mA for 3 minutes for the first treatment. At the end of the treatment the current is reversed at 2 mA for 1 minute to release the electrode and packing. The electrode gel or packing is gently removed, and the nasal cavity inspected. The nasal mucosa should have a white covering. A metallic taste may be experienced.

Progression of dosage and results
Increase the dose by 1 mA and 1 minute at each treatment until a final dose of 8 mA for 8 minutes is given. Generally 6 treatments at weekly intervals are sufficient to produce some form of relief. The zinc sulfate forms an insoluble proteinate called zinc albuminate when it reacts with the protein of the mucosa. The layer of zinc albuminate protects the nasal mucosa from allergic reactions and promotes reduction of the congestion. When the protective layer exfoliates, it leaves the mucosa decongested and with reduced secretions.

4.   RENOTIN ION TRANSFER

Renotin is used as a counter-irritant. It is placed under the anode and, because it bears a positive charge, is repelled into the tissues when a direct current is applied.
The effects are:
Local
Capillary vasodilatation, in the skin only, due to the direct effect of the chemical on the capillary walls.

Increased exudate, due to increased capillary permeability.

Flare, due to a reflex, possibly an axon reflex, by which the walls of the arterioles are influenced. Flare occurs in the skin only.
General
Generalised effects are rarely seen with the use of renotin.

Indications
Ligamentous lesions such as of the medial or lateral ligament of the knee.

Tendinous lesions such as in tennis elbow or golfer's elbow where there is strain of the common extensor tendon origin or common flexor tendon origin.

Contraindications
Because of the possibility of general vasodilatation, treatment is contra-indicated where there is any source of bleeding, for example gastric ulcers or haemophilia.
Patients with any allergy-based disorder, for example asthma, hay fever, or dermatitis.

Heart disease.
Arteriosclerosis.
Pregnancy.
Skin lesions.
Infection.
Acute inflammation.

Equipment required
Normal requirements for direct current treatment, plus:
Renotin 2% cream
wooden spatula
a single piece of lint the same size as the folded active pad, which must not be larger than 100 mm × 100 mm

Position the patient in half lying, fully supported. Take the patient's pulse before and after treatment, and record it.

Explain to the patient the nature and purpose of the treatment. In addition to the usual direct current warnings the patient should be warned that the prickling under the anode will be intense and will persist.

Also if the patient feels sick, or experiences a generalised warmth, a feeling of blushing, prickling behind the eyes, dizziness, drowsiness or a headache, he must let the therapist know *immediately*, as these are possible symptoms of a general reaction.

The dispersive (cathode) is applied first, placed away from the active and not bandaged on by the same bandage.

Use the spatula to spread a layer of renotin on the moistened separate piece of lint and bandage with the folded lint pad and metal electrode on the part to be treated. It is necessary to apply this quickly as renotin starts to take effect as soon as it is placed on the skin. The size of pad must be the exact size of the lesion with an excess of 10 mm all around.

When it may be necessary to remove the application quickly, the active electrode can be secured by a sandbag.

Turn the intensity up slowly to the required dose and check for symptoms of an adverse reaction to the renotin, for example if the pulse rate rises by more than 8 beats/minute, or if there is flushing of the throat or ears.

At the completion of the treatment, turn down the intensity and remove the active electrode. Any trace of renotin is wiped off, the patient's skin is washed with soap and water, and then dried vigorously with a towel. The single piece of lint is thrown away.

Leave the patient lying down for 5 to 10 minutes, sit the patient up for a few minutes, then check the area and take the pulse again before allowing the patient to leave.

In the event of a general reaction, leave the patient lying down for half an hour, to allow the blood pressure to return to normal, then sit the patient up for 5 to 10 minutes, before allowing the patient to stand up. Keep checking the pulse rate. If concerned call a doctor.

Record the size and location of the area treated, current intensity and duration of treatment, description of local reaction, and any general reaction if experienced.

Dosage
The maximum dose is half that of anodal galvanism, but at the first visit, as a
test, only half that dose (that is 0.25 anodal galvanism) is given, as some people
are hypersensitive to renotin. If the anodal folded lint pad measures 60 mm × 50
mm the dose for renotin ionisation would be

$$\frac{6 \times 5 \times 0.15}{2} = 2.25 \text{ mA}.$$

The test dose is half that dose $= \dfrac{2.25}{2} = $ 1.125 mA for 3 minutes.

With no adverse reaction, the time can be increased by 1 minute at successive
treatments to a possible maximum of 5 mA for 10 minutes.

Treatment is usually given on alternate days, but daily for a few days is not
contra-indicated. If after 12 treatments the patient shows no, or only slight,
improvement, the treatment should be discontinued.

7.3 Summary of Direct Current Treatment

Direct current has little use today, except for the introduction of specific drugs
into areas of superficial lesions. With the development of more effective
analgesic drugs, its use as a counter-irritant for the relief of pain has been
minimised.

Care must be taken when using direct current for iontophoresis, as not only do
the drugs used have possible side effects, but there is also the risk of producing a
chemical burn on the skin. This will be avoided if the techniques and precautions
described are strictly adhered to.

References

Clayton's Electrotherapy and Actinotherapy, P M Scott, 6th ed, *London: Balliere*, 1969.

Cornwall, M W, 1981, Zinc iontophoresis to treat ischaemic skin ulcers, *Physical Therapy*, 63, 3, 359–360.

Friedenberg, Z B, Harlow, M C and Brighton, C T, 1971, Healing of non-union of the medial malleolus by means of direct current: A case report, *J Trauma, 11*, 10, 833–835.

Ganne, J M, 1964, Some aspects of treatment of pain by counter-irritation, *Aust J Physio, 10, 90.*

Gordon, A H, 1969, Sodium salicylate iontophoresis in the treatment of plantar warts, *Phys Ther, 49*, 869.

Grice, K, 1980, Hyperhidrosis and its treatment by iontophoresis, *Physiotherapy, 66,* 2, 43–45.

Morgan, K, 1980, The technique of treating hyperhidrosis by iontophoresis, *Physiotherapy*, 66, 2, 45.

Savage, B, 1954, Preliminary electricity for the therapist, *London: Faber.*

8 Low Frequency Currents

Some Key Points in this Unit

Full wave rectification is the reversal of the direction of alternating current during alternate half-cycles. The current is unidirectional and pulsed.

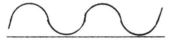

Half wave rectification is the use of a rectifier to allow current to pass in one direction only, as the flow is blocked during alternate half-cycles of the alternating current. The current produced is a pulsed direct current.

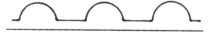

Faradism denotes tetanic currents which have a pulse duration of 1 ms and a frequency of 50 Hz. The currents may be alternating currents or interrupted pulsed currents. They also have a surging modulation.

Faradic current is an uneven alternating current with each cycle consisting of two unequal phases. The first phase has a peak EMF of 1 ms followed by a train of damped oscillations with a frequency of 1000 Hz.

Faradic-type currents are surged modular pulsed currents with a range of pulse durations from 0.02 ms to 1 ms and a frequency of from 50 to 100 Hz. These currents stimulate nerves and produce tetanic-like contractions.

Tetanic currents are short duration interrupted direct currents and alternating currents which are capable of producing a tetanic-like contraction of muscle.

Interrupted direct current is a unidirectional current which is regularly interrupted or pulsed.

Short duration interrupted direct currents are currents which range from a pulse duration of 0.02 ms to 1 ms and basically stimulate normally innervated muscles.

Long duration interrupted direct currents are currents which range from 10 ms to 2000 ms pulse duration. They are used in the stimulation of partly or completely denervated muscle.

Frequency is expressed in hertz. One hertz (1 Hz) is one cycle per second.

The **motor point** is the region where the greatest density of terminal motor end plates are found near the surface of the muscle. It is not necessarily the point where the nerve enters the muscle.

Exponential progressive currents are pulsed currents which reach their maximum peak intensity slowly. The speed of rise of currents is variable, as is seen in rectangular, trapezoidal, triangular, and saw-tooth pulses.

Catelectrotonus is the state of increased excitability of a nerve or muscle near the cathode.

Anelectrotonus is the state of diminished irritability of a nerve or muscle produced in the region of the anode during the passage of an electric current.

8.1   Kinds of Electric Current

Medical electricity has been practised in Europe from the start of the eighteenth century, where it was used for a wide variety of conditions from arthritis to paralysis. Since the discovery that electricity stimulates irritable tissues, particularly nerve and muscle, it has been used clinically as both a diagnostic and therapeutic agent. The physiological and therapeutic effects of electric currents are due to the chemical and physical changes produced in the tissues.

Low frequency currents are those currents in which the direction of electron flow changes periodically with a frequency which varies from 1 Hz to 2000 Hz. At this low frequency, the current can stimulate both sensory and motor nerves, and meets a skin resistance of at least 3200 ohms when the frequency is 50 Hz. *High frequency currents are those of 500 000 Hz and above.* At this frequency they are termed *oscillations*, and have no effect on sensory or motor nerves.

Alternating currents. These currents are also known as *sinusoidal currents.*

In an alternating current the direction of electron flow periodically changes in a rhythmic manner, and at a specific frequency or cycles per second. One cycle (1 Hz) represents a complete sequence of change in amplitude at each polarity. The frequency of sinusoidal current used medically is 50 Hz. When an alternating current flows in a conductor, the total number of electrons that move in one direction equals the total number that move in the reverse direction. Thus ions in a solution energised by the alternating current will migrate to and fro between the electrodes, and no net ion transfer will occur.

Surged alternating currents have the magnitude of the intensity of each pulse gradually increased or decreased. The pulse is the sine wave on each polarity. The length of the surges can be varied from 1 s to 10 s. The cycling of the intensity is graded from zero to the desired maximum.

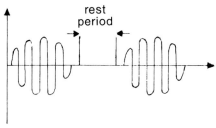

There are two types of surged alternating current used in medical electricity.

Faradism is an uneven alternating current with a frequency of 50 Hz and a pulse duration of 1 ms. *Pulse duration* is the time taken for the pulse wave to reach its peak and then subside to the baseline.

Surged sinusoidal current is an even alternating current with a frequency of 50 Hz and a pulse duration of 10 ms.

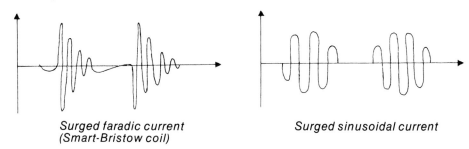

Surged faradic current
(Smart-Bristow coil)   *Surged sinusoidal current*

Interrupted direct currents flow in the same direction intermittently, with the strength of the current reducing to zero between each period of flow. In modern electronic machines the AC from the mains is decreased in voltage and converted into a direct current which is then interrupted and smoothed by an appropriate choice of resistors and capacitors, to give the desired triangular, saw-tooth, or square wave pulse forms.

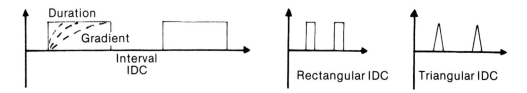

A *pulsed current* is a series of DC impulses with a repetition rate. It is similar to interrupted DC. The pulse durations are from 0.02 ms to 2000 ms and the frequency varies from 1000 Hz to 5 Hz.

A pulse duration of 1 ms has a frequency of 50 or 70 Hz.

A pulse duration of 10 ms has a frequency of 50 Hz.

A pulse duration of 100 ms has a frequency of 1.5 Hz.

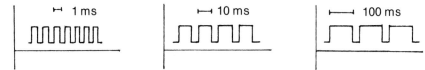

Surged interrupted direct current has the peak intensity increase and decrease brought about gradually. In treatment with AC or interrupted DC, there is no fixed current intensity. Often the intensity is cyclically reduced to zero, and such currents are described as being *modulated*.

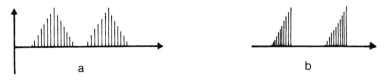

Surged IDC

Depolarised interrupted direct current — the interrupted DC has a definite positive polarity, but when using long duration pulses it is desirable to have depolarised impulses. A current of low intensity flows in the reverse direction during the interval between the impulses in order to reduce the chemical effect that may occur.

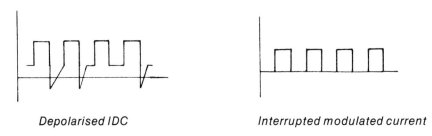

Depolarised IDC   *Interrupted modulated current*

Interrupted modulated — here the intensity is cyclically reduced to zero at regular intervals.

8.2   Physiology of Muscle Fibre and Neurons

The neuron can be seen from a functional point of view as an integrator, conductor, and a transmitter of coded information. It has three basic functions:

(*a*)   a specialised ability to react to stimuli;

(*b*) an immediate and rapid transmission of excitatory stimuli to other parts of the cell;

(*c*) the influencing of other neurons, muscle cells and glandular cells.

The neuron consists of a cell body and processes that are termed *axons* and *dendrites*.

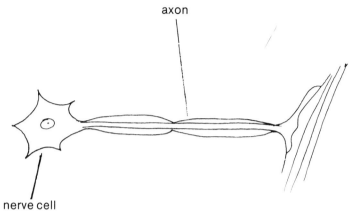

axon

nerve cell

The neuron

A neuromuscular synapse is the contact portion between an axonal twig and a muscle fibre. As the motor axon approaches the muscle fibre, it loses its myelin sheath and divides into several small branches. The branches lie in shallow grooves on the surface of the muscle fibre. The region of the muscle fibre under these twigs is termed the *motor end plate*. It includes the sarcolemma, a raised area containing *sarcoplasm*, and the *sole plate*. The membrane of axon terminal is separated from the sarcolemma by a distinct gap termed the *synaptic clefts*. The motor end plate possesses highly specialised functional features which enable the impulse in the nerve fibre to be translated into an impulse in the muscle fibre,

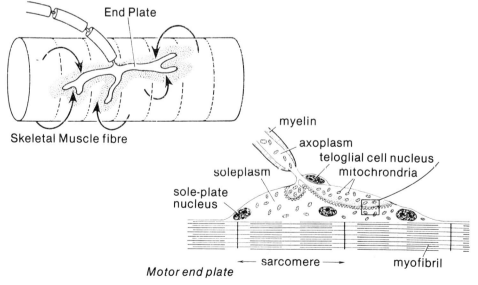

End Plate

Skeletal Muscle fibre

myelin

axoplasm

teloglial cell nucleus

mitochrondria

soleplasm

sole-plate nucleus

←— sarcomere —→   myofibril

Motor end plate

through the action of a chemical link, *acetylcholine*, in the presence of calcium ions. Only the motor end plate of the muscle is sensitive to acetylcholine, the rest of the muscle membrane being insensitive. The contraction of a muscle fibre results from the excitation and propagation of the nerve impulse through the neuron and its termination in the muscle membrane via the motor end plate.

The peripheral nerve consists of an *axon*, a *myelin sheath with neurolemma cells and connective tissues*. A varying number of nerve fibres form a peripheral nerve. Generally all nerve fibres over 2 μm in diameter are *myelinated*. Some nerve fibres are non-myelinated. The myelin sheath consists of fine concentric lamellas of protein and lipid, which are interrupted at regular intervals by the *nodes of Ranvier* and are derived from *Schwann cells* which lie in the neurolemma. The *neurolemma sheath* surrounds the nerve fibre.

The mixed peripheral nerves consist of myelinated and non-myelinated nerve fibres, enclosed in a sheath of connective tissues or *endoneurium*. Within the nerve trunk, the fibres are collected into bundles bound by a condensation of connective tissue, termed the *perineurium*, and finally a thick coat of connective tissue surrounds the whole nerve trunk and is termed the *epineurium*.

The functions of the connective tissue are:
(a)   support of the nerve fibres;
(b)   nutrition through the network of blood vessels which lies in the connective tissue;
(c)   the conductive activity of the nerve fibre through its electrolytes.

The functions of the axon are to act as a communication pathway between the spinal cord and muscle. The nature of the axoplasmic transport provides both a slow signalling system, which enables messages coded in the form of chemicals to be sent in both directions between the neuron and the muscle fibre it innervates, and a rapid signalling to the periphery when required.

The conduction of an impulse in a myelinated nerve is saltatory, in that the nerve impulse skips along the nerve fibre from one node of Ranvier to the next. The active generation of current occurs at the node of Ranvier and the myelin sheath acts as an insulator with considerable electrical resistance. Higher speeds of conduction are obtained when the nodes of Ranvier are further apart.

Types of nerve fibres. The nervous system responds promptly to all kinds of stimuli. The nerve fibres have different rates of transmitting the impulse depending on the diameter of the nerve fibre and other factors. There are three main types of fibres:

A fibres: Large, myelinated, fast conducting, motor and sensory nerve fibres. Group A fibres are divided into alpha α, beta β, gamma γ, and delta ∂ neurons.

B fibres: Smaller and slower conducting myelinated, efferent, pre-ganglionic fibres of the autonomic nervous system.

C fibres: Unmyelinated post-ganglionic fibres of the sympathetic nervous system. Unmyelinated or poorly myelinated afferent fibres of the peripheral nerves. Group C fibres are small and slow conducting.

Classification of the functional characteristics of nerve fibres according to Erlanger and Gasser

TYPE OF FIBRE	FUNCTION	DIAMETER μm	SPEED OF CONDUCTION m.s^{-1}
GROUP A (myelinated) alpha α	efferent to motor end plates	12–22	70–125
beta β	afferent to Meissner's corpuscles; Pacinian corpuscles; Golgi neurotendinous endings, monitoring fast touch-pressure, joint position and movement sense, and secondary stretch to spindle	5–12	30–70
gamma γ	efferent to intrafusal fibre in spindle		
delta ∂	afferent monitoring quick pain, temperature and light touch	2.5	12–30
GROUP B (myelinated)	pre-ganglionic autonomic efferent	less than 3	3–15
GROUP C (non-myelinated)	post-ganglionic sympathetic	0.3–1.3	0.5–2.3
	afferent fibre of peripheral nerves and dorsal roots; free nerve endings	0.4–1.2	0.5–2.0

The motor unit is the functional unit of centrally controlled muscle function and it consists of (1) an anterior horn cell, (2) a neuron, and (3) a number of muscle fibres innervated by that neuron. A skeletal muscle with its motor nerve will consist of a variable number of motor units depending upon its functions.

The number of muscle fibres served by one axon varies from 108 (first lumbrical) to 1934 (medial head of gastrocnemius). The fibres of the motor unit are arranged randomly in the muscle. The motor units differ from each other, depending on the size, and biochemical and physiological properties of the muscle fibres.

There are thought to be three types of muscle fibres in man, with varying muscle-twitch speeds. There are histochemical differences between these muscle

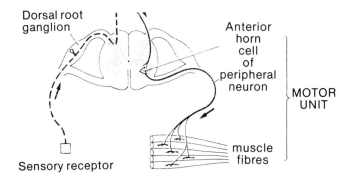

fibres. The myosin-ATPase activities of the fibres and the aerobic and anaerobic metabolism contribute to the classification, shown in the following table.

Classification by Peter and others 1972

GENERAL FEATURES	FAST TWITCH OXIDATIVE GLYCOLYTIC	FAST TWITCH GLYCOLYTIC	SLOW TWITCH OXIDATIVE
red coloration	dark	pale	dark
myoglobin	high	low	high
capillary network	rich	poor	rich
mitochondria	many large	few	small
Z line	wide	narrow	intermediate
fatigue	resistant	sensitive	very resistant

Many muscles contain both types of motor units, though muscles such as soleus have a predominance of red fibres with a slow twitch. It has also been found that it is possible for one type to convert to another, for example after tenotomy or joint immobilisation and disuse an alteration is seen which brings to the fore the importance of the trophic influence of the motor neuron activity.

Since motor units exhibit striking differences in terms of size, speed of contraction and biochemistry, the recruitment of motor units during voluntary electrical, or reflex contractions will depend upon the task demanded of them and the structure of the muscle fibre.

ELECTROPHYSIOLOGY

Therapeutic and diagnostic techniques using low frequency currents are dependent upon the electrical activity of the motor unit. The three main electrical properties of nerve and muscle are *electrical excitability, refractory period*, and *accommodation*.

Nature of stimulus. Any change in the environment of an irritable tissue may be regarded as a stimulus. Because electrical currents are highly effective in stimulating muscle and nerve, and they can be graded finely and measured accurately, they are more suitable than other stimuli in producing contraction of muscles directly or by way of nerves for diagnostic or therapeutic purposes.

Electrical excitability. In looking at the electrical basis of the function of neurons, it must be remembered that muscles and nerves can be excited by different kinds of stimuli, and the response of a motor neuron to a stimulus can be measured, either by the strength of contraction of the muscle fibres it supplies or by the conduction process along the nerve fibre expressed by its *action potential*.

The stimulus for a muscle contraction evokes the large anterior horn cells in the spinal cord and brain stem to send nerve impulses (action potentials) through the axons and motor end plates to the muscle membrane, and then excite it to contract. Before it can be excited to conduct an impulse, a nerve cell has to have a potential difference of 50 to 100 millivolts between the inside and outside of the cell. In the resting state a neuron is a charged cell not conducting a nerve impulse. The cell membrane acts as a boundary between the interstitial fluid outside and the intracellular fluid inside. Outside there is a high concentration of sodium and calcium ions.

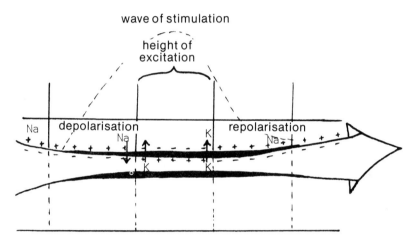

In the intracellular fluid, potassium and protein are kept in higher concentrations. The concentration differential between sodium and potassium ions is produced and maintained by the metabolic activity of the neuron. Sodium is pumped out of the cell, and the potassium is pumped into it. Calcium ions contribute to maintaining the physiological state of the plasma membrane. The plasma membrane is more permeable to potassium than sodium, but at equilibrium the inside of the resting cell reaches an electrical negative potential relative to the interstitial fluid.

The resting membrane potential is generally between 70 and 100 millivolts. Excitation of a nerve cell causes the affected area of the cell membrane to become momentarily permeable to sodium ions. A rapid influx of sodium ions reverses the polarity of the cell and the interior changes to a critical threshold of 25 to 50 mV for about 1 ms. The sodium pump then restores the resting situation.

The change of membrane potential is the action potential. The threshold stimulus to trigger off the action potential must be over 12 mV depolarisation. These electrical changes increase the permeability of neighboring regions to sodium ions so that action potentials are propagated throughout the nerve cell.

Action potential. If a nerve is stimulated by electrical means, a conducted impulse occurs, and a characteristic series of potential changes is observed as the impulse passes from the exterior electrode.

(*a*) First there is a brief irregular deflection of the baseline stimulus artifact due to current leakage.

(*b*) The stimulus artifact is followed by an isopotential interval of a latent period, which ends with the next potential change, and corresponds to the time it takes the impulse to travel along the axon from the site of stimulation to the other electrode.

(*c*) The first manifestation of the approaching impulse is a beginning of the depolarisation of the membrane. After an initial 10 mV depolarisation, the rate of depolarisation increases. The lowest voltage at which a single nerve fibre will fire is called the *minimal stimulus*, which is about 0.8 mV. The point at which there is a change of the rate of depolarisation is called the *firing level*. There is now a voltage difference of 30 mV. It then reverses and falls rapidly towards the resting level. When repolarisation is about two-thirds completed, the rate of repolarisation decreases and resting level is approached more slowly. The sharp rise and fall of the impulse and the slow return is a sequence of potential changes called the *action potential*.

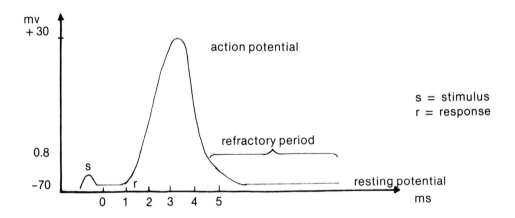

The conduction of the excitation is propagated at a velocity of 25 to 100 m.s^{-1} depending on the nerve fibre. Each stimulated nerve needs a short period of recovery before it can be excited again. This *refractory period* is necessary to re-establish the resting potential. The conduction of excitation is generally a biological process, with chemical changes (molecular changes), thermic effects and accompanying electrical (action potential) phenomena.

Neuromuscular transmission. Let us look at the synaptic events that enable excitation to spread from the motor neuron to the muscle fibre. When the impulse invades the motor end plate, it depolarises the axon membrane in the usual way, but of greater importance is the entry of calcium ions from the extracellular fluid.

It has been shown that neuromuscular transmission will cease if calcium ions are absent. The presence of the calcium ions is necessary for the release of the transmitter substance *acetylcholine* (ACh), which is contained in the synaptic vesicles. Once the acetylcholine is discharged it diffuses to combine with receptors in the muscle membrane. The fall in muscle membrane potential is called *the end plate potential*. The end plate potential arises from an increase in the permeability of the membrane to sodium and potassium. When the critical excitory potential has been exceeded, an action potential takes place and the impulse is propagated in both directions along the fibre. The transmission is concluded by the hydrolysis of acetylcholine into choline and acetate by the enzyme *cholinesterase*.

Steps in neuromuscular transmission

axon terminal	action potential ◄──────────── synthesis of ACh
	calcium entry
	release of ACh
cleft	diffusion of ACh ──────► hydrolysis of ACh
muscle membrane	increased permeability to Na⁺ and K⁺
	depolarisation (end plate potential)
	action potential

Electrical characteristics of skeletal muscle. The electrical events which occur in muscle are the same as in nerve with quantitative differences in timing and magnitude. The resting membrane potential of skeletal muscle is –90 mV. The action potential lasts 2 to 4 ms and is conducted along the muscle fibre at about 5 $m.s^{-1}$. The absolute refractory period is 1 to 3 ms and the repolarisation with its related changes is slower.

Contracticle responses — The muscle twitch
A single action potential causes a brief contraction followed by relaxation. This is called a muscle twitch. 'Fast' muscles concerned with fine movements have twitch durations as short as 7.5 ms. 'Slow' muscles involved with gross movements have a twitch of up to 100 ms duration.

Summation — Tetanus
When a single maximal stimulus is delivered to a motor nerve or directly to a muscle, all the fibres of the muscle are activated and the maximum twitch is

developed. If repeated stimuli are given before relaxation has occurred, additional activation of the contractile elements is produced and a *response of a tetanic contraction is added to the contraction already present*. This is known as summation of contractions, or tetanus. The tension developed in a tetanic contraction is 4 times that obtained in a single muscle twitch.

A rate of 350 stimuli per second is necessary to produce a complete tetanus in the internal rectus of the eye, while a rate of 30 per second is enough for the slow soleus muscle, and about 100 stimuli per second for a fast limb muscle.

Electrical excitability of nerve and muscle. The electrical excitability of nerve and muscle membrane is variable, and is governed by the following three factors:

  intensity of current;
  duration of current flow;
  speed at which the current reaches peak intensity.

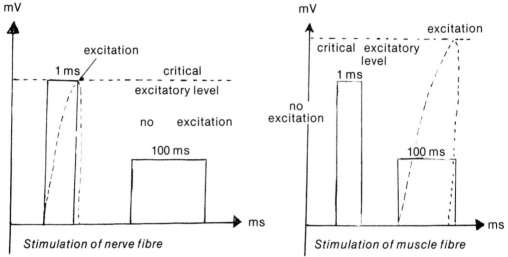

Nerve fibre. Stimulation of a nerve fibre with *short duration pulses from 0.02 ms to 1 ms* interrupted pulsed current will immediately reach the critical excitatory level, cause depolarisation, generate an action potential, and induce a muscle contraction. If *longer pulse duration of 100 to 1000 ms* is used, the intensity of current required to produce a muscle contraction is decreased. It is generally close to that required by a 1 ms pulse duration. More current is needed when the pulse durations are less than 0.1 ms as the duration of current is very brief. More current is needed for 100 ms pulse durations if the shape of the pulse is saw-tooth or triangular.

Muscle fibre. Stimulation of a muscle fibre with a short duration pulsed current from 0.02 to 1 ms will not cause excitation and muscle contraction unless given at very high intensities. If a bipolar technique is used when the muscle is stimulated at both ends of its muscle belly, then less current will be needed. If a longer duration pulse from 100 to 1000 ms is used, less current will be required to produce a muscle contraction. *The longer time provided offsets the need for higher intensities*, and so muscle contraction occurs with intensities less than that required by a short pulse duration.

Polarity. If a nerve fibre is stimulated directly by the *cathode*, the surface of the membrane nearer to the cathode becomes more negative in relation to the opposite side, and the surface nearer the anode becomes more positive. As the outer surface of the resting membrane potential is positive, the side nearer to the cathode reduces the potential difference more rapidly, causes depolarisation and initiates a nerve impulse and muscle contraction. If the anode is placed nearest to the nerve fibre it will still initiate a muscle contraction by activating the nerve membrane from the further surface, but it would not be as effective as the cathode in stimulating the nerve fibre.

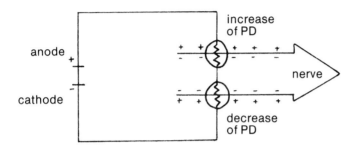

Electrical stimulation of a nerve fibre

Accommodation. The power of accommodation is the property of nerve or muscle tissue to adapt itself to slowly increasing stimulation intensities. If long duration pulses from 100 to 2000 ms are used to excite a nerve or muscle fibre, there is a decrease in excitability of the membrane. As the current slowly passes through the tissue, the level of excitation is raised and a longer time is needed to trigger off the *critical excitatory level*. This change in critical excitatory level is called *accommodation*.

Nerve fibre has a high accommodation rate, and long duration pulses do not readily excite a nerve. A slow-rising triangular, saw-tooth or trapezoidal pulse causes more accommodation and higher intensities will be needed to excite the nerve membrane.

In a rectangular pulse the current is turned on abruptly, maintained constant for the duration of the stimulus and turned off abruptly.

In exponential progressive impulses with triangular, saw-tooth or trapezoidal shapes, the peak intensity is reached slowly and reduced slowly or abruptly.

Muscle has a much lower accommodation rate.

The refractory period of a nerve or muscle fibre is the length of time following an impulse during which there is a depression of membrane excitability. At first for a period of 2.2 to 4.6 ms, and for large axons 0.5 ms, there is an *absolute refractory period* where all sodium channels are closed and no impulse can pass through. This is followed by a *relative refractory period* where the fibre can fire an action potential provided the stimulus is greater than the initial threshold value. Full recovery normally takes 10 to 15 ms.

8.3   Sinusoidal Currents

PHYSICS

A sinusoidal current is an evenly alternating low frequency current. The sinusoidal currents used for therapeutic purposes have a frequency of 50 Hz and a pulse duration of 10 ms providing 100 stimuli per second. The graph of the current is seen in the following diagram. It is a sine curve. Sinusoidal currents may be used as surged or unsurged currents. The surges can be regulated from 6 to 30 surges per minute. The rate of surging varies with different generators.

The sinusoidal currents produced in low voltage generators are usually sine wave alternating currents produced by multivibrator circuits. The sine wave-shaped output generally has a peak of 80 volts. The pulse duration is 10 ms and the frequency is 50 Hz. This means that the current stays in the tissues for a period of 10 ms. The meter will register the intensity of the peak voltage in the sine position. The maximum reading on the meter in the sine position will vary with different apparatus.

In treatment it is important to reduce currents cyclically to zero. When the *peak current intensity* is increased and decreased gradually, this type of modulation is called 'surging'. If it is necessary to stimulate muscle, then a surged sinusoidal current applied over the nerve to a muscle will produce a muscle contraction. The generators have a dial which will continuously adjust the surge to the required rate, for example 6 to 30 per minute, or a 1 to 2 second surge.

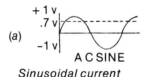

(a)   A C SINE
Sinusoidal current

(b)
Surged sinusoidal current

PHYSIOLOGICAL EFFECTS

When an electric current is passed through the body, a change of concentration of ions occurs at the cell membranes. The change in ionic concentration is the actual cause of stimulation of the tissue. If it occurs at the nerve membrane, muscle contraction occurs. If it occurs in other tissues of the body, then there is ionic movement of tissue fluid and other constituents. In the case of the alternating current, we must remember that each individual half wave negates the electrolytic effect of the previous half wave, having an opposite direction of current flow. For this reason, any stimulating effect is achieved at the peak intensity of the wave, if the intensity is high enough to reach the threshold value to cause depolarisation and stimulation.

It is not possible to cause a burn with an alternating current, unless high intensities are given for a long time, or if the bare metal is in close contact with the skin for a long period of time. In medical sinusoidal currents, the pulse duration is 10 ms, long enough to cause irritation of the sensory nerves.

Effect on motor and sensory nerves. The short pulse duration of 10 ms and the frequency of 50 Hz is adequate to stimulate nerve. If the sinusoidal current is positioned on the motor nerves of the muscle, over the motor points and surged, then a muscle contraction and relaxation will be produced. It will also irritate the sensory nerves and cause a prickling sensation which is not very comfortable. Nevertheless there will be muscle contraction, with superficial cutaneous vasodilatation due to the irritation of the sensory nerves occurring simultaneously. The surged sinusoidal is a tetanic current.

Effects on the tissues of the body. If there is any swelling or inflammatory exudate, an unsurged sinusoidal current will help absorption of the exudate by channelling the excessive fluid to the lymphatic and venous channels.

Stimulation of the sensory nerve will cause superficial vasodilatation by the axon reflex and, if continued for a longer period, there will be some capillary vasodilatation from the release of histamine-like metabolites. The hyperaemia lasts for at least half an hour after the treatment has ended.

INDICATIONS

Pain. The use of unsurged sinusoidal current is sometimes tried to relieve pain and tenderness. Wall and Sweet's investigations on pain have shown the effect of electrical stimulation of large diameter nerve fibres originating from a painful region. The stimulation interferes with the perception of pain. The effect of 10 minutes of stimulation lasts for at least half an hour.

There is also clinical evidence that unpleasant painful sensations are associated with loss of conduction in some of the efferent fibres. Cases such as causalgia from partial nerve lesions, post-herpetic syndrome, paroxysms of pain from amputation stumps are characteristic of cases where there are abnormal behavior patterns in the conduction of the efferent neuron. These patients usually have pain triggered of by mild stimuli, which last for varying periods. So for these particular patients the unsurged sinusoidal current would stimulate the large efferent fibres and inhibit pain at the spinal level through the pre-synaptic inhibitory mechanism.

Cases of referred pain and psychosomatic pain do not respond to sinusoidal current.

Pain and swelling. The accumulation of excessive exudate compressing the tissues and causing pain can be helped sometimes by sinusoidal current. Stimulation of the muscles over the painful area, with the limb in elevation, can be effective. Not only is the circulatory muscle pump acting, but superficial vasodilatation will help in the removal of waste products. If the patient is given 10 minutes of un-surged sinusoidal, and this is then followed by surged sinusoidal current, alteration of the semi-permeability of the cell membrane, allowing diffusion of ions, will also help in the absorption of the exudate. It is not a comfortable treatment, and patients must be able to tolerate the discomfort.

CONTRA-INDICATIONS

Skin lesions. In order to prevent a burn, large cuts and abrasions, or open areas which cannot be insulated with vaseline, must not come into the pathway of the current. Dermatological conditions such as eczema, psoriasis, acne, dermatitis, and other such conditions are exacerbated by electrical currents.

Infection can be aggravated by electric currents and it is also possible to spread the infection.

Impaired sensation. The sensation of the part being treated must be checked. If there is complete loss of sensation, it could be dangerous if long periods of current with too high an intensity were given. The density of current in the part is governed by the patient's subjective feeling of current tolerance.

LOW FREQUENCY GENERATORS OFFERING SINUSOIDAL CURRENTS

Essential features

An *output selector* which clearly indicates a sine wave. Generally these machines do not require a selection of pulse duration and frequency.

An *output meter* which is switched automatically to the sine wave selected, and reads the peak voltage on the sine position being delivered to the patient.

Some machines do not have an adequate output for therapeutic use. For example, although the Faradic-Galvanic unit is labelled as producing up to 120 volts sinusoidal current, it rarely produces more than 80 volts.

A *surge control dial* which is continuously adjustable to the required speed. Some generators have 8 different surge rates, that is a frequency between 6 and 30 surges per minute (such as the Neurotron), while others have a dial which is continuously adjustable from a 1 second surge to a 5 second surge (such as the galvanic faradic unit).

A mains ON/OFF control switch

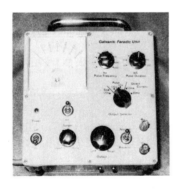
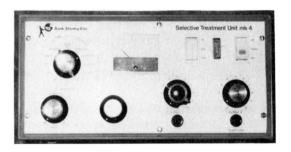

The galvanic-faradic unit   the selective treatment unit

TECHNIQUE OF APPLICATION OF UNSURGED SINUSOIDAL CURRENT

Equipment required

electronic stimulator

two metal electrodes

pad and plastic to cover the active electrode; the pad should be of absorbent material, 10 mm thick when compressed

two leads
a bandage
soap
cotton wool
towels
a small basin with warm water
a bath filled with warm water
vaseline
wooden spatula

Position the patient comfortably with the limb supported on a pillow covered with plastic and a towel. Cover a stool with plastic for the bath.

Explain to the patient the purpose of the treatment (counter-irritant effect).

Skin test the patient for pain sensation.

Select the settings on the machine for a sinusoidal current with a pulse duration of 10 ms and a frequency of 50 Hz. Generally the selector switch shows this specific current, and no other frequency or pulse duration dials need be adjusted.

Connect the leads firmly to the metal electrodes and the machine terminals.

Place the active electrode on the folded pad which should be 10 mm thick when compressed. *The pad should be moistened evenly, with all excessive water wrung out.*

Test the machine on yourself. Put your elbow into the bath and hold the moist active pad and electrode in your hand. Watch the meter to see that it goes up and down smoothly.

Explain to the patient the sensation that you are feeling and that he will experience.

Examine the area of skin under both active and indifferent electrodes for any cuts or abrasions and if present insulate with vaseline using a spatula.

Wash the skin and leave wet, but ensure that the water is not dripping all over the part.

Bandage the active electrode firmly into position, with the electrode in the middle of the pad.

Place the foot in the bath with the indifferent electrode.

Turn the current up slowly until the patient experiences an intense stinging sensation under the active electrode (you must increase the intensity up to the patient's pain limit).

The response decreases after 20 to 30 seconds when the intensity should be again increased to obtain a similar stinging. Continue this sequence.

After 4 minutes' treatment, assess the result.

If the stinging has been adequate, there is immediate marked numbness to touch and pressure, and all pain is lost in the treated area. Immediate or partial improvement with numbing is required for successful results, so the first treatment is a useful guide. If no numbness, or only partial numbness is present, repeat for another 4 minutes. The erythema and numbness persist for about 1 hour.

If the patient complains of any uncomfortable feeling in the leg at the water line, use a spatula to apply vaseline around this area.

DOSAGE

Daily treatments for 4 to 6 days may be given, although few patients require more than 4 treatments. If there is no improvement with 3 treatments, discontinue.

DANGERS

Burns may be caused by:

(*a*)   overdosage by too great an intensity for a long period of time;

(*b*)   bare metal electrode on the skin, due to loose bandaging of the electrode and pad, when high intensities are given;

(*c*)   metal in the path of the current.

Shock. The current should be increased slowly. If increased or decreased too quickly, the patient gets a mild shock which is uncomfortable.

Switching on a machine set at a high output may cause a shock.

A dry scaly skin will suddenly conduct when the moisture has seeped through after a few minutes of soaking, causing a shock.

Pain. Overdosage could cause intense discomfort and pain to the patient.

Small raised edges or tiny cuts missed out on observation cause a burning type of pain as current tends to collect at these points.

8.4   Faradic Currents

One of the first muscle stimulating currents to be used in medicine was the faradic current, an uneven alternating current with a pulse duration of 1 ms, frequency of 50 Hz followed by damped oscillation of 1000 Hz. The current was also hand surged. The apparatus used to produce this current was the *faradic or induction coil*.

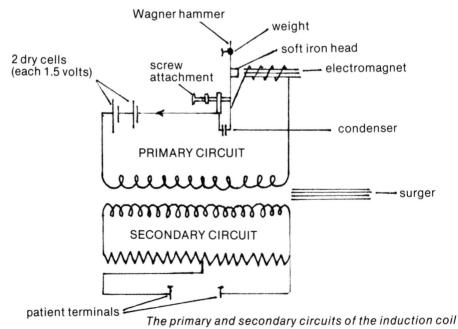

The primary and secondary circuits of the induction coil

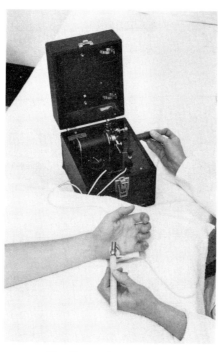

The Smart-Bristow Coil

The current is surged by an iron core which slides in and out of the primary coil. The gradual increase and decrease of peak intensity is called a *surging current*.

The peak current at 1 ms pulse duration stimulates the nerve fibre to produce a muscle contraction. The current is comfortable, and has the advantage of being hand surged, thus enabling the physiotherapist to control the strength and duration of the contraction.

Today the induction coil is an obsolete instrument, and few departments own a machine. Yet it is the most comfortable faradic current available. The word *faradism* is associated with the current produced by the induction coil — an uneven alternating current. It is a word used loosely by many physiotherapists to cover all faradic-type currents.

PHYSICS

The current produced is an uneven alternating current with a spike wave form generated by a battery voltage source by means of an induction coil. The spike wave has a 1 ms pulse duration, and with sufficient current intensity produces a contraction of muscle. The control of peak intensity by surging the current produces a near normal tetanic-like contraction and relaxation of muscle. Output wave form, frequency and intensity are unstable in the faradic coil and will vary with contact spring tension, output current and battery strength. *There is no polarity to be considered with the alternating current produced by the induction coil.*

PHYSIOLOGICAL EFFECTS

The physiological effects and uses of the original faradic current — the so-called term 'faradism' — are the same as those produced by the faradic-type currents or the short duration interrupted direct current, and will be considered in the following section.

8.5   Faradic-Type Currents

A faradic-type current is a short duration interrupted direct current with a pulse duration of 0.02 to 1 ms and a frequency of 50 to 70 Hz. The current is also surged at a variable controlled speed, ranging from 4 to 30 surges per minute with varying rest periods, thus showing modulations of pulsed or interrupted direct currents. The faradic-type currents and the original faradism are muscle stimulating currents acting directly on nerve fibres. These currents are normally used therapeutically for stimulating muscles with an intact nerve supply.

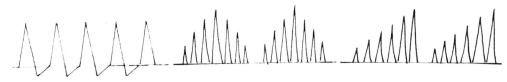

Faradic-type current   *Surged faradic-type currents*

PHYSICS

Faradic-type currents are short duration interrupted direct currents ranging from a 0.02 ms to a 1 ms pulse duration. They are unidirectional currents basically with a depolarised impulse, obtained by including a capacitor and resistor in the output of the circuit. Some machines have only a definite positive polarity and are not depolarised. The effect of stimulation is the same whether the current is depolarised or not, as the pulse durations are too brief to have any chemical action on the skin, unless they are used for excessively long periods, with a dry skin.

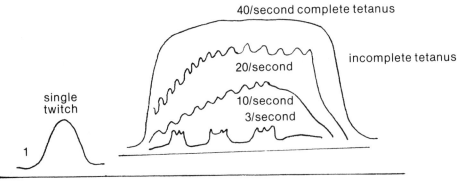

Summation and tetanus

All faradic-type currents must be surged to produce a near normal tetanic-like contraction and relaxation of muscle. In normal muscle contraction there is a series of rapidly repeated stimuli (a tetanus) to the muscle fibre, so that the effects of successive active states can add together.

Contraction time is the time elapsing from the start of contraction to the moment of peak intensity in an isometric contraction (McComas and Thomas, 1968).

In different apparatus varying surge speeds are available. Surges can be adjusted continuously from a 2 second surge to a 5 second surge, or, as in a Siemens' Neurotron 626, can be selected by a regulator selecting frequencies from 6 to 30 surges per minute.

Pause durations. Some machines have a dial for selection of pauses. As a rule the pause duration should be at least 2 to 3 times as long as that of the pulse to give the muscle sufficient time to recover. In the Siemens' Neurotron machines, an automatic blocking system prevents the patient current from being switched on if the pause in relation to the pulse duration is too short. This is indicated by a red pilot light.

Frequency. Some machines have controls for frequency selection. The selection range is 0.5, 1.5, 10, 50, 75, 100, 500 and 1000 pulses per second. Other machines have the frequency adjusted automatically when the faradic-type current is selected.

Pulse durations. In stimulating a normally innervated muscle, the choice should be made from pulse durations of 0.02, 0.05, 0.1, or 1 ms. Generally the most comfortable pulse is either 0.1 ms with a frequency of 70 Hz or 1 ms pulse with a frequency of 50 Hz. A rectangular shaped pulse is more comfortable than a triangular pulse, though if the muscle has disuse atrophy a triangular 1 ms pulse could be used to initiate a contraction. It is best to select a pulse duration which gives the most comfortable near-normal muscle contraction.

Faradic-type currents are always surged when used for therapeutic purposes.

Polarity. The active electrode should always be connected to the cathode, as a muscle contraction will be more easily produced with less current.

PHYSIOLOGICAL EFFECTS

The effects of electrical stimulation on normally innervated muscle tissue has been recognised for more than a century. The basis of the physiological effects of faradic-type currents is their ability to stimulate nerve by producing a change in the semi-permeability of the cell membrane, by altering the resting potential of the membrane, and when the cell membrane potential reaches the critical excitory level, the muscle supplied by the nerve is activated to contract. A single brief stimulus is associated with a single contraction.

In order to achieve a constant contraction, the stimuli must be applied at a rate of at least 30 stimuli per second to produce a tetanic-like contraction. A faradic muscle contraction is seen as a tetanic-like contraction of muscle. The number of motor units brought into action will depend on the strength of current and the placement of the electrodes. The electrodes are placed on the nerve trunk supplying the muscle and the motor point of the muscle. The cathode is connected to the electrode over the motor point.

The motor point is the region in a muscle where a great density of terminal motor end plates is found near the surface. It does not necessarily correspond with the entrance of the nerve into a muscle. At these motor points there is a zone of low threshold excitability, and the skin is very sensitive to electrical stimulation by faradic-type currents.

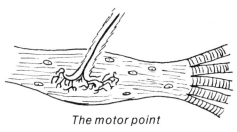

The motor point

Again it must be remembered that motor points are not the only sensitive areas in the skin, since there are several areas in the body where the motor nerves become so superficial that the application of current will produce depolarisation, an end plate potential change, and activate all muscles supplied distal to the point of stimulation. Stimulation of a motor point isolates the particular muscle or segment of a muscle, whereas stimulation of other superficial motor nerve fibres affects several muscles simultaneously.

All muscles have an exact location of the motor point in the muscle, which will vary slightly from patient to patient. It is generally situated in the middle of the longitudinal axis of the muscle. It is difficult to locate the motor points of deep muscles, and location is hampered if the skin is dry, scaly, or rough. Swelling will also mask the location of the area. Charts of the motor points are shown on the following pages.

Sensorimotor effects. By stimulating the motor nerves of a muscle, faradic-type currents can produce either an isometric or an isotonic contraction of a muscle or muscle groups without any volitional control. It is also possible to co-ordinate a volitional control with an electrical contraction of muscle. The strength of contraction, the duration of contraction and relaxation can be carefully monitored. Faradic stimulation of muscle can be used for the treatment of any clinical problem that can be solved by the use of isotonic or isometric con-tractions of muscles. It is pain-free, comfortable, and ensures a constancy in the selected strength of contraction at a specific duration of contraction and relaxation which cannot be guaranteed with voluntary contractions.

Thus one can produce a working hypertrophy of muscles, prevent atrophy, or re-activate a forgotten muscle action. *The stimulation of sensory nerves is minimal*, as the pulse duration is too brief to cause any sensory irritation. A mild prickling feeling is felt when the current first breaks down the skin resistance and, after a few minutes of treatment, a mild reddening may be seen under the active electrode.

Faradic-type currents will not stimulate denervated muscles. It is essential that there is an intact nerve supply to the muscle being treated. The intensity of current needed to depolarise muscle membrane, in the absence of nerves, with faradic-type currents is too great to be comfortably tolerated by the patient.

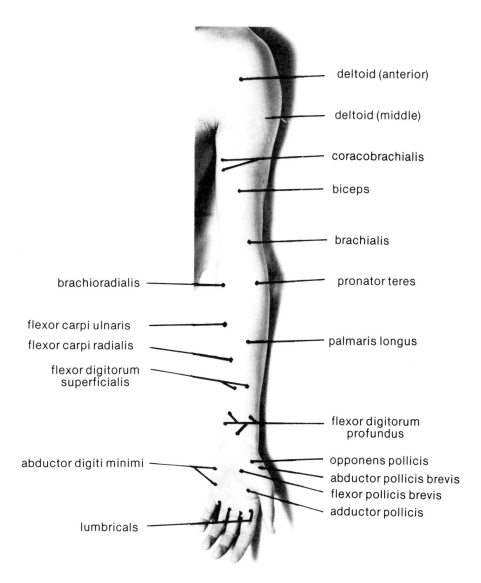

Motor points on the flexor aspect of the arm

Ionic movement of intracellular substances and extracellular tissue fluid. Since body tissue which is electrically permeated largely represents an electrolyte, it is possible that, when an electric current is passed at the interfaces of two electrolytes, such as tissue fluids and the protoplasm of biological entities — that is, at the cell membrane, a change in the concentration of ions will occur. The change in ionic movement will produce a stimulation of a muscle if it is applied on the nerve, but if the current is passed through any biological tissue there is bound to be some ionic movement.

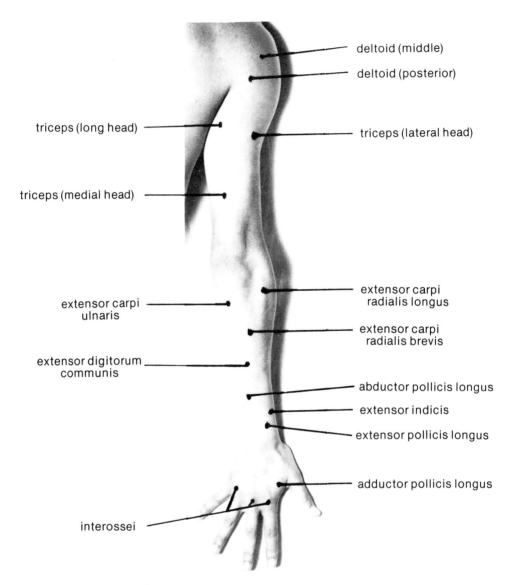

triceps (long head)

triceps (medial head)

extensor carpi ulnaris

extensor digitorum communis

interossei

deltoid (middle)

deltoid (posterior)

triceps (lateral head)

extensor carpi radialis longus

extensor carpi radialis brevis

abductor pollicis longus

extensor indicis

extensor pollicis longus

adductor pollicis longus

Motor points on the extensor aspect of the arm

When faradic-type currents are given over a large painful and swollen area, with no selection of motor nerves in the pathway of the current, it is possible to reduce the swelling and the pain. It is necessary to use as great an intensity of current as can be tolerated by the patient. It has been tried and proven successful for any chronic painful swelling which has not yielded to other measures. It is often termed 'through and through faradism'. The physiological basis for the reduction of swelling is the alteration in the permeability of the cell membrane by the faradic-type current, and thus the acceleration of fluid movement in the swollen tissues. It also causes arteriolar dilatation, which removes all metabolites and waste products.

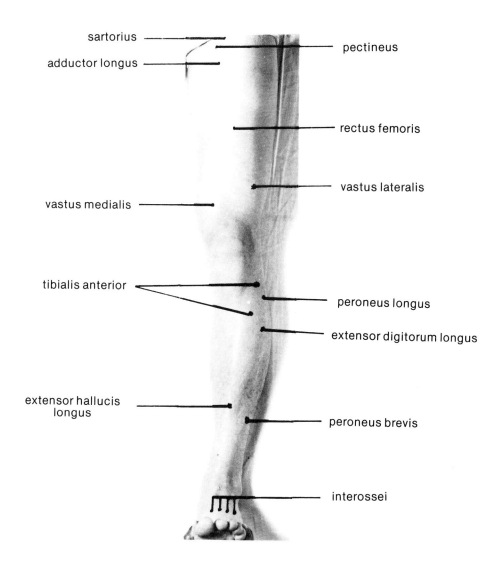

sartorius

adductor longus

pectineus

rectus femoris

vastus lateralis

vastus medialis

tibialis anterior

peroneus longus

extensor digitorum longus

extensor hallucis longus

peroneus brevis

interossei

Motor points on the anterior aspect of the leg

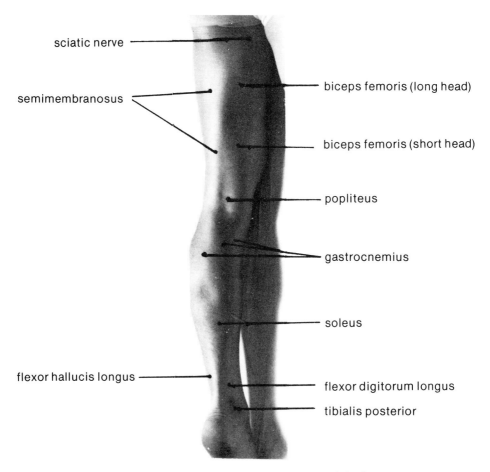

Motor points on the posterior aspect of the leg

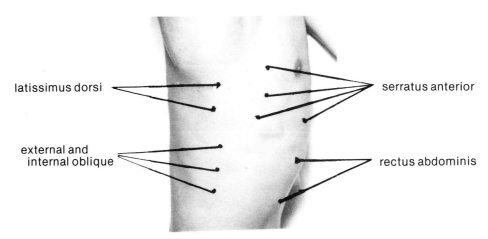

Motor points on the trunk

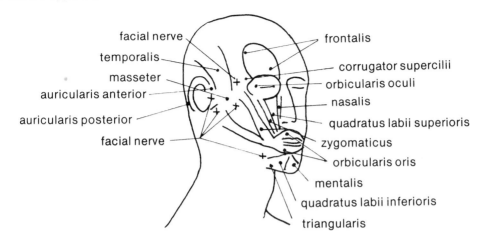

Motor points on the face

INDICATIONS

Facilitation of muscle contraction when inhibited by pain. Controlled muscle contraction results from a sequence of events involving at least 3 neurons: excitation of the small efferent fibres which merely cause contraction of the intrafusal fibres; stretching of the muscle spindle which sends information to the anterior horn neurons where recruitment of motor units is followed by the contraction of muscle; and from the internuncial neurons, there is inhibition of the anterior horn cells supplying the antagonistic groups. If this servo-mechanism works efficiently, there is no need to stimulate the muscles electrically. Various factors may produce imbalance:

(*a*) Pain and muscle spasm during exercise causes central inhibition and limits movement.

(*b*) Muscle wasting impairs afferent impulse production and makes restoration of muscle power a slow process.

(*c*) Over-activity of the antagonistic group results from a deficiency of afferent impulses from the wasted muscles, and a deficient inhibition of antagonistic muscles.

(*d*) Muscle imbalance may be due to disuse or faulty postural habits, as seen in the intrinsic foot muscles and the back muscles.

(*e*) Old age renders some patients too senile to follow instructions regarding active exercise and causes further muscle weakness as a complication of the lesion.

(*f*) Tenacious exudate following trauma may limit movement and obstruct circulation.

In 1962 Smilie demonstrated that knee joint injuries produced reflex inhibition of the quadriceps muscle. This results in a loss of tone, bulk and voluntary control.

Also the pain factor leads to decreased exercise tolerance which further exacerbates the problem. More atrophy occurs and the knee joint becomes susceptible to further injury.

Physiotherapists use many types of procedures in attempting to facilitate a motor response. They can use exteroceptive stimuli such as touch, cold, heat, and electricity, or use proprioceptive stimuli such as stretch, resistance, and vibration. Hypotonic muscles which do not readily respond to stretch present problems to those who attempt to facilitate a muscle contraction.

Normal 'muscle tone' is maintained by constant fusimotor activity which serves to keep spindle receptors sensitive to stretch. If fusimotor fibres are deprived of this stimulation by injury to central pathways, the internal stretch on the spindle is removed, the muscle becomes flaccid and does not resist external stretch. Any effort to increase the activity of fusimotor fibres in the weak muscle and thus increase muscle tone is termed 'biasing the spindles'. One can bias the spindles by a combination of touch over the skin of the affected muscle, an active contraction and resistance. This increases the fusimotor discharge to muscle as well as increased alpha neuron activity.

Physiotherapists over the years have used faradism to re-educate the quadriceps muscle when it is inhibited by pain, particularly in patients who have had knee surgery, such as the menisectomy operations. It is thought that the removal of the menisci could interfere with normal proprioceptive mechanisms. Today it is still used as an effective measure when techniques of voluntary activity have failed to produce an effective muscle contraction to stabilise the knee joint.

Inhibition of pain by faradism. Pain and muscle spasm can be inhibited by the use of faradism. Pain has an inhibitory effect on the large anterior horn cells, so that electrical stimulation of the afferent nerve fibres would reduce the inhibition and influence the alpha motor neuron pool, and facilitate transmission to the extrafusal fibres with inhibition of the antagonists, thus allowing a more natural sequence of movements.

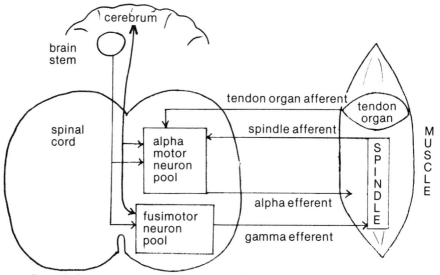

Some influences on motor neuron pools and muscle activity

The painful knee syndrome. Physiotherapists are often faced with the problem of a painful knee following trauma with inhibition of contraction in the quadriceps muscle. It appears that the inhibitory mechanism which leads to muscle wasting may cause loss of proprioceptive feedback so that the patient is unable to feel the quadriceps contracting properly.

The classical symptoms in patients with knee problems are:
atrophy of the quadriceps muscle with a noticeable different in the region of vastus medialis;
inability to extend the leg for the final 15°;
inability to flex the hip with the knee joint fully extended;
a flexed knee gait;
an unstable knee which gives way without warning.

According to Hallen and Lindhall (1967) *the extensor lag could be due to one or more of the following factors:*
mechanical disadvantage;
physiological disadvantage;
inhibition by pain;
contractures of the joint capsule;
adhesions between the quadriceps and the femur.

Current opinion today is that the whole quadriceps mechanism is important in obtaining a good contraction of the quadriceps muscle, particularly to control the last 15° of extension. The greater electrical activity recorded in the vastus medialis at the end of extension is due to working at its greatest mechanical and physiological disadvantage.

Criteria for the selection of faradic-type currents to produce a muscle contraction

(*a*) A muscle contraction that is inhibited by pain.
(*b*) The patient should not have any capsular contractures or adhesions in the muscles around the joint.
(*c*) There should be no gross effusion of the knee as it will cause difficulty in obtaining the motor points of the muscle.
(*d*) The presence of muscle atrophy and diminished muscle tone.

Some conditions successfully treated with faradism for the problem of inhibition of quadriceps contraction by pain include:
menisectomy;
chondromalacia patellae;
chronic effusion of the knee joint;
rheumatoid arthritis;
recurrent subluxation of the patella.

CONTRAINDICATIONS

Skin lesions. Any large open area which is in the direct pathway of the current, particularly under the electrodes, will cause intense discomfort and pain, as current tends to collect at that point or on raised areas. Small skin lesions can be insulated with vaseline.

Certain dermatological entities, such as eczema, tinea, ring-worm, psoriasis, fungus growths and similar conditions, should not be in the pathway of the current.

Low frequency currents tend to exacerbate the condition, and if it is infectious it will help to spread the infection further in the patient himself, or to other patients using the same apparatus. Particularly in hot humid climates, care must be taken to inspect the part.

Oedematous areas with a fine paper-like skin must be avoided to prevent breakdown.

Infections. An infection must not be treated with low frequency currents because of the danger of spreading the infection or exacerbating the condition.

Inflammation. Any acute inflammation with an underlying danger of infection or with thrombosis as a complication is a contra-indication.

Thrombosis. Patients with deep vein thrombosis or with atherosclerosis of the arterial vessels must not be treated with faradic-like currents because of the danger of causing an embolus.

Marked loss of skin sensation. If there is total loss of sensation in the limb being treated, a low frequency current must not be given for a long period of time. Even with short duration pulses a chemical burn is possible if the treatment is given for over 20 minutes with a high intensity.

Active tuberculosis or cancer in the area may be exacerbated.

Cardiac pacemakers. It is not advisable to apply a low frequency current in the region of the thorax or the pacemaker control unit (shoulder or abdomen), as it may interfere with the function of the pacemaker.

Thrombophlebitis. The dislodgement of a small thrombus may result.

Unreliable patients. Patients who cannot co-operate or understand the dangers of the treatment, for example, very old or very young patients.

Superficial metal. Metal in the pathway of the current will concentrate it and may cause a burn.

SELECTION OF APPARATUS FOR FARADIC-TYPE CURRENTS

Essential features of low voltage stimulators necessary for the selection of suitable faradic-type currents include:
(a) a range of *pulse durations* from 0.02 to 1 ms, or a standard faradic current with a 1 ms pulse duration and a frequency of 50 Hz;
(b) controls for *intensity/dose*; the controls should read zero at the OFF position;
(c) a *meter* for reading intensity; this is generally expressed in voltage unless it is a constant current circuitry where there is current control, as in the Siemens' Neurotron;
(d) optional *frequency and rest period control*; some machines have a frequency control which requires the therapist to select the correct frequency with the pulse duration; make sure that the rest between pulses is at least twice the pulse duration;

(*e*) there should be adequate continuous control of the speed of *surged currents*; there is generally a range of from 6 to 30 surges per minute;

(*f*) clearly marked *patient terminals* indicating both a *cathode and anode* pole; in the tetanic alternating currents, as in the Smart-Bristow coil, there is no need for polarity markings;

(*g*) a *polarity reversal switch* is incorporated in most electronic equipment, thus facilitating selection of polarity;

(*h*) a clearly marked Mains *ON/OFF switch*;

(*i*) the ability to select the *shape of the pulse* — rectangular, triangular, trapezoidal;

(*j*) a *safety mains plug* which must have an earth socket.

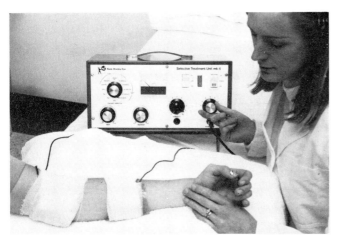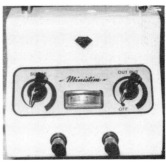

Examples of machines producing faradic-type currents

FARADISM FOR STIMULATION OF INNERVATED MUSCLES

Faradism can be used to obtain either a group action or the contraction of an individual muscle.

Equipment required
a Smart-Bristow coil (faradism) or a low frequency electronic stimulator
two leads
two suitably sized metal electrodes
two moist pad electrodes, 5 mm thickness compressed when using Smart-Bristow coil or 10 mm thickness compressed when using electronic stimulators
two pieces of plastic to cover the pads
a sandbag
a bandage
two small basins of warm water
towels
soap
insulating cream (petroleum jelly, vaseline, or lanolin)
spatula

Position the patient comfortably with a plastic sheet and towel under the limb. Support the muscle in the pain-free position with the area to be treated adequately exposed. The knee should be flexed slightly over a rolled up towel, and the ankle stabilised to prevent hyperextension if the quadriceps muscle is being treated.

Advise the patient as to:

(*a*) the rationale for treatment;

(*b*) the sensation to be experienced — when the current is turned on a prickling sensation is felt; as the intensity is increased the muscle will contract, and relax as intensity decreases.

Check that there are no contraindications to treatment.

Examine the area to be treated. Note any cuts, skin lesions and inflammation. Small cuts and abrasions need to be insulated with sterile vaseline. Inflammation impedes the penetration of the current. Large open areas and extensive inflammation may contraindicate treatment. Measure the girth of the muscle for wasting.

Test the ability of the muscle to contract fully isometrically. Note the patient's particular problems in doing so.

No skin test for sharp-blunt discrimination is necessary when using the Smart-Bristow coil as there are no chemical effects with the faradic current, but the test must be carried out when an electronic low frequency stimulator is used.

With soap and water wash the patient's skin where both the electrodes are to be placed to remove any grease. Rinse with clean water.

Place a warm, moist pad over these areas to decrease skin resistance.

Connect the leads *firmly* to the machine.

Check that all the controls on the machine are in the correct position.

Plug into the mains power supply and switch on, if applicable.

Select the settings for faradic-type current, if applicable.

Soak the pads in water.

Connect the leads firmly to the metal electrodes.

Cover the metal electrodes with the pads and test the application on yourself by placing the flexor surface of the forearm on one pad electrode and holding the other in the hand. Describe to the patient the sensation you feel and make sure the patient can see the muscle contraction produced.

Remove the hot soak and if there are any breaks in the patient's skin insulate these with a small amount of vaseline, using the spatula.

Moisten the skin where both the electrodes will be placed.

The group action is obtained by placing one electrode over the nerve trunk. Cover with plastic and hold in position with a sandbag or bandage on firmly. If this is not possible, this electrode can be placed over the nerve roots at the spine. The other electrode, also covered with plastic, is placed across the motor points and held in position by the therapist or bandaged on firmly. The principle is that, wherever possible, the impulse is passed via the nerve, therefore one electrode is positioned on a suitable superficial nerve trunk and the other electrode over the motor point.

Warn the patient

(*a*) that there should be no sustained intense prickling or burning sensation under the entire area of either electrode, or in one spot, when using an electronic stimulator;

(b)   not to touch any of the equipment, if power from the mains supply is being used.

(c)   not to move

(d)   that a mild, prickling sensation will be felt, increasing as the intensity increases, and accompanied by a muscle contraction.

The therapist should be seated facing the patient, and with the machine placed conveniently for manipulating the controls. Where the surge is controlled manually, the therapist's forearm should be supported with the shoulder relaxed.

Check that all the controls on the machine are in the correct position.

Give a few gentle contractions until the patient becomes accustomed to the current. Then increase the intensity gradually until he sees and feels quite a strong contraction. This gains the patient's confidence as he realises that the muscle will contract painlessly.

Keep repeating the electrical stimulation while instructing and encouraging the patient to contract voluntarily with the current. As he feels the current increasing in intensity, instruct him to tighten up his muscle and to relax the contraction as the current intensity decreases, until gradually he superimposes his voluntary contraction over the electrically-produced one.

The patient then progresses to contract the muscle strongly as the current intensity increases and to hold the muscle in its contracted position against the decreasing intensity of current. Allow a relaxation phase between each contraction.

Finally test if the patient can voluntarily initiate, hold and relax the contraction. Once this is achieved, discontinue the electrical stimulation. This is often achieved with just one or two treatments.

The entire emphasis of the treatment is on the active participation of the patient.

If it is necessary to stimulate muscles *individually*, for example the vastus medialis to overcome a quadriceps lag, place one metal electrode with a pad over the nerve as above. Using a suitably sized button electrode (large in this instance), covered with 5 mm thickness of absorbent material and secured with a rubber band, locate the motor point and give the necessary number of contractions.

At the conclusion of treatment, remove the electrodes, wash the skin thoroughly and check for any excessive erythema which could indicate a chemical burn.

FARADISM IN THE TREATMENT OF CHONDROMALACIA PATELLAE

Recently in Canada, and for a long time in the Soviet Union, the use of faradism for the treatment of chondromalacia patellae has been found effective, particularly to obtain hypertrophy of the weak muscle groups.

The patient is positioned with the knee flexed to 5° with a restraining strap placed over the ankle to prevent hyperextension of the knee joint. Patients are given 20 maximum tetanic contractions within the patient's pain threshold. Selection is made of a pulse which gives a 10 second contraction, with a 50 second rest period, at a frequency of 65 cycles per second. The triangular current is used for the first 2 to 5 treatments and then progressed to the rectangular wave form. Treatment is given daily or three times a week.

FARADISM WITH COMPRESSION FOR CHRONIC SYNOVITIS

Cases of painful and chronic effusion of the knee with a quadriceps lag have been treated successfully by stimulating the quadriceps group in elevation with a pressure bandage around the knee and quadriceps muscle. The treatment is carried out with the patient's knee held flexed to 5° with a restraining strap placed over the ankle to prevent hyperextension of the knee joint. No other exercises are given.

SEQUENTIAL FARADISM IN QUADRICEPS REHABILITATION

This method of faradism uses simultaneously an electronic low voltage stimulator and an induction coil to obtain maximal contractions of the total quadriceps mechanism. The problem of reduced proprioception with inability of the vastus medialis to co-ordinate with the rest of the quadriceps group to maintain the leg in full extension, may be treated by this method.

Position the patient in long sitting with a pillow or block under the heel. The other leg rests on the floor or stool over the edge of the bed.

Attach the indifferent electrode (120 mm × 80 mm) of the electronic stimulator over the femoral nerve trunk in the groin. The active electrode is placed over the common motor points approximately two-thirds of the way down the thigh.

Attach the induction coil apparatus (Smart-Bristow coil) or a scond surge controllable electronic stimulator to the patient by placing an indifferent electrode under the thigh (120 mm × 80 mm). The active electrode (50 mm × 50 mm) is placed on the motor point of vastus medialis. The electronic stimulator is positioned to obtain the longest hold of the current obtaining a good maximum tetanic-like contraction with a reasonable rest period between each contraction.

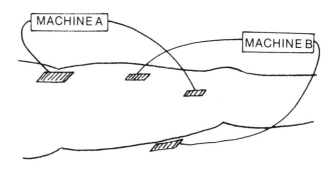

Sequential faradism to quadriceps.
(Machine A is operated by the patient;
machine B is operated by the therapist.)

The rest periods are reduced to a reasonable minimum, allowing the muscle time to relax. Before commencing treatment make sure that the electrode positions enable the quadriceps muscle to contract fully with no fibrillations and discomfort.

The main bulk of the quadriceps is stimulated with the electronic stimulator, initially for about 10 to 20 contractions. The patient is then instructed to work the induction coil, using the surger. The vastus medialis, which is connected to the induction coil, is made to contract just before the main bulk of the quadriceps contraction starts. The surger in the induction coil is kept in, maintaining the contraction of vastus medialis, until the main quadriceps contraction is completed. It is then withdrawn ready for the next sequential set of contractions.

The sequential groups of contractions are given in sets of 10 with a rest in between. The treatment lasts about 20 minutes. The patient is encouraged to contract the vastus medialis voluntarily in time with the electronic stimulation as he feels and controls the contraction. Thus proprioception is re-educated, pain of muscle contraction is inhibited and the patient obtains a more satisfactory voluntary contraction of the total muscle bulk. The strength of contraction should be as maximal and comfortable as possible. A course of daily treatments for 2 to 3 weeks is given.

FARADIC FOOT BATH

Equipment required

a Smart-Bristow coil or a low frequency electronic stimulator with faradic-like duration and frequency

two metal electrodes (100 mm × 30 mm)

two leads

a small table and trolley for the machine

a stool covered with plastic and a towel for the bath

two baths with warm water

towels

vaseline

a wooden spatula

a chair or stool for the operator

Position the patient comfortably in high sitting on a plinth with the back well supported with pillows, and the feet on a stool covered with plastic and a towel.

Patient orientation should explain the rationale for treatment and the sensation to be experienced.

Check that there are no contraindications to treatment with faradism.

Examine the area to be treated. Note any cuts, skin lesions, inflammation or swelling. Small cuts and abrasions need to be insulated with sterile vaseline. Inflammation and oedema impede the penetration of the current. Large open areas and extensive inflammation may contra-indicate treatment.

No skin test for sharp-blunt discrimination is necessary when using the Smart-Bristow coil as there are no chemical effects with the faradic current, but the test must be carried out when a low frequency electronic stimulator is used.

Place the patient's foot in a bath of warm water to decrease the skin resistance.

Connect the leads firmly to the machine.

Check that all the controls on the machine are in the correct position.

Plug into the mains power supply and switch on, if applicable.

Select the settings for faradic-type current, if applicable.

Connect the leads firmly to the metal electrodes and place the metal electrodes into the bath.

Test the application on yourself by placing your hand across the two electrodes. Describe to the patient the sensation you feel and make sure he can see the muscles contracting and relaxing.

Remove the patient's foot from the hot soak and if there are any breaks in the skin insulate them with a small amount of vaseline using the spatula.

To stimulate the *lumbricals*, position the patient's foot in the bath with one electrode obliquely under the metatarsal heads and the other under the heel.

Warn the patient

(*a*)   when using an electronic stimulator there should be no sustained intense prickling or burning sensation under the entire area of either electrode, or in one spot;

(*b*)   if using power from the mains supply, not to touch any of the equipment because of the danger of shock.

The therapist should be seated, facing the patient, and with the machine conveniently placed for manipulating the controls. When the surge is controlled manually, the therapist's forearm should be supported with the shoulder relaxed.

Check that all the controls on the machine are in the correct position.

Give a few gentle contractions while the patient becomes accustomed to the current. Then increase the intensity gradually until quite a strong contraction is produced, so the patient can see the movement required and can feel the muscle action which helps to re-establish the movement pattern.

Keep repeating the electrical stimulation while instructing and encouraging the patient to contract voluntarily with the current. As he feels the current increasing in intensity he should tighten up his muscles, and relax the contraction as the current intensity decreases, gradually superimposing his voluntary contraction over the electrically-produced one.

The patient then progresses to contract the muscles strongly as the current intensity increases and to hold the muscles in the contracted position against the decreasing intensity of current. Allow a relaxation phase between each contraction.

Finally test whether the patient can voluntarily initiate, hold and relax the contraction. Once this is achieved, discontinue the electrical stimulation. The entire emphasis of the treatment is on the *active* participation of the patient.

To stimulate the *plantar interossei*, place one electrode under the medial and the other under the lateral border of the foot and repeat the above technique. The water level in the bath must not be higher than the web of the toes, as with the resistance of the dorsum of the foot being so much less than that of the sole, contraction of the dorsal interossei will occur.

To stimulate *abductor hallucis*, place one electrode under the heel and the other on the motor point (obtained most easily by using a button electrode), and repeat the above technique.

RE-EDUCATION OF A MUSCLE ACTION DUE TO PROLONGED DISUSE OR INCORRECT USAGE

The painful foot

Sometimes patients present physiotherapists with a specific problem of pain on activity, in a specific group of muscles, which is caused by disuse atrophy or incorrect usage of the muscle group. This problem is often associated with *'pain in foot' syndrome*.

Pain in the feet is a common complaint, and often the insidious nature of the onset of pain and the patient's assumption that little can be done to relieve the pain makes it a chronic condition. In order to identify the cause of the painful foot one must understand the mechanical and physiological considerations.

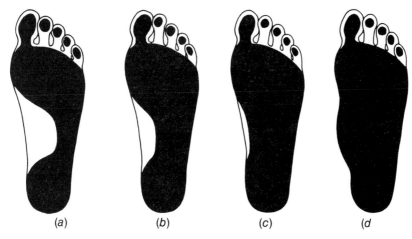

    (a)   (b)   (c)   (d

Footprints showing (a) a normal foot; (b) 1st degree pes planus; (c) 2nd degree pes planus; (d) 3rd degree pes planus.

The foot has two main functions:

(*a*)   *Static function* — On standing it can be observed that in the normal foot the calcaneum lies vertically under the tibia. The lateral border of the foot, which is made up of the lateral cuneiform and the fifth metatarsal, is weight-bearing as seen in a normal footprint. The lateral cuneiform rests on the cuboid, the cuboid rests on the base of the fifth metatarsal and the latter rests on the ground. The lateral border of the foot is built like a rough wall leaning slightly medially. The top course of the wall overhangs the region of the medial and intermediate cuneiforms and these, with the first and second metatarsal bones, produce the appearance of an arch on this side of the foot. On standing, the load is transmitted from the talus to the posterior tubercles of the calcaneum and its fibro-muscular attachments, and to the heads of the first and fifth metatarsals.

As a rule the cuneiforms are bound firmly together and to the navicular, so that the overhanging top course of the wall cannot fall vertically downwards. It can collapse only when the talus is rotated medially carrying the navicular and cuneiforms medially, with the result that the whole foot leans over to the medial side as is seen in a painful flat foot. *Thus in a flat foot the arch does not collapse vertically, but the foot leans over to the medial side.* The condition of flat foot can only be diagnosed by observing and palpating the extent to which the calcaneum is leaning over, that the patella should be pointing in the direction of the feet, and the navicular should not be prominent.

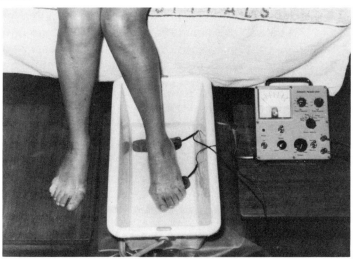

Faradic foot bath for a painful foot.

(*b*)   *Dynamic function* — the dynamic function of the foot is concerned with *propulsion and stabilisation*. In the course of propulsion it is important to look at the integration of the calf muscles, the peroneal muscles and the flexors of the toes. The foot can be looked upon as a spring which compresses under load and resets itself on removal of the load. The Stabilisation of the foot during locomotion is the restoration of equilibrium in the longitudinal and lateral directions. The peroneus longus muscle is important in that it stabilises the lateral arch by raising the cuboid once it stops lowering the metatarsals. It is important to maintain the length of the peroneus longus, and maintain the strength of the calf muscles, posterior tibials, the lumbricals and the interossei, flexor hallucis longus, and the abductors and adductors of the big toe, as these muscles, with the ligaments, support the plantar arches.

Pain in the foot can be due to the following factors:

muscle imbalance with mechanical dysfunction;

traumatic origin;

arthritic origin;

infection;

tumors;

dystrophic origin;

referred pain from the lumbar spine, L4, 5 nerve roots or the knee joint.

The pain could be localised in the ankle and tarsal region, forefoot, plantar aspect of foot, or the toes.

Examination of the foot must determine the exact location and cause of the pain.

If the cause of the painful foot is due partly or wholly to weak muscles, and this is identified clearly by testing the specific muscles concerned, then a decision is made to use the faradic-type currents for the re-education of its action, and to hypertrophy the muscles if atrophied.

The use of faradic-type currents to produce a maximal contraction of weak muscles in the foot is mainly *to act as a means of proprioception, to allow the patient to feel the precise nature of the contraction, and its specific action on the foot.* It could also be used solely to hypertrophy the muscles with or without the aid of exercises. If pain and swelling exist together with weak muscles, then the use of faradic stimulations for a longer period of time will activate the circulatory pump, which is one of the basic functions of the intrinsics of the foot.

Some common conditions treated with faradic-type currents include:
pes planus (flat foot);
metatarsalgia;
plantar digital neuritis (Morton's metatarsalgia);
plantar fasciitis;
calcaneal spur;
Sudek's atrophy;
hallux valgus;
hallux rigidus;
osteochrondritis;
rheumatoid arthritis.

The main aim of these treatments is to retrain the action of the weakened muscles of the foot to perform their normal functional activity in propulsion, dynamic and static posture and balance. It is also used to facilitate normal circulatory activity in the foot when the problem of swelling exists.

Treatment is generally given by means of a foot bath.

RE-EDUCATION OF WEAK PELVIC FLOOR MUSCLES

Methods using faradic-type currents to re-educate the pelvic floor muscles have been used by physiotherapists for many years. Today better post-natal care has reduced the demand for the treatment, nevertheless it still remains an effective treatment for patients who are unable to control micturition or defaecation, and when exercise methods have failed.

Indications
Stress incontinence of micturition or defaecation
Frequency symptoms with lack of control of micturition
Damaged anal or urinary bladder sphincter
Insidious occurrence of involuntary and intermittent loss of urine

Causes
In females, following childbirth some complications such as cystocele, rectocele, or minor prolapse of the uterus may occur causing stress incontinence. A

retroverted uterus may be the cause of a subjective frequency feeling. It may also be caused by anatomical changes in the fibro-muscular support of the proximal urethra, bladder neck and bladder base, due to advancing age and parity. Provided the changes are not too advanced, surgical repair is performed.

In males, following prostatectomy, particularly perineal prostatectomy, or sometimes after transurethral or retropublic procedures, damage to the sphincter may cause stress incontinence of urine. Most patients recover after a period of time, but some cases are left with the option of wearing a portable urinal. Repair of the anal sphincter which has been damaged is occasionally performed using a muscle transplant, using the gracilis muscle, and re-education of the new action is taught.

Technique I

The patient lies in prone-lying position with a pillow under the hips to keep the hips well flexed. The side-lying position with a pillow between the lower legs may be used if the patient cannot tolerate prone lying. Place a plastic sheet under the patient. Make sure no fluids have been taken for 2 hours prior to treatment.

The rectal electrode is a small 75 mm electrode (insulated). Other equipment required includes lubrication jelly (sterilised), a low frequency stimulator, a large indifferent electrode and pad (150 mm × 100 mm electrode).

Rub jelly on to the rectal electrode and insert into the anus. It should not be inserted too deeply or else it will stimulate the deep rotators of the hip and the gluteus maximus. Place the large electrode and pad over the lumbosacral region.

Select a faradic-type current (0.5 to 1 ms pulse duration, 50 to 70 Hz frequency). Faradic surges of 2 seconds duration at a repetition rate of 12 surges per minute are given in three groups of 12 contractions with a rest period of up to 3 minutes in between. The contractions must be as strong as the patient can bear. The number of groups of contractions may be increased as the muscle becomes stronger. The patient can superimpose an active contraction on top of the electrical contraction. At the end of the treatment the patient must do some exercises for regaining tone in the pelvic floor. The synergists of the pelvic floor muscles are the gluteus medius and the adductors.

Technique II

Position the patient in lying position with 3 pillows under the knees and a small rubber ball between the legs. The legs are slightly abducted and rotated externally. This is to encourage the action of gluteus medius, which is a synergist for the levator ani and pubo-coccygeus muscles.

Select a faradic pulse (1 ms duration, 50 Hz frequency). A large indifferent electrode and pad are placed in the lumbosacral region. A rectal electrode is placed in the rectum. Faradic surges at a moderate rate are given as strongly as the patient can bear. The patient compresses the rubber ball between the legs when the current contracts the pelvic floor muscles, and relaxes with the cessation of the current. If no rectal electrode is available, place a large button electrode on the perineal body.

Four groups of 15 contractions are given. Give less for the first two treatments, and gradually increase the number of contractions. Generally one course of treatment is sufficient to improve muscle tone. (One course is 6 to 10 treatments.)

This is followed by active exercises. Proprioceptive neuromuscular facilitation techniques such as bilateral extension adduction patterns with slow reversal of the pattern or repeated contractions of the same pattern are useful for the younger patients.

REDUCTION OF LIMB OEDEMA

Oedema in part or the whole limb could be caused by many factors:

Soft tissue trauma. The presence of high protein oedema in the tissues of the limbs following tissue damage produces excessive fibrosis and adhesions unless it is removed before organisation of the exudate occurs. Cases like crush injuries of a foot, hand or the whole limb produce oedema that would impair function.

Gravitational oedema. This can be caused by prolonged immobilisation of a limb following trauma. Traumatic oedema is either produced by the original injury or by mechanical factors following the injury. Extravasation of blood and tissue fluid into the soft tissues may result in swelling and interference with normal circulation.

Lymphoedema of the extremities may be primary or secondary. Secondary lymphoedema may be due to the removal of lymphatic vessels and nodes by surgery, or obstruction of the lymphatic system by infection, malignant disease, or tumors. In any case the water and protein balance across the capillary membrane is disturbed, resulting in the accumulation of extravascular, extracellular fluid. When lymphatic vessels are obstructed, the retention of protein in the tissue spaces increases colloidal osmotic pressure and stimulates the production of fibrosis in the tissue spaces.

Post-phlebitic syndrome. Oedema of the limb following deep vein thrombosis of the leg.

Varicose ulcers. Oedema of the lower leg with chronic venous ulcers.

METHODS FOR THE REDUCTION OF LIMB OEDEMA

(a)   Compression units

Today there are pressure pumps available which provide intermittent compression to the limbs. The pumps simulate the function of the physiological muscle pump without movement of the muscle or joints. It is also similar to the milking action produced by the massage technique of squeezing kneading. The overall effect is the removal of the exudate in the direction of the venous and lymphatic channels.

(b)   Jobst extremity pump

This pump applies intermittent compression to the limb by means of a pneumatic appliance that is alternately inflated and deflated according to a prescribed time cycle. Pressures are from 60 to 100 mm Hg for 45 seconds and off for 15 seconds. Once the limb oedema is reduced, a custom-built elastic stocking or arm-sleeve is worn, acting as an external fascial sheath.

The intermittent pressure is applied to the whole limb. Some units have a sectionalised splint, so that inflation of each section occurs rhythmically and consecutively as a milking action from the distal to the proximal end. The method is useful in the early acute stages of limb oedema.

(c) Ame units of intermittent pressure therapy

The Ame units are compressor cycling units using the principles of automatic gas cycling devices. The unit consists of two parts: the cycling valve which is connected to an air compressor, and an inflatable cuff which is affixed over the limb. The Ame-3 unit incorporates a sensitive pressure gauge calibrated from 0 to 200 mmHg. Pressures from 10 to 40 mmHg are useful for acute and early cases, while up to 60 mmHg is useful for chronic cases (Masman and Conolly). It also has a variable timing phase between 5 seconds and 60 seconds. Small areas in the acute stages could have 5 second pressure phase and a 6 second resting phase at a pressure of 30 mmHg for 20 minutes.

A chronic condition involving the whole limb could have a 40 second pressure phase and a 30 second resting phase at 60 mmHg for 30 minutes. Treatments should never exceed 40 minutes, as maximal benefit has been reached in this time period. Treatment is given with the limb in elevation, followed by a firm bandage and instructions to patients to use the muscle pump and prevent prolonged gravitational causes of oedema by keeping the limb elevated at rest.

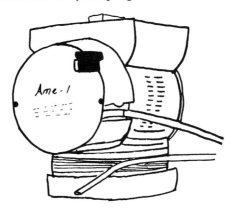

The Ame Compressor cycling unit

(d) Massage of the limb in elevation

A time-honored technique for limb oedema is massage, using the techniques of effleurage, kneading, and petrisage. The overall effect does not remain for as long a period as that gained by the compression units. Furthermore massage is time-consuming. The compression units are more quickly effective, and maintain the effects for a much longer time. Occasionally it is useful to do massage after faradism under pressure or after the use of a compression unit, to accelerate absorption of exudate.

(e) Faradism under pressure in elevation

The use of faradic-type currents to stimulate the muscles that generally act as the muscle pump of the affected limb, in conjunction with compression and elevation, has been practised for many years. The use of the electrical compression unit has cut down the need for this technique. Today it is used particularly for the woody type of oedema which is resistant to other methods, and also if the muscles which generally work the circulatory muscle pump are weak and show hypotonicity, then the added result of the treatment will produce a working hypertrophy of the muscles concerned.

The circulation pumps in the arm are the long flexors of the hand and wrist and the biceps muscle, as most of the larger lymphatic and venous channels are in the flexor aspect of the arm and forearm. The muscle pump of the lower leg is the calf muscles, and the quadriceps and hamstrings group are important for the knee and thigh.

Technique of treatment

Examine the patient for cuts, abrasions, and any areas of skin breakdown. Ensure that the skin is not thin and fragile. Measure the limb at fixed points before and after treatment. Suggested points for measurement are:

fingers	— distal and proximal interphalangeal joints
	— base of finger
hand	— heads of the metacarpals
	— thumb web
	— line of wrist joint
arm	— thumb web
	— line of wrist joint
	— 100 mm, 200 mm, and 300 mm above the wrist joint
foot	— head of first metatarsal
and ankle	— base of fifth metatarsal
	— 50 mm proximal to the metatarsal
leg	— base of knee joint
	— 100 mm, 200 mm, and 300 mm above apex of medial malleolus

Test the patient for sharp and blunt sensation.

Make sure that there is no infection present and no thrombi in the venous system.

Check the strength of the muscles to be stimulated.

Note any atrophy of muscle, which is generally masked by the oedema.

The apparatus needed includes a low voltage electronic stimulator; two electrodes to place over the motor points of the muscles to be stimulated; plastic; elastic compression bandage or air-splint; and leads.

Test the machine to see that it is working. Demonstrate the contraction to the patient on yourself.

To treat the arm:

Position the limb in elevation with the patient comfortably supported. Place the electrodes on the flexor aspect of the forearm over the motor points of flexor digitorum superficialis and profundus, and over the motor points of the biceps and brachialis. Keep the arm elevated at 45° to take advantage of gravity flow. Strap the electrodes lightly and check that the muscles are contracting correctly with the machine. Now firmly wrap a compression bandage starting distally until the shoulder is reached. Make sure that there are no gaps between each turn of the bandage. *Do not bandage so firmly as to occlude the circulation.* As an alternative to a bandage, use an inflatable air-splint with moderate inflation. It acts as a good compression aid against which the muscles contract.

If the hand is grossly swollen and 'woody', place one electrode on the dorsum of the hand and the other electrode on the palmar aspect of the hand. This will stimulate the intrinsics. The active electrode is on the palmar aspect of the arm. The size of pad and electrode should be large enough to cover the palm of the hand (50 mm × 40 mm).

To treat the leg:
Place the active electrode on the calf muscles (90 mm × 50 mm). Place the indifferent electrode on the dorsum of the foot (120 mm × 50 mm). Ensure that the calf muscles are contracting well. Apply a firm bandage to the leg starting at the toes and finishing at the knee joint, or as an alternative use an air-splint.

Having fixed the electrodes and ensured that the muscles are contracting and well bandaged, obtain a fairly strong contraction within the patient's tolerance and give a treatment for 20 minutes. Select a rectangular pulse with a duration from 1 to 10 ms and a frequency of 50 to 70 Hz, with a 3 or 4 second surge if using a galvanic-faradic unit, or a 10 second contraction with a 50 second rest period at a frequency of 65 Hz if using the Siemens' Neurotron.

Treatment should be given daily. There must be reduction of oedema immediately after treatment, of which at least 50% should be maintained. If there is no improvement after 2 or 3 treatments, it is best to stop.

8.6   Long Duration Modular Pulsed Currents

INTRODUCTION

It is just over 200 years since Luigi Galvani first discovered the use of the interrupted galvanic current to stimulate nerves and muscles in frogs. Later, in 1804, the galvanic current found support in Europe for the treatment of paralysis. In 1883 Duchenne in France worked with induced currents which were transmitted to the body by moist electrodes. Until then the current had been introduced by bare lead electrodes or acupuncture needles. Acupuncture techniques using electricity had been brought back by missionaries from China as far back as 1750. Since the introduction of the portable electronic low frequency generators in the early twentieth century, long duration pulsed currents with pulse durations varying from 100 ms to 2000 ms in varying shapes, such as rectangular, saw-tooth, triangular and trapezoidal, have been used extensively for the treatment of denervated muscles.

Synonyms
Interrupted galvanism (an old historical term)
Exponential progressive currents (a term popular in Europe)
Interrupted direct current (IDC) (this term covers both short and long duration pulsed currents)

PHYSICS OF LONG DURATION MODULAR PULSED CURRENTS

Long duration pulsed currents are unidirectional currents, interrupted at regular intervals with a specific regular *Pulse duration* varying from 100 ms to 2000 ms.

The period of a long interrupted pulse duration is the sum of the duration and the interval.

Pulse durations from 1 ms to 100 ms are connected loosely with both long and short duration pulses. A muscle must have a partial nerve supply to be stimulated

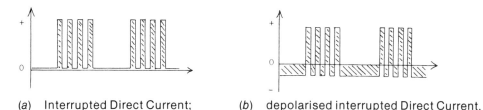

(a) Interrupted Direct Current;   (b) depolarised interrupted Direct Current.

Long duration pulses

by pulses of 10 ms, 30 ms or 50 ms duration. These are often called long duration pulsed currents by physiotherapists. Nevertheless it will be seen later that stimulation by these pulses definitely indicates the integrity of some of the fibres in the affected nerve.

The *intervals* of the pulse wave are generally at least 2 to 3 times the length of the pulse duration. A pulse of 100 ms must have an interval of 200 to 300 ms.

The *frequency* is generally from 5 Hz to 10 Hz, depending on the pulse duration.

A pulse duration of 100 ms has a frequency selected of 1.5 Hz with an interval of about 500 ms.

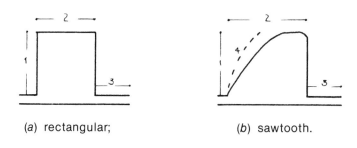

(a) rectangular;   (b) sawtooth.

(1 — intensity; 2 — pulse duration; 3 — rest phase.)

Long duration pulses

Varying modulations are sometimes designed into circuits. One form of modulation in IDC is when the intensity of the current is cyclically reduced to zero. In *interrupted modulation* the current is turned on and off. The modulation rate is stated as cycles per minute, with the off period between the periods of current flow termed the *rest period*. The frequency of an interrupted direct current is always higher than its modulation rate. Long duration pulses are never used with a surging modulation as they are generally used for denervated muscles which need the intensity for stimulation.

The shapes of pulsed waves are variable.

The *rectangular pulse* has the current turned up abruptly, maintained constant for the duration of the stimulus, and turned off abruptly.

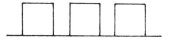

The *exponential progressive currents* use pulses which reach their maximal intensity slowly. Each time the speed of rise of current is slowed, an increase of intensity will result in a renewal of the current's ability to depolarise muscle membrane and cause a contraction. There are different ways of gradually increasing the speed of rise of current intensity within the selected pulse duration.

The *saw-tooth pulse* has a gradual rise of current followed by an abrupt turning off.

The *triangular pulse* has an equal phase of slow rise and then slow falling off in intensity.

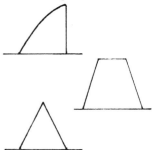

The *trapezoidal pulse* rises slowly, stays on a plateau for a short period and then gradually declines.

The use of varying pulse shapes in the selection of currents for denervated muscles is important, as there is a definite relationship between the extent of the nerve lesion, the speed of rise of current, the pulse duration and the intensity of current needed to produce a contraction of muscle.

PHYSIOLOGICAL EFFECTS

The basis of the physiological effects of long duration modular pulsed currents is the ability of the currents to stimulate denervated muscles, whether they are completely or partially denervated.

Responses of muscle and nerve to long duration pulses

As discussed earlier in Unit 7, at rest both nerve and muscle membrane have a high intracellular potassium and low calcium content giving rise to a resting membrane potential of –90 mV. A propagated nerve impulse consists of a wave of depolarisation spreading down the nerve fibre causing a release of acetylcholine at the neuromuscular junction. This causes a further wave of depolarisation over the muscle fibre membrane resulting in physical contraction. The velocity of conduction of nerve fibres is proportional to the fibre diameter and is influenced by factors such as compression, age, and temperature. Fast precision muscles conduct at about 7.5 ms. Slow postural and gross movement types of muscle conduct at about 100 ms.

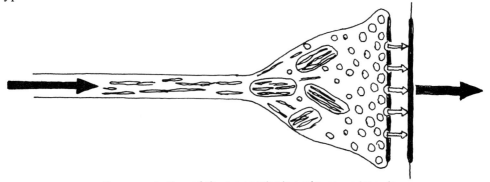

Representation of the transmission of a nerve impulse

A localised constriction of a peripheral nerve or a diffused thinning of its fibres will cause a reduction of nerve conduction velocity of the nerve. Not all fibres are affected equally, and this produces a scatter in the response of the muscle shown by the electrical contraction generated. So, if a muscle is denervated and the muscle is directly stimulated by an electrical stimulus, provided the pulse duration is long, then a certain minimum of current intensity will cause excitation at the muscle fibre by producing depolarisation directly, or it may act indirectly on the neuromuscular junction of the motor neuron. Whether the response results from one or the other depends on the state of the nerve, on the state of the muscle, and to some extent on the distribution of the electric field. In complete denervation, it acts directly on the muscle fibre.

Quantitative assessment of neuromuscular activity with long duration pulses. Two factors of importance in the quantitative assessment of neuromuscular excitability are:

(*a*) the strength of the stimulus required to produce excitation;

(*b*) the duration of the applied stimulus.

The threshold response or *rheobase, is the minimal voltage of prolonged pulse duration necessary to excite a muscle and produce a bare minimal perceptible and palpable contraction.* It is measured in volts or milliamperes. Normal rheobase values are from 5 to 35 V.

The *chronaxie is the minimal time required to excite the tissue for a stimulus of twice the strength of the rheobase.* It is measured in milliseconds. Normal chronaxie values are from 0.05 to 0.5 ms.

During the passage of a current through a tissue, the critical level of excitation (that is the change in its resting potential) is raised slowly to a threshold potential of between 5 and 15 mV more positive. Therefore a longer time is needed to build up the threshold stimulus to the critical level of $+30$ mV from the -90 mV of resting potential. *This change in excitatory level is called accommodation.* Accommodation, which is the apparent decrease in excitability, develops more rapidly in nerve fibres than in muscle fibres.

The rheobase of a denervated fibre may be less than that of the nerve fibre, but the chronaxie is much longer, and the muscle will not respond to tolerable currents of shorter duration. Muscle has less powers of accommodation than nerve, which is an irritable tissue, and therefore muscle is easily tetanised by currents that are slightly higher than the rheobase. To tetanise nerve tissue needs a higher intensity than to produce a rheobase. The tetanus-twitch ratio for nerve is 5:1 to 6:1.

Physiological effects of the exponential progressive currents

Du Bois-Raymond and Nernst realised that the threshold value required to produce a minimum twitch in a sound voluntary muscle is smallest when the current rises to a peak value almost immediately, that is in a minimum of time, as in the rectangular pulses. If, however, the current rises slowly to its fullest value as in trapezoidal, triangular, and saw-tooth pulses, normal muscle tissue sets up a resistance which increases the threshold for stimulus, and greater intensity has to be given to produce a contraction. *So a rectangular pulse of 1000 ms needs less current than that required by a triangular pulse of 1000 ms.* But if the muscle is denervated, a long duration progressive pulse such as a triangular pulse needs less intensity and selectively picks up the denervated muscle, without picking up normal muscles. *This is because denervated muscles have lost all power of accommodation*, and the slow interrupted currents give ample time for depolarisation, producing a good muscle contraction with less intensity.

Advantages of exponential currents

The ability to stimulate denervated muscle selectively will at once suggest advantages in the use of these currents for therapeutic purposes. The phenomena of leakage to normal muscles does not occur so readily. As the pulse is selective in itself, a button or disc electrode is not necessary. A fairly large electrode can be used, allowing more passage of current for a given amount of skin tolerance. The patient is able to tolerate enough intensity to produce a strong contraction as the sensory nerves also are accommodating to the stimulus.

In summary, a normal motor unit is stimulated via the nerve and has the property of accommodating itself to long duration pulsed currents. A denervated muscle has lost the property of accommodation and is more easily tetanised by currents of longer duration and an intensity slightly greater than rheobase. Denervated muscle has a longer chronaxie and is not stimulated by tolerable currents with pulses of shorter duration.

CAUSES OF DENERVATED MUSCLES

Motor unit lesions

In 1939 Sherrington appreciated that the varied reflex and voluntary contractions of a muscle are achieved by the different combinations of motor units. In other words, all movements are planned by the central nervous system in terms of

Anatomical and functional site of involvement including possible aetiology

SITE	AETIOLOGY
motor neuropathy anterior horn cell with central connections	poliomyelitis; motor neuron disease, such as progressive muscular atrophy and amyotrophic lateral sclerosis; syringomyelia
peripheral neuropathy — nerve root	prolapsed intervertebral disc; traction injury; trauma
— plexus	penetrating wounds; traction injury
— peripheral nerve	idiopathic peripheral neuritis; polyneuritis; Guillain-Barre syndrome; Landry's paralysis; tumors; trauma
myopathy muscle fibre	myopathies; polymyositis; myotonia; infection; endocrine dysfunction; connective tissue disorders
neuromuscular junction	myaesthenia gravis; myotonia congenita; electrolytic disturbances; toxins

motor units and not individual muscle fibres. If we consider the lesions that affect the muscle fibre and its nerve supply, causing denervation and paralysis, we will see a wide variety of disorders.

Some lesions are determined genetically, others are acquired. Some diseases progress rapidly, others progress insidiously or resolve spontaneously. Some are associated with gross derangements of muscle structure, and some affect the nerve structure and function. It is now customary to classify lesions according to the site of greatest functional or structural abnormality. The signs and symptoms of the lesion depend on whether it occurs at the level of the central nervous system or the peripheral nervous system. The questions asked of a paralysed muscle are: Is it spastic or flaccid? Does it show a poverty of movement or rigidity? And so on.

Nerve compression
(a) Acute lesions
The delicate structure of the nerve fibre makes it susceptible to mechanical injury. The type and severity of the resulting lesion will depend on many factors, such as the mechanics of the injury: was it stretched, divided or compressed? If compressed, what was the extent and duration of the compression? The severity of the lesion will depend on the healthiness of the neuron. Cases of metabolic or toxic neuropathies are more vulnerable to compression.

Nerve lesions have been classified by Seddon (1948, 1972) and by Sunderland (1951, 1968).

SEDDON's CLASSIFICATION
Neuropraxia   Axonotmesis   Neurotmesis
SUNDERLAND
Five degrees of nerve injury.

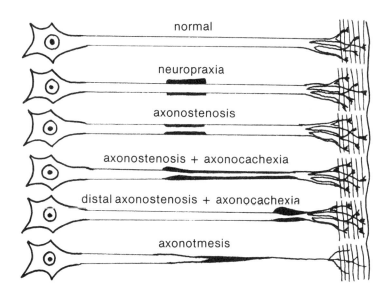

normal

neuropraxia

axonostenosis

axonostenosis + axonocachexia

distal axonostenosis + axonocachexia

axonotmesis

Sunderland's classification of nerve lesions

Neuropraxia is a temporary loss of function without discontinuity of the axon, often a simple local interruption of the conductivity of nerve fibre due to pressure or crushing. In this situation stimulation proximal to the injury will not result in contraction, but stimulation distal to the injury will cause contraction. Sometimes not all the nerve fibres are neuropraxic, so stimulation proximally might produce a small response. There is no Wallerian degeneration.

Axonostenosis is localised compression of the axon which is prolonged and severe. The excitability and conduction velocity are reduced over the affected stretch, but are normal or near normal below it.

Axonocachexia is reduction of calibre over the whole distal portion of the axon. There is decrease in excitability and conductivity over the whole affected portion. Threshold values are sometimes high.

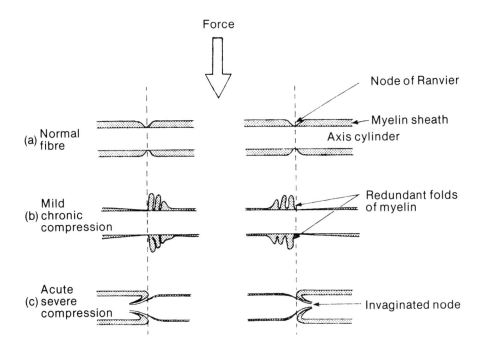

Compression of an axon. The severity of the lesion will determine the results of compression. (Fowler, 1975)

Axonotmesis is total interruption of the axons and their myelin sheaths with preservation of the neurolemma sheath and the connective tissue stroma. No contractions follow nerve stimulation. A contraction can only be stimulated via the muscle using long duration pulses. It is always followed by Wallerian degeneration. Signs of denervation are picked up readily by the various methods of electrodiagnosis.

Neurotmesis is discontinuity of the whole nerve following complete section. There is no stimulation response. Wallerian degeneration takes place. The nerve has generally been completely severed or else seriously disorganised by scar tissue so that spontaneous regeneration is impossible.

The changes which constitute (Wallerian) degeneration in nerve cells and their processes may be initiated by transection, crushing of the nerve fibre, local injection of toxic substances, or interference with their blood supply.

Injuries to nervous tissues are of different orders of severity. Sunderland classifies them as follows:

First degree injuries. These are the most common and are caused by
(*a*)   Interruption of conduction in the axons with preservation of their anatomical continuity, such as by pressure being applied to a nerve for a limited time, thus occluding its blood supply and resulting in a local anoxia sufficient to impair the nerve's function.
(*b*)   The direct effect of pressure on axons causing local injury. Damage of this kind will be repaired so that function returns within a few hours to a few weeks. The axon is not destroyed but merely loses its functional properties for a short time.

Second degree injuries. Loss of continuity of the axons without a breach of the endoneurium. These are the result of prolonged and/or severe pressure being exerted on some part of the nerve, such as was formerly carried out deliberately, in crushing the phrenic nerve to paralyse one half of the diaphragm in tuberculosis.

Death of the axon at the site of pressure is followed by death of the axon distal to it because the axon is separated from the cell body on which it depends for its nutrition and, therefore, its existence. Chromatolysis occurs in the cell body.

Regeneration of the axon is facilitated by the presence of uninterrupted endoneurial tubes, down which the regeneration axons grow to effect their former connections. The axoplasm grows down the endoneurial tubes at the rate of 2 to 3 mm per day. Remyelination of the axon follows closely its growth down the endoneurial tubes.

Third degree injuries. They are characterised by complete loss of continuity of the nerve fibres with preservation of the epineurium.

Fourth degree injuries. There is interruption and disorganisation of the nerve fascicles including the perineural sheaths.

Fifth degree injuries. There is severance of the nerve trunk.

(*b*)   Chronic lesions

The entrapment neuropathies

Consideration must be given to the consequences of chronic injury on peripheral nerves and in particular to the effects of prolonged compression of nerves by adjacent tissues. Nerves are likely to be damaged at certain vulnerable positions along their course through 'wear and tear'. These disorders are known as entrapment neuropathies. Some common entrapment neuropathies include:

carpal tunnel syndrome   —   a lesion of the median nerve at the wrist.
ulnar nerve entrapment   —   this occurs as the ulnar nerve runs behind the medial epicondyl at the elbow.

radial nerve lesion   — this occurs as the radial nerve winds around
                                          the spiral groove of the humerus; it is
                                          popularly known as 'the Saturday night
                                          palsy'.

common peroneal nerve lesion   — this nerve is vulnerable to pressure as it
                                          crosses the head of the fibula, for example
                                          in prolonged squatting or the wearing of
                                          tight high boots.

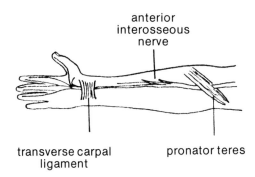

Sites of compressive lesions which may produce pain in the territory of the median nerve

Some less common entrapment neuropathies include:
the median nerve as it passes through the pronator teres muscle below the elbow;
the anterior interosseous branch of the median nerve;
the posterior interosseous branch of the radial nerve;
the lateral cutaneous nerve of the leg (also known as 'meralgia paraesthetica');
the posterior tibial nerve within the tarsal tunnel.

The double crush syndrome
Upper limb paraesthesis with muscle weakness can be due to two crushed areas in
one nerve. Upton and McComas (1973) established the hypothesis. They considered that, for example, patients with cervical involvement of C_6, C_7, and C_8
roots would be predisposed to the development of both cubital and carpal tunnel
syndrome. There is sufficient data available to support the double crush
hypothesis as a possible way of explaining unusual clinical observations.

WALLERIAN DEGENERATION
The stability of the axon depends on its connection with the cell body. If the axon
is injured with neurotmesis (interruption of the endoneural continuity) or with
axonotmesis (no interruption of the endoneural continuity), degeneration of the
peripheral nerve occurs. When the axon commences to break up, it is termed
Wallerian degeneration.

Nerve degeneration is breakdown of the myelin sheath and disintegration of
the axis cylinder, together with proliferation of the Schwann cells resulting in the
formation of neurolemmal bands and shrinkage of the endoneural sheaths.

Injured axons will conduct for 72 hours after injury. There is loss of conduction in the axon 71 to 79 hours after injury. 8 days later the destruction of the

myelin sheath takes place. Chemical changes occur in the myelin sheath with disappearance of the lipids. This takes 8 to 23 days after section. 25 days after nerve section there are maximal proliferative changes in the Schwann cells of the peripheral stumps, and an increase in RNA and DNA occurs. These changes begin minimally in the first few days.

Fragmentation of the motor end plates takes place 32 hours after nerve section, but they retain their excitability for up to 10 days. Breakdown of axon and myelin sheaths takes place faster in the muscle than in the nerve trunk. Degeneration is usually completed in 2 weeks. When degeneration is complete, the electromyograms will show fibrillation potentials.

Nerve regeneration will occur in axonotmesis, and in neurotmesis if there is good apposition of nerve endings by surgery. The rate of outgrowth of axons is 4 to 5 mm a day in favorable conditions. The average is 3 mm a day after crushing, 2 mm a day after suture. The rate of functional regeneration is slower than the rate of outgrowth of axons. A gradual deceleration of 0.5 mm a day has been seen in injury to big nerve trunks. The rate of growth in the hand and foot is 0.5 mm per day (Guttman, Cajal and Sunderland). *Tinel's sign* of a painful response on percussion of the nerve trunk distal to the injury is useful to determine rate of growth.

MUSCLE DENERVATION

Efficient motor and sensory function depends upon muscles and adjoining soft tissue which are normally innervated and vascularised, tendons that move freely in their sheaths and across other structures with which they are in contact, joints and periarticular structures that permit a free and unrestricted range of movement, and normal sensory mechanisms in the skin, articular, periarticular, and muscular structures. Interference with any of these systems will adversely affect motor function, the extent of the disturbance depending on the nature and magnitude of the lesion.

In order to evaluate the effects of low frequency currents on denervated muscles, let us summarise the changes in general that occur with lesions of the motor unit.

We have seen earlier in this unit the wide variety of disorders that affect the muscle fibre and its nerve supply. For more than a century it has been known that the muscle fibre and the motor neurons exert a sustaining influence on each other. The sustaining action of nerve on muscle, which includes a certain regulation of tissue (or cell) metabolism, and depends on the integrity of the connections between the muscle and the nerve, is said to be *trophic*.

In general, severance of any section of the motor unit will result in:

(*a*) morphological, physiological, and biochemical changes in muscles, bones, joints, and periarticular structures due to denervation;

(*b*) changes in normally innervated structures which are introduced indirectly by the immobilisation of a limb, and by vascular and lymphatic stasis;

(*c*) disturbance of the sensori-motor function.

Denervation atrophy. Bearing in mind that 10 to 25% of normal muscle is connective tissue, following severance of a nerve to muscle, the muscle will gradually waste over a period of weeks. The atrophy can be detected at about the third day sometimes, and is rapid in the first 2 months. At the end of 3 months, only 30 to 40% of the original muscle remains. Much of this will be the connective tissue content. Further atrophy is slower and less in quantity. This marked atrophy is known as *denervation atrophy*, and the *trophic influence* of muscle and nerve plays an important part in denervation atrophy. It has been shown that several substances are transported from the nerve to the muscle. They provide a possible explanation for the trophic influence of nerve on muscle.

Morphological changes. In the early stages of denervation, we see reduction of sarcoplasm, changes in sarcolemmal nuclei, reduction of myofibrils, and disintegration of the axon terminal at the neuromuscular junction, with a complete disruption of the motor end plate, though the end plate nuclei are not altered in the early stages. Disorders of the neuromuscular junctions form a specific group of conditions which are the cause of muscular weakness, such as myaesthenia gravis and neuropathies from toxins. The pathological changes of the motor end plates in these cases are different from that caused by a lesion of the peripheral nerve.

According to Guttman, muscle spindle nuclei are not affected for a year at least.

Degenerative changes begin after about 70 days, and a variable proportion of muscle fibres undergoes degenerative changes after several months have elapsed. There is also an increase of connective tissue. Collagen content decreases in the first month and then increases between 8 and 12 weeks.

Changes in joints, periarticular structures, tendons and ligaments. Changes in tendon, tendon sheaths, joints, ligaments and capsule are generally due to disuse. These structures show fibrosis from disuse. The accumulation of tissue fluid in the fascial planes between muscles leads to the formation of adhesions and fibrosis and restricts free movements of muscles. There is also joint instability due to muscle weakness.

Changes in bone. Bone is a living tissue which has innervation from sensory and sympathetic fibres to the periosteum, medullary cavity and cortex. Changes in bone occur in adults if there is a long period of denervation and if extensive areas are denervated. There is some decalcification of the cortex, and the appearance of osteoporosis. It is more marked in the bones of the hands and feet.

In *growing bones* the nature of involvement depends on the period of immobilisation, the period of denervation, and the extent of denervation. There is reduction in the texture of the bone as well as some interference in the growth.

Biochemical and energy changes. There is a reduction in creatinine, adenosine triphosphate, and potassium accompanying the loss of muscle fibre, while increases in collagen, chloride, sodium, and calcium follow the increase in connective tissue.

The energy metabolism of denervated muscle is upset. The best known sources of energy in muscle are carbohydrates — blood glucose and muscle glycogen. Muscle stores lipids, carbohydrates, and proteins as sources of energy and utilises them according to the function of the muscle and the type of work it does. Denervation alters the capability of the muscle to draw on its energy stores.

Disturbances in substrate utilisation. The blood flow through denervated muscles is increased during the initial period (1 to 5 months), and decreased later after periods longer than 5 months. There is increased blood flow in the capillary bed of the muscle yet, even though the muscle is supplied with sufficient blood, *it is unable to use the substrates*. This causes metabolic and functional disturbance and is one reason for the marked denervation atrophy that occurs. The trophic influence of the nerve affects the regulation of metabolism which ensures the morphological and chemical composition of the muscle and its capacity of adaptation to external stimuli. The reasons for the inability of the denervated muscle to utilise the substrates are still being studied. Reports dealing with metabolic loads state that:

(*a*) the role of carbohydrates as the substrates of energy for oxidative metabolism increases after denervation;

(*b*) the rate of glycogen synthesis is retarded due to the reduction in its breakdown during starvation;

(*c*) the consumption of energy in denervated muscles is increased for fibrillation activity and synthesis of lipids, but fibrillation activity is not the cause of denervation atrophy; so the main problem of denervation atrophy is due to disturbance of substrate utilisation by muscle, and loss of the trophic influence of nerve on muscle.

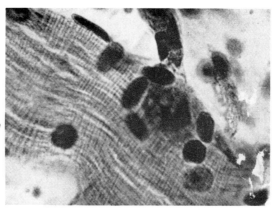

Human muscle fibre 69 days after denervation. End-plate sarcoplasm is still conspicuous and a single Schwann sheath may be traced to the end-plate.

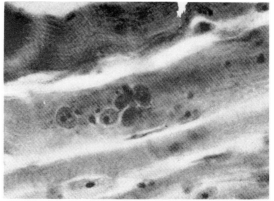

Muscle 250 days after denervation. The end-plate is preserved.

Physiological changes. Section of a peripheral nerve or lesions of the motor unit will cause a variety of physiological changes in the muscle. Each cause of the lesion will have to be studied separately to determine the specific physiological changes. If the peripheral nerve is severed, then the following changes are expected:

Flaccidity and paralysis of movement. There is loss of muscle tone partly or completely and inability of the muscle to respond to voluntary effort or reflex influences.

Fibrillations are the spontaneous activity of muscle that takes the form of fine rapid asynchronous rhythmic contractions of muscle fibres. They impart a faint rippling movement to the surface of the muscle. Fibrillation occurs in nerve lesions with loss of axonal continuity.

Altered excitability to electrical stimulation. There is loss of the response of normal muscle to a faradic-type current stimulation (a pulse duration of 1 ms) with a brisk contraction when a muscle is denervated. It will respond only to a pulse with longer durations and a slow increase of intensity, as the muscle would have lost is property of accommodation. As muscle atrophy increases, there is reduction in excitability of the muscle membrane by electrical stimulation. Longer pulse durations with a slower rise of intensity have to be used to produce a contraction. The electromyogram will diagnose the altered action potentials in denervated muscle. In normal muscle at rest there is no electrical activity, but in lesions of the peripheral nerve, spontaneous electrical activity termed *fibrillation potentials* are picked up by the electromyogram (EMG).

EFFECTS OF ELECTRICAL STIMULATION ON DENERVATED MUSCLES

The use of electrical stimulation on denervated muscles has been a controversial subject. It has been practised since the first half of the last century (Reid 1841, Guttman 1942, Egen 1958, Wakim 1958). To date electrotherapy represents the most effective method of influencing the rate of denervation atrophy. Differences of opinion about the clinical results of electrotherapy in influencing denervation atrophy and other effects are due, to a certain extent, to the fact that almost every author used a different electrotherapeutic method at varying times, and many experiments were done on animals. Today there are a few authors (for example, Seddon, Sunderland, Guttman, and Wakim), who describe the most important conditions for obtaining positive results with electrotherapy. Let us look first of all at the possible effects of electrotherapy in the treatment of denervated muscles.

Retardation of denervation atrophy. Experiments have shown that if electrical stimulations are started early and under the optimal conditions, using maximal isometric contractions, they will *retard the rate of denervation atrophy*. The physiological mechanism underlying the effect is still being debated, but it is thought that a group of repetitive stimuli producing contractions will normalise the rate of glycogen synthesis and enhance the role of carbohydrate oxidation (Bass, Fischer). The findings of Guttman were concerned with the increasing content of proteins, after repeated stimulation, without a corresponding increase of nucleic acids in the denervated muscle. This may be the answer to the fundamental question associated with the mechanism of electrotherapy (Zak and Guttman, 1960). It is important not to give supramaximal contractions at high intensities as it will have unfavorable effects on regeneration of the peripheral nerve (Beranek and Guttman, 1953), as well as adverse effects on metabolism and trophic states of the muscles (Guttman and Vodicka, 1953; Vodicka, 1955). Most authors agree that strong contractions should take place under isometric conditions, so that the muscle must be positioned in such a way as to prevent isotonic movement.

Utilisation of substrates. Blood flow in denervated muscles is increased after denervation, particularly in the first 3 months, but as there is disturbance of muscle metabolism and cell permeability, muscles are unable to utilise the substrates, and denervation atrophy is marked. Electrically-produced contraction and relaxation would aid the muscle in utilising its substrates and thus maintain nutrition.

Venous and lymphatic stasis. Owing to the failure of the muscle pump which activates venous and lymphatic circulation, there is accumulation of tissue fluid in the fascial planes in and around muscles. This will predispose to causing contractures of the muscle and of the soft tissues around the muscle. Electrical stimulation is thought to aid absorption of the exudate by the pumping action of the muscles.

Working hypertrophy. Electrotherapy does not produce a weight increment in denervated muscles, but it helps to retard the rate of denervation atrophy. However in cases of partial nerve lesions when some of the muscles supplied by the nerve escape damage and get disuse atrophy, electrotherapy will produce a working hypertrophy of these muscles.

Maintenance of muscle extensibility. Passive length-tension relationships of muscle and the adhesive forces between muscle fibres and connective tissue in denervated muscles have been the subject of experiments (Stolov). It has been found that, on denervation, there is elongation of the tendon and an increase of adhesive forces due to the increased collagen activity in the chronic stages. The changes do not occur in the acute stages. Isometric maximal contractions with resistance retard the collagen activity in the chronic stages.

SELECTION OF TREATMENT FOR DENERVATED MUSCLES

Time. It is important that if electrotherapy is to retard the rate of denervation atrophy it should be started in the acute stage, as maximal atrophy occurs in the first 3 months after onset.

Pulse duration, shape of pulse, frequency and rest pause. If there is loss of axon continuity and Wallerian degeneration has set in, the use of long duration exponential progressive currents will produce a good brisk contraction with minimal intensity. The use of progressive currents isolates the denervated muscles and does not pick up any of the surrounding normal muscles. Long duration pulses of up to 2000 milliseconds will help to obtain a brisk contraction with less intensity and less discomfort to the patient.

Neuropraxia — 100 ms rectangular pulses

Axonostenosis and mild axonotmesis — 100 to 600 ms triangular or trapezoidal pulses.

Denervation and degeneration (axonotmesis and neurotmesis) — 100 to 2000 ms triangular or saw-tooth pulses.

Regeneration — Do not use faradic-type currents with maximal contractions. Continue using long duration rectangular pulses, taking care not to overstimulate with high intensities.

Type of contraction. Many workers have agreed that 2 or 3 brief periods of maximal isometric contractions each day will effect maximum benefits in the retardation of atrophy. It is important not to overstimulate with too great an intensity for too long a period as it will have detrimental results on the metabolism and trophic states of the muscle (Guttman and Vodicka). It has been found that 20 to 30 strong isometric contractions at least twice a day is the optimal level of treatment. 90 to 200 moderately strong contractions daily is an alternative method.

It is important to have a rest phase between contractions. An interval of 1 minute should be given between groups of contractions. If 25 to 40 maximal contractions are being given, they should be done in groups of 10 with a 1 to 2 minute rest in between the groups. Great care should be taken to watch for fatigue which will be seen if there is a need to increase the intensity, or if there is obvious fibrillation of the muscle. If 90 to 200 moderate contractions are used, there should be a 1 to 2 minute interval between groups of 30 contractions.

Frequency. The effectiveness of electrotherapy is proportional to the frequency of treatment. Many workers in the past have advocated 2 to 3 treatments per day. It is possible to select simple equipment and teach the patient's family to operate the machine, thus reducing the number of visits to be made to the physiotherapy department. The treatment should be carried out until voluntary activity returns.

Selection of muscles. *Stimulation should be used if there is a strong indication for recovery.* It is of particular value if the lesion will take a year or more for neurotisation to occur since fibrotic differentiation in muscle fibres may be well advanced by this time. Recently early and frequent stimulation of cases with neuropraxia of the common peroneal nerve has proved successful in shortening the recovery period. Maximal contractions are more easily induced in small muscles than in large muscles. It is essential to maintain the function of the small distal muscles particularly, as they tend to fibrose more easily and will take the longest time to recover. Deeper muscles are more difficult to isolate and may need a higher intensity. Large proximal muscles are less likely to fibrose than the small distal muscles.

Length-tension relationships. The starting position of the muscle should be in the lengthened position and well supported to prevent over-stretch and isotonic movement on contraction. The use of the lengthened position of the muscle together with moderate resistance ensures the development of maximal tension, which has been proved as a necessary optimum factor for the retardation of the rate of denervation atrophy. Furthermore isometric maximal contractions in the lengthened position also help in the inhibition of fibrosis. This reduces the extent of the fascicular and intrafascicular fibrosis and agglutination that develop with complete inactivity.

Assessment. Assessment should be carried out by means of voluntary muscle tests, sensory assessment, SDC and EMG reports, chronaxie values and galvanic tetanus ratios to assess recovery or regression. The selection of pulses must depend on electrodiagnosis. Utilisation time obtained from the SDC and chronaxie values can help to determine the pulse duration to be selected for treatment.

Temperature. In order to make sure that minimal intensities are used for maximal contractions, it is necessary to warm the muscles before stimulation. Warming can be done with a warm bath or towel. A raised temperature lowers the rheobase value for the muscle.

Skin resistance. It is important to break down skin resistance by washing the skin and removing all dry scales. A high skin resistance will produce pain and discomfort to the patient as intensities for stimulation are increased.

Oedema. It is necessary to reduce oedema of the denervated area before giving stimulation to the muscles, because higher intensities will be needed to produce a muscle contraction if oedema is present.

CONTRA-INDICATIONS

Oedema. It has been found that gross swelling makes it impossible to stimulate the muscle membrane to obtain depolarisation and muscle contraction. Large intensities of current will be required which will be too painful for the patient to tolerate. A slight swelling can be ignored.

Pain. If the patient has pain in the area to be treated, due to any reason, it is best to investigate the pain and not stimulate the muscle. The underlying pain would make it difficult for the patient to tolerate any intensity.

Scar tissues and contractures. Large amounts of scar tissue in the skin over the muscles to be stimulated and adhesions in the muscle will make it impossible for the current to pass through and produce depolarisation of the muscle membrane.

Temperature. Cold will reduce conductivity of the current into the tissues and heat will aid conductivity, so stimulation is not given to cold muscles.

Skin lesions. Any dermatological conditions will cause pain and discomfort to the patient, as the current will not enter the tissues smoothly. Any large cuts and abrasions that cannot be insulated by vaseline will offer less resistance to the pathway of the current, causing accumulation of current at these points and the possibility of a burn.

Lack of pain sensation. Any gross lack of pain sensation over the entire region of the denervated muscles must be considered as a contra-indication, to avoid the possibility of a burn through overdosage.

Active tuberculosis or cancer. These conditions may be exacerbated by electrical stimulation in the area.

Cardiac pacemakers. The pacemaker function may be inhibited by stimulation in the region of the thorax or the area where the control unit has been inserted.

Thrombosis and thrombophlebitis. Stimulation of muscle contraction may dislodge clot resulting in embolus formation.

Unreliable patients. Patients who are unable to understand instructions or appreciate the dangers of the treatment, for example very old or very young patients.

Superficial metal. Metal in the pathway of the current will concentrate the current and may result in a burn.

Infections. There is a grave danger of spreading infection to adjacent areas via the blood stream if stimulation is given to infected muscles.

SELECTION OF APPARATUS FOR THE TREATMENT OF DENERVATED MUSCLES

The following features are essential to obtain the maximal benefits of electrotherapy for the treatment of denervated muscles.

Choice of pulse duration from 0.02 to 2000 ms. The basic range of pulses needed for denervated muscles is 10 to 100 ms pulses. Some stimulators offer 100 and 600 ms pulses only in a portable generator, as it has been found that these two pulses are most commonly used.

Choice of pulse shape. Generators may or may not give you a choice of the various progressive currents. The following are some of the choices available.

Neurotron 627

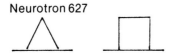

Selection of triangular or rectangular pulses.

Neurotron 626

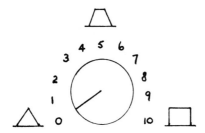

Selection of triangular, trapezoidal and rectangular pulses.
In position 0 the apparatus gives triangular pulses; in position 10 it gives rectangular pulses; from 1 to 9 it gives trapezoidal pulses in which the rise becomes steeper.

The Rank Stanley Cox machine

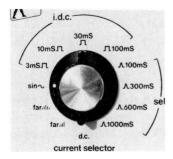

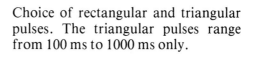

The galvanic-faradic unit

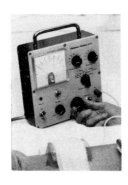

Choice of rectangular and triangular pulses. The triangular pulses range from 100 ms to 1000 ms only.

This offers rectangular pulses only, up to 200 ms.

The pause duration between the pulses can be altered in some generators. In other apparatus the frequency selector switch determines the rest phase in accordance with the pulse duration. It is important that the *rest phase is at least twice the pulse duration* so as to give the muscle time to recover between pulses.

Measuring instruments. It is important to determine whether the circuitry of the stimulation apparatus is a constant voltage circuit or a constant current circuit, that is, whether it is voltage stabilised or current stabilised.

A constant voltage circuit (voltage control, low internal resistance). Here a defined voltage impulse is administered to the skin via the electrodes. The current that flows in the tissues depends upon their resistance. Owing to a capacitor effect in the skin, a current deflection occurs at the beginning of each pulse which falsifies the intended impulse form. Terminal voltage is maintained regardless of variations in patient resistance, but variations in output current to accommodate patient resistance changes can be made.

In constant voltage machines, the measuring instruments read in volts. The galvanic-faradic unit and the Both have constant voltage circuits.

Constant current circuits (current control, high internal resistance). These enforce in the tissue the desired current impulses by correspondingly controlling the voltage during the impulse. Distortion of the impulse is avoided. Constant current apparatus will maintain a pre-set value of output current when the load changes, but its output voltage will vary with the load resistance. In both cases

Ohm's law is satisfied ($U = IR$). The Neurotron apparatus is a constant current machine and the meter is read in milliamperes.

The following figure is a diagrammatic representation of the form of voltage applied to the electrodes and the current flowing in the tissues with constant current (CC) and constant voltage (CV) circuits. The shaded areas indicate distortion of the current impulses compared with the voltage impulses delivered.

It is also important to check the measuring ranges. In the Neurotron the measuring ranges go up to 5, 20, and 80 mA. In the galvanic-faradic unit there are two ranges: 1 to 30 volts and 1 to 120 volts. The ranges can be selected by control buttons or knobs which should be clearly identified.

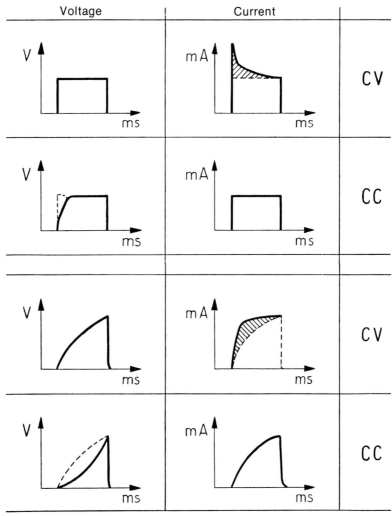

Schematic representation of the form of the voltage applied to the electrodes and the current flowing in the tissue in the case of constant-current (cc) and constant-voltage (cv) circuits, for rectangular and exponentially progressive current impulses. Shaded areas: distortion of the current impulses actually flowing compared with the voltage impulses delivered by the apparatus. (Siemens)

Polarity reversing switch. It is usual with a bipolar technique to see that the cathode is placed distally. Occasionally a better excitation effect may occur if the cathode is applied proximally, so it is always useful to have a polarity reversal switch to see which position is the most excitable. Most generators have a polarity reversal switch.

Mains on/off switch. It is important to ascertain the position of the mains switch and see if it is the only means of cutting off the power supply to the patient. Occasionally the output control for intensity does not cut off the current to the patient when the control is at zero. This must be ascertained before connecting the patient to the terminals. A light generally indicates if the machine is connected to the mains.

Patient terminals. It is important to identify the cathode and the anode terminals. *RED* generally indicates the anode and *BLACK* indicates the cathode.

TECHNIQUE OF APPLICATION

Equipment required
a low frequency stimulator offering long duration pulses and progressive current pulses
two leads
two metal electrodes to fit the muscle to be stimulated if a bipolar technique is to be used, or a metal electrode and a disc or button electrode to fit the muscle to be treated if a monopolar technique is selected
a small table or trolley for the equipment
two bowls of water
soap
towels
protective plastic
bandages or rubber straps to secure the pads and electrodes
pads which are made of absorbent material, such as sponge, Wettex cleaning cloth, lint or gauze pads, all of which must be 10 mm thick when compressed, and 12 mm larger in length and breadth than the electrodes
pillows
vaseline and a wooden spatula
an instrument to test for sharp and blunt

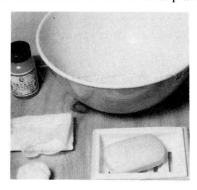
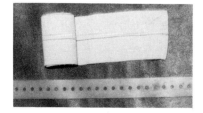

Place the patient in a position that gives the part to be treated support and comfort. Thoroughly wash the part to be treated. Note if lotions, creams or oil have been used. The electrode area should be cleansed by rubbing firmly with alcohol to remove any dry scaly skin. Be careful not to break down the skin when rubbing a flaccid area or a recently healed scar. Insulate all minor cuts, abrasions, and raised edges with vaseline. Protect the patient's clothing from water. Place the muscles to be treated in a stretched position, but also supported.

Do not over-stretch. Ensure that stretch is in the direction of the longitudinal axis of the muscle. In two joint muscles, relax one joint and stretch the muscles over the other joint. As an alternative, the muscle can be positioned in the neutral resting state.

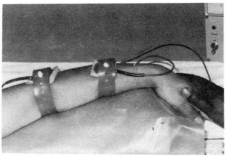

(a) with muscles stretched;   (b) neutral position.

Position of the limb

Explain the basic physiological effects of the current on the denervated muscles as the prevention of marked denervation atrophy, the maintenance of extensibility of muscle, the prevention of contractures, and the maintenance of the nutrition of the muscle.

Explain the sensation to be experienced — a mild prickling sensation followed by muscle contraction and relaxation.

Check that there are no contraindications to treatment with low frequency currents.

Check that the patient can differentiate between sharp and blunt. Check the return of any voluntary activity.

Warm the part to be treated with a hot towel or a warm bath. Check the temperature of the towel or hot soak before applying it to the patient.

Test the integrity of the leads and machine terminals. Ensure that the leads are not broken inside the insulation. Also check the safety of the machine plug and wall socket.

Test the polarity of the terminals by placing the terminal ends into a bowl of water and connecting the terminals to the direct current circuitry, using the maximum intensity possible. After about 2 minutes bubbles of gas will appear at the cathode.

Check that the meter needle is going smoothly through its whole range.

Ensure firm connection of the leads to the terminals.

Check the smooth working of the knobs and switches in all the controls of the machine, with no breakages in the insulation of the controls.

Check the patient's assessment data. Look at the strength-duration curve and identify the *utilisation time*. Look at the electromyogram report or nerve conduction tests if available. Assess the extent of denervation and follow the guidelines for selection of suitable pulses.

Demonstrate the current on yourself. Place the two electrodes and pads on the table, position your forearm on the pads, position the dials on the current selected and demonstrate to the patient the muscle contraction that will occur. *Do not fake the contraction*. Be completely relaxed when you demonstrate. If using a pad electrode and button electrode, place your supinated forearm on the pad and hold the button electrode in your hand.

Position the apparatus so that the controls can be reached comfortably, while simultaneously holding the electrodes on to the patient and facing the patient. Ensure that all dials are at zero and the leads firmly fixed at the terminals.

Soak the pads in warm water. Squeeze the water out of the pads, leaving sufficient moisture to make a wet pad. Take care that it is not dripping all over the patient, as this will mean that current will pass to other muscles.

For large muscles the bipolar technique is selected by positioning the two electrodes and pads on either end of the muscle belly. Ensure that the electrodes are not on the tendinous parts but lie at the poles of the muscular belly or the ends of the muscular region. The cathode is generally placed at the distal end.

For small muscles use the monopolar technique. The indifferent is generally placed away from the muscle either on the opposite side of the part or on a nerve trunk, provided it does not stimulate another nerve. The safest place is one which is not connected to the denervated muscle groups. The cathode is placed on the muscle belly slightly distally.

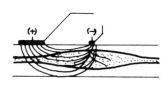

Monopolar technique

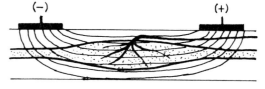

Bipolar technique

Ensure that the electrodes are firmly connected to the skin via the pads. There should be 12 mm of pad visible around the electrode when it is positioned on the pad. A piece of protective plastic should cover the pad before bandaging with a crepe bandage or a perforated rubber strap. Ensure that there is firm but not too strong a contact between the pad and the skin, to prevent occlusion of the circulation.

Warn the patient to tell you if the area under the electrodes gets too uncomfortable, hot or painful. Request the patient not to move or touch any of the apparatus. This is to ensure that the electrodes do not get dislodged and cause a burn.

The controls of the machine should be positioned at the selected pulse wave. Increase the intensity dial slowly until a muscle contraction occurs. Keep asking the patient if the sensation he experiences is comfortable and tolerable.

Dosage
If the muscle is in a stretched position give 30 to 40 strong contractions with resistance. Give a 2-second rest between each contraction. Treat the patient daily. Stop when voluntary contractions occur.

If the muscle is in the neutral position, then give 200 contractions in groups of 30 contractions. There should be at least a 2-minute rest between each group of 30 contractions. Treat the patient daily. Stop when voluntary activity returns.

Progression
Check each day if the selected pulse duration and shape are still suitable, to obtain the best near-normal active contraction with the least amount of intensity. For example, if the patient was reacting to a 1000 ms triangular pulse and the strength duration curve shows some signs of recovery, the patient will probably react better to a 600 ms triangular pulse. Progressively as recovery takes place, there will be a need to change the pulses to 100 ms triangular, then down to 100 ms rectangular, until shorter durations are seen to be the most satisfactory currents. By this time voluntary activity has generally returned, and all electrical stimulation can be stopped.

Recording of treatment
The following items must be recorded each time the patient is treated:

Description of pulse wave selected	— pulse duration, shape, rest pause or frequency.
Position of muscle	— stretched with resistance, neutral resting position.
Strength of contraction	— strong, moderate, minimal.
Number of contractions	— 40 in groups of 10, 200 in groups of 30.
Quality of contraction	— brisk, slow, worm-like and slow, fibrillations from fatigue if and when it sets in.
Time	— time taken to give the prescribed number of contractions.
Rheobase	— measured in volts or amperes.
Signs and symptoms	— pain, oedema, dry scaly skin, sensory function, temperature.

DANGERS

Burns (electrical and chemical)
The following precautions must be taken to prevent burns.

Do not position the electrodes over abrasions, cuts, new skin or recent scar tissue. Current tends to collect over these points or raised edges, thus precipitating a burn.

Remove all metal in the pathway of the current. The metal against the dry skin will tend to concentrate the current and cause a burn.

Do not stimulate muscles through a dry scaly skin with high resistance, as current will accumulate on the dry skin and cause discomfort, pain and a burn.

Ensure that there are no impurities or chemicals in the pads, as this could produce a chemical burn, particularly if long-duration pulses are being given.

Make sure that the pad is 10 mm thick when compressed, or it will be possible to get a chemical burn with long duration pulses if treatment is given at the same spot for long periods of time.

Make sure that the electrode is in the center of the pad and bandaged on firmly to prevent the electrode slipping and touching the bare skin, causing a burn.

Shock

The following precautions must be taken to prevent shocks to patient or therapist:

Make certain that the mains plug has an earthed socket. Do not use a two-pin plug.

Make sure that the output control is at zero before connecting the machine to the patient or the patient will receive a shock if the output is high on connection.

Dry scaly skin will require time for moisture to penetrate the tissues, and the patient will get a shock when a large intensity suddenly penetrates the tissues. So it is necessary to moisten the skin and remove all dry scales before increasing the current intensity.

Ensure that the metal casing of the equipment is not damaged.

Tissue damage

The following precautions must be taken to prevent any harm to the muscles stimulated.

It is important *not to over-stimulate a denervated muscle* to the point of fatigue. Fatigue will retard the progress of recovery.

Do not stimulate over recent fracture sites or if non-union of fractures is present. Contractions of muscle groups could cause displacement, and in recent fractures the healing process could be disturbed.

Do not over-stretch the muscles or give too strong a resistance while treating patients with the stretch and maximal contraction technique, as it will produce irreversible damage to the tendon.

Do not treat a recovering nerve after denervation and degeneration changes have occurred, as it is thought *to hamper re-myelination of the nerve*.

Do not treat a patient with an *external or implanted pacemaker* as it will interfere with the circuit of the pacemaker.

In treating geriatic patients, ensure that the patient does not fall asleep. Be aware that they may have a high skin resistance, poor sensation and may be hard of hearing.

In treating deaf patients make sure that they have understood all instructions and warnings.

8.7   High Voltage Galvanic Stimulation

Physical Properties

High voltage galvanic generators produce a high voltage current with a high peak intensity but a low average current, and a very short pulse duration.

The high peak intensity, usually produced as a twin pulse, can reach a maximum of 300 to 400 milliamperes. These peaks are safe, however, because of the short pulse duration, and have the advantage of penetrating deeper than the currents produced by low voltage generators. Thus direct stimulation of deep nerves and muscles can be very effective, and, using appropriate techniques, a muscle can be stimulated to contract in isolation or as part of a total pattern of movement.

The short pulse duration, ranging between 50 and 100 microseconds, permits selective stimulation of sensory and motor axons with little effect on the pain fibres, so is more comfortable to the patient. With such short pulse durations, the chemical effects of low voltage interrupted direct current have not been demonstrated, and stimulation can safely be maintained for longer periods of time.

High voltage galvanism will not produce contraction in denervated muscles as the pulse duration is too short to depolarize the muscle membrane. However partially or totally innervated muscles will respond to high voltage galvanism.

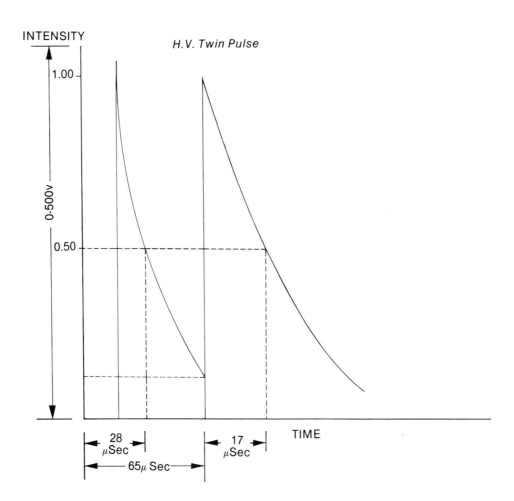

INDICATIONS

At present there are no published results of clinical studies of the use of high voltage galvanism. However it may be assumed that high voltage galvanism will achieve the same results as low voltage stimulation, with the exception of the treatment of denervated muscles. Studies are currently being conducted and their findings are awaited with interest. The following effects are claimed, based on unsubstantiated clinical observations.

Pain reduction. It is suggested that pain may be reduced by either of two methods.

(*a*)   By providing supra painful stimuli in a very narrow area, using very very small electrodes closely spaced.

(*b*)   By minimizing pain fibre stimulation and providing for maximal sensory fibre stimulation using larger electrodes with careful intensity control so that sensory fibre stimulation which is not painful occurs.

These methods are thought to stimulate the release in the central nervous system of an opiate substance (endorphins) which acts to suppress pain. This effect has yet to be demonstrated on humans.

In particular, high voltage galvanism has been found to be effective in the relief of pain in arthritis, radicular pain, bursitis, sprains and strains.

Increased joint mobility. The reduction of pain by high voltage galvanism may increase joint mobility. Other mechanisms may include the direct effect on blood vessels, increasing circulation, or other effects on joint connective tissues which are yet to be proven. In particular, high voltage galvanism has been found to increase range following fractures, menisectomy, osteoarthritis and frozen shoulder.

Increase in peripheral circulation. This may be achieved by stimulating intermittent muscle contractions simulating the muscle pump effect on the venous circulation.

Alternatively, the deeper penetration of the high voltage current may stimulate the sympathetic neurons directly causing vasodilatation.

Healing of ulcers. There are two possible explanations:

(*a*)   a positive electrical potential exists in the ulcer and by adding external positive current the repair process is accelerated; it is also suggested that electrical stimulation with the negative pole will destroy any bacteria present.

(*b*)   healing may be hastened by the increase in superficial circulation stimulated by the high voltage current.

Decreased muscle spasm. The strong muscle contractions produced by the high voltage stimulation may result in greater muscle relaxation. Alternatively, the relief of pain may result in reduction of muscle spasm.

Reduction of post-traumatic oedema. Clinical observations in U.S.A. have found that immediately after treatment with high voltage galvanism there was a significant reduction of oedema. However the mechanism of this effect may be complex and no attempts have been made to explain the observed effect.

CONTRAINDICATIONS

Although the literature fails to recommend any contraindications, it would be advisable to observe the contraindications for the use of low frequency currents, in particular interrupted direct current.

DOSAGE

Intensity. The intensity is governed by the patient's tolerance and therefore intact pain sensation must be ensured. In cases of oedema, muscle spasm and reduced joint mobility the intensity should be high enough to produce a muscle contraction.

Pulse Rate Setting. 80 pulses per second.

Switching Rate Setting (surge). The current may be applied continuously or in a surged manner.

Electrodes. The electrodes should generally be selected as follows:
(*a*)   active electrode (usually the anode) — large enough to cover the entire painful or oedematous area, or affected joint; in the case of muscle spasm, two active electrodes are used, one on the muscle belly and the other on the musculo-tendinous junction.
(*b*)   the dispersive electrode (usually the cathode) is positioned in the lumbar region.

Treatment Time. Treatment is usually applied for 20 minutes, although in cases of oedema 30 minutes may be more effective. It is recommended that high voltage galvanism be preceded by the use of hot packs in cases of pain, reduced joint mobility and muscle spasm, and followed by ultrasound, joint mobilization and mild stretching techniques in cases of pain, reduced joint mobility and muscle spasm.

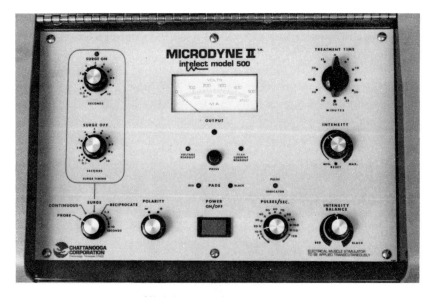

High Voltage Galvanic Unit

8.8   Diadynamic currents

Diadynamic currents have been used in Europe for many years and have recently been introduced in Australia. The majority of the literature available is in European journals and is rarely translated into English, therefore local clinical studies will be welcomed to confirm the benefits of these currents.

PHYSICAL PROPERTIES

There are generally five different currents available for diadynamic therapy.

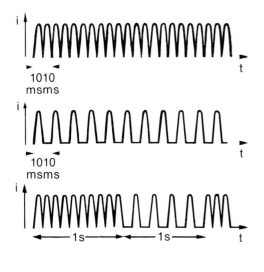

Fixed Diphase (DF) This is a full wave rectified alternating current with a frequency of 50 Hz.

Fixed Monophase (MF) This is a half wave rectified alternating current with a frequency of 50 Hz.

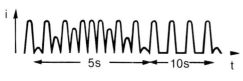

Short Periods (CP) Equal phases of DF and MF are alternated without intervening pauses.

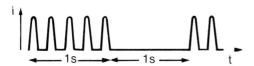

Long Periods (LP) This consists of a 10 second phase of MF followed by a 5 second phase of DF in which the peak intensity is varied, with a general tendency to rise and then fall.

Syncopal Rhythm (RS) This consists of a 1 second phase of MF followed by a 1 second rest phase.

Thus diadynamic currents are basically a variation of sinusoidal currents.

PHYSIOLOGICAL EFFECTS

Diadynamic currents have been shown to be primarily effective in the relief of pain. According to Henke (1958) this effect is due to a combination of the following physiological reactions.

Masking. Stimulation of a sensory nerve may not always cause excitation, but its excitability is altered so that the stimulation threshold is raised. Bernard recommends the DF current as being particularly effective in producing masking.

Vasomotor effects. Stimulation with diadynamic currents produces vasodilatation and hyperaemia as a result of the release of histamine in the tissues. As the current flows primarily in the superficial tissues, this effect is unlikely to occur in deeper structures except perhaps by reflex activity.

Muscle stimulation. Particularly when the CP and LP currents are used, muscle contraction will be stimulated, resulting in an increase in the blood flow to the muscles.

Stimulation of vibration sense. This is said to cause central masking of pain.

INDICATIONS

Diadynamic currents are recommended for the relief of pain and oedema in the following types of conditions:

Soft tissue injury — sprains, contusions, epicondylitis
Joint disorders — post-immobilisation, arthritis
Circulatory disorders — raynaud's disease, migraine
Peripheral nerve disorders — neuralgia, neuritis, herpes zoster, radiculopathies

CONTRAINDICATIONS

Diadynamic currents should not be used in the presence of any condition which is a contraindication to the use of low frequency currents. These have been detailed earlier in this unit.

METHODS OF APPLICATION

The choice of application should be based on the clinical problems presented. Various methods may be selected.

Pain spot application. The two electrodes may be applied as a bipolar technique, with the anode applied over the pain spot and the cathode adjacent to it. Alternatively, the cathode may be applied proximally on the limb, or over the nerve root supplying the painful area (monopolar technique).

Nerve trunk application. The two electrodes are placed along the course of the appropriate peripheral nerve where the nerve is superficial. The patient should feel a tingling sensation in the area supplied by the nerve stimulated.

Paravertebral application. The electrodes may be applied on both sides of the spine at the level of the nerve root supplying the painful area. If several nerve roots are involved, the electrodes may be applied alongside the spine at the highest and lowest nerve root levels.

Vasotropic application. The electrodes are applied along the vascular paths affected in the circulatory disorder being treated.

Myo-energetic application. To produce muscle stimulation the two electrodes are positioned at each end of the muscle belly. Alternatively, a monopolar technique may be used with one electrode on the motor point of the muscle and the other proximally to it.

Transregional application. To treat a joint, electrodes may be positioned on opposite sides of the joint.

Electrodes are generally available in a variety of sizes, as metal plate electrodes, yoke electrodes, and suction electrodes. The electrodes should be separated from the skin by moist sponge pads.

DOSAGE

Current type

DF is primarily used for the initial treatment and before the application of other currents. It is also used in the treatment of circulatory disorders. The patient feels a prickling sensation which subsides after a short time. Muscle contraction only occurs at high intensities.

MF is used for the treatment of pain without muscle spasm, following a preliminary application of DF. The patient feels a strong, penetrating vibration which persists for longer than the sensation of DF. Muscle contraction occurs at lower intensities than with DF.

CP is used for the treatment of traumatic pain. In the DF phase the patient feels a fine tremor which rapidly diminishes, and in the MF phase, a strong, constant vibration. With sufficient intensity rhythmic contraction of muscles occurs.

LP has a long-lasting analgesic effect, particularly in the treatment of myalgia. It is also used in combination with CP in the treatment of neuralgia. The patient is aware of the strong vibrational MF phase giving way to the prickling of the DF phase which rises and falls slowly.

RS is used for faradic-type stimulation of muscles and can be used to test the excitability of motor nerves.

Intensity

The intensity should be increased slowly until a definite vibration or prickling is felt, but without any pain or burning sensation. Continuous (tetanic) muscle contraction should not occur.

Duration

It is recommended that the total application should not exceed 10 to 12 minutes. Most single applications are given for 3 minutes.

Frequency

Generally 6 or 7 treatments are necessary and these are given daily or every second day.

8.9 Summary of the Use of Low Frequency Currents

Nerve and muscle are both excitable tissues and when stimulated by electric currents respond in a characteristic manner. The degree of response depends on the strength of the exciting stimulus and its duration. Abnormality of muscle function is often met, and it is important to determine the specific underlying neurological dysfunction that produced the abnormality. A study of the lesions that occur in the control of the motor unit is important to enable the physiotherapist to assess the patient and formulate treatment.

Electric currents are effective in stimulating nerve and muscle, and can be graduated accurately. They are the most suitable type of stimulation for producing contraction of muscles directly or by way of nerves for therapeutic and diagnostic purposes. Low frequency currents are used as a means of electro-exercise, electro-analgesia, electrodiagnosis, and electro-osmosis of medications.

The factors influencing the effectiveness of a stimulus are the magnitude of the change and the rate of change. The rate of change of the stimulus is important because of the phenomenon of accommodation. Nerve accommodates well and cannot be stimulated by a change of several volts or milliamperes if the change is gradual over a period of 100 to 1000 milliseconds. Muscle does not accommodate as well and is stimulated by a stimulus that is increased gradually in intensity and has a duration of 100 to 1000 ms.

Muscle loses what little accommodation it has in denervation, and hence long duration, slow-rising pulses can be used effectively for exercising the muscle to delay atrophy, maintain its extensibility, and to maintain the nutrition of the muscle by encouraging muscle metabolism through its contractility. The use of short duration pulses from 0.02 ms to 1 ms, sharply rising to a maximum intensity is used for exercising weak muscles to initiate remembrance of the pattern of movement when lost, or to hypertrophy a weak muscle. If used effectively with exercise, it reduces the rehabilitation period of the patient.

High voltage galvanism is currently gaining popularity in America, though there is no documented evidence of its effectiveness. It may be a useful tool in the treatment of pain, oedema, joint stiffness and muscle spasm, and is more comfortable for the patient than many low frequency currents in use today.

Diadynamic currents are a variation of sinusoidal currents. The various forms of currents produced are useful in the relief of pain and oedema in a variety of conditions.

References

Amrein, L and others, 1971, Use of low voltage electrotherapy and electromyography in physical therapy, *Phys Ther*, December, 1283.

Anderson, S A et al, 1976, Evaluation of pain suppressive effect of different frequencies of peripheral electrical stimulation in chronic pain conditions, *Acta Orthop Scand*, 47, 14.

Bernard, P D, 1950, La Thérapie diadynamique, *Les Editions Naim*, Paris.

Bowman, Harry D and Shaffer, Kathryn L, 1957, Physiological basis of electrical stimulation of human muscle and its clinical application, *Phys Ther Rev, 37*, 207-223.

Brain, R, 1969, Diseases of the nervous system, *Oxford University Press*.

Brand, P W, 1928, The care of insensitive feet, *Proc XII World Cong Rehab Internl*, 3, 6, 9, and 10.

Clayton's Electrotherapy and actinotherapy, P M Scott, 6th ed, *London: Balliere*, 1969.

Collins, E D, Montgomery, E and Stanton, S L, 1972, Treating incontinence electrically, *B M J*, July 3: 112-113.

Collins, E D, Urethral incontinence in women. Observations on the effect of electrical stimulation, *Roy Soc Med — Proc*, 1972, 832.

Darling, Robert, MD and Downey, John, MD, 1971, Physiologic basis of rehabilitation medicine, *W B Saunders Co, Philadelphia*.

Davey, Conolly and Masman, 1976, Clinical evaluation of the Masman pressure unit, *Aust J Phys,* 4 Dec.

Downer, A H, 1970, Physical therapy procedures, Selected techniques, *Springfield, Ill, Thomas*.

Dumoulin, J and others, 1971, Treatment of peripheral neurogenic disorders of excitatory motor currents, *Electrodiagn Ther, 8,* 28-43 (in French).

Erb, W, 1868, Zur Pathologie und pathologische Anatomie peripherischer Paralysen, *Deut Arch Klin Med, 4*, 535.

Furness, M A, 1972, Prevention of dehabilitation in leprosy, *Proc XII World Cong Rehab Internl*.

Gerrish, H H and Brown, W C, 1964, Electricity, *Woodheart-Willcos, Homewood, Ill*.

Gilbert, Esther, 1974, Kinesitherapy of the flat valgus feet, *Proc WCPT, Montreal*.

Glen, E S, 1972, Treating incontinence electrically, *BMJ, July*, 1972, 292

Gracanin, F et al, 1975, Optimal stimulus parameters for minimum pain in the chronic stimulation of innervated muscle, *Arch Phys Med Rehab*, 56, 243, 249.

Greguis, J and Pfefferova, H, 1973, Comparison of various types of physiotherapy with reference to the specific effects of the sonodynator, *Fysiatr Rheum Vestn*, 56, 4, 215-222.

Groenewald, J M, 1973, The treatment of rectal incontinence by surged faradic-type current stimulation, *S Afr Med J*, 16/6/73, 1005.

Haslam, L M, 1973, Electrotherapy '72, Report of a survey, *Physio Can*, October.

Henke, G, 1958, The mode of action of diadynamic currents according to Bernard, *S R W News*, 7, 13-15.

Johnson and others, 1977, The Russian study of faradism in the treatment of chondromalacia patellae, *Physio Can, December, 29,* 5.

Kiesswetter, H, 1972, Treating incontinence electrically, *BMJ*, 1972, 768.

Licht, S, ed, 1967, Therapeutic electricity and ultraviolet radiation, *New Haven, Conn, Licht*.

Livenson, A R, 1974, Aspects of the electrical hazards of electrical equipment, *Biomed Eng, 7*, July, 277–280.

McQuire, 1975, Electrotherapy and exercises for stress incontinence, *Physio*, October.

Moore, T, 1972, Treating incontinence electrically, *BMJ*, 589.

Morozova, G P, 1969, Treatment of Dupuytren's contracture with diadynamic current in combination with paraffin applications, *Vopr Kurortol Fizioter Lech Fiz Kult*, 34, 1, 78–9.

Nikolova-Troeva, L, Feb, 1968, The modern electrotherapeutic methods in the therapy of endarteritis obliterans, *Ther der Gegan*, 190–198.

Nikolova-Troeva, L, 1969, Physiotherapeutic rehabilitation in the presence of fracture complications, *Münch Med Woche, 111:11,* 592-599.

Photiades, D P, 1972, Pulsed electrical energy for soft tissue injuries, *BMJ*, August, 417.

Schach, R P, 1972, Urinary stress incontinence, *S Afr Med J*, 845.

Shaffer, D V, Branes, G K, Wakim, K G, Sayre, G P and Krusen, F H, 1954, The influence of electrical stimulation on the course of denervation atrophy, *Arch Phys Med, 35*, 491.

Smeralova, V et al, 1975, Clinical experience with combined therapy of ultrasound and diadynamic currents, *Fysiatr Rheum Vestn*, 53, 5, 304–8.

Vodovnik, L et al, 1965, Pain response to different tetanizing currents, *Arch Phys Med Rehab*, 46, 187–192.

Wakim, K G and Krusen, F H, 1955, The influence of electrical stimulation on the work output and endurance of denervated muscle, *Arch Phys Med, 36*, 370.

Walker, 1976, Sequential faradism on quadriceps re-education, *Physiother, 62*, No 8.

Werner, J, Electrical stimulation for peroneal palsy, *Phys Ther, 48*, 12.

Wheeler, P C, Wolcott, 1969, Accelerated healing of skin ulcers by electrotherapy, *South Med J, 62*, 795.

Wynn Parry, C, 1973, Rehabilitation of the hand, *London: Butterworth*.

9 Medium Frequency Currents

9.1 Interferential Currents
9.2 Transcutaneous Nerve Stimulators
9.3 Summary of Medium Frequency Currents
References

Some Key Points in this Unit

Medium frequency currents alternate the direction of the flow of electrons at a frequency between 3000 and 6000 Hz. They stimulate sensory and motor nerves, and meet with little skin resistance.

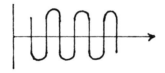

Interference therapy uses two medium frequency currents around 4000 Hz to evoke interference currents between 1 and 100 Hz.

Transcutaneous nerve stimulation is a technique of neuromodulation that affects the sensory pathways by modifying the impulses. It leads to the relief of pain.

9.1 Interferential Currents

The use of medium frequency currents selected within a range of 3900 and 5100 Hz for therapeutic purposes was originated in Austria by Nemec of Vienna and has been in use in Europe for the last twenty years. Nemec overcame the difficulty of applying low frequency alternating currents to deeper tissues by using medium frequency currents around 4000 Hz to overcome skin resistance. Two such currents when properly applied evoke an interference current between 1 and 100 Hz. The use of interferential therapy is gaining popularity internationally, and it merits careful examination of its selective usage today.

PRINCIPLES OF INTERFERENCE THERAPY

Interferential therapy is a method of producing low frequency alternating currents selectively at any tissue depth, without the problem of skin resistance.

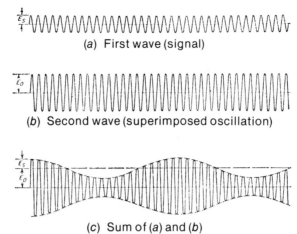

(a) First wave (signal)

(b) Second wave (superimposed oscillation)

(c) Sum of (a) and (b)

The result of superimposing two waves of different frequencies. The frequency of the envelope pulsation (heterodyne wave) is the difference between the original frequencies.

The problem of skin resistance. Low frequency stimulators used today produce currents with frequencies which vary from 0.5 to 1000 Hz. These currents meet resistance from the skin, allowing only a small proportion of the current to enter the tissues. High frequency currents such as short wave diathermy and microwave diathermy are too high in frequency to stimulate skin or muscle, and have mainly thermal effects.

Skin impedance diminishes with increase of frequency according to the formula:

$$Z = \frac{1}{2\pi FC} \quad \text{where } Z = \text{impedance in ohms}$$

F = frequency in Hz

C = capacity of the skin in microfarads

The above formula gives values for measurement of skin resistance of

at   50 Hz = 3200 ohms per 100 cm^2

at 4000 Hz = 40 ohms per 100 cm^2

So it becomes evident that it should be possible to irradiate the tissues more deeply and accurately without polar effects at the skin if medium frequency currents are used.

The interference effect. When two differing unmodulated medium frequency alternating currents are applied simultaneously to the tissues, through paired electrodes, a vibration is generated in the tissues where the currents cross. In this area where the two currents are heterodyned, the intensity of the combined currents will increase and decrease rhythmically. This is the *interference effect*. The combined current has a beat frequency which is the difference between the two medium frequencies. If the incoming frequencies are 4000 Hz and 4100 Hz, then the beat frequency is 100 Hz. *The beat frequency is thus a modulated alternating current* with a surge speed which is varied at will. The intensity of the beat current is the sum of the two currents.

In the interferential therapy units one circuit is kept constant at one frequency and a beat frequency can be selected by altering the frequency of the second circuit. For example, if one circuit is 4000 Hz and a beat frequency of 50 Hz is required, the second circuit is selected at 4050 Hz.

Principles of production of the interference effect. Interferential apparatus is equipped with two oscillators which produce a fixed frequency in one circuit, and a variable frequency in the other circuit. The apparatus in use today utilises frequencies from 4000 to 5100 Hz.

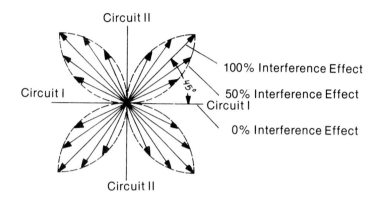

Static Interferential Field

It is possible to let the interferential frequency make a frequency swing allowing a rhythmical progression covering the entire frequency range. A *frequency range* means that the actual interferential current continuously changes between two limiting values following a certain pattern, for example, from 20 to 80 Hz. The biological effects in the tissues are due primarily to low frequency currents which can be varied in many ways to gain the desired physiological effects.

The medium frequency currents are applied to the tissues of the body by means of a pair of electrodes for each circuit, generally using a quadripolar technique. An unmodulated sinusoidal AC signal of fixed frequency is applied to one pair of electrodes, and another pre-selected frequency within the given range is applied to the other pair of electrodes.

The four electrodes are positioned so that the area where the two currents cross each other, or are heterodyned, is directly over the lesion. It is easy to detect the polarity of the electrode by the color of the knob, and to identify the electrodes carrying one circuit. The wires are colored red and white.

Variations of interference. Interference frequencies come in automatic pre-selected modes with the desired intensity at a constant level. The following basic modes are found in all apparatus:

Frequency scale: 1 to 100 Hz constant frequency
1 to 10 Hz rhythmic frequency
90 to 100 Hz rhythmic frequency

The word 'rhythmic' indicates that the frequency swings continuously, changing the frequencies from the lower value to the higher value. It may take 10 seconds to go up and 5 seconds to come down. 'Constant frequency' indicates that the interference current is as indicated by the scale.

Frequency swings by two control knobs. The Bosch and the Endomed have two controls whereby any variation of a lower and higher value can be selected. The Bosch has pre-selections varying from 0 to 100 Hz, and the Endomed has pre-selections varying from 0 to 150 Hz. For example in the Endomed, if a frequency swing from 20 to 70 Hz is required, adjust the steady frequency control to 20 Hz and the frequency swing control to 50 Hz.

Skin current compensations. A skin current tends to occur when the electrodes of two separate circuits are close together if these are of opposite polarity. The current tends to take the easy pathway presented along the skin between the two electrodes of the two separate circuits instead of going through the tissues. This can be avoided by ensuring that like poles lie adjacent to each other. The Endomed is equipped with an indicator which signals the onset of skin currents, and has a control knob which eliminates them.

Interferential vector system. One of the advantages of the interferential field is that specific areas of tissues at any depth can be treated with the pulsed low frequency stimulator. The interference currents set up across the field are distributed unequally. In patients who have a diffuse area of pathology, and where the accuracy of lesion within the static interferential field is doubtful, the Nemectrodyn 5 and 8 have developed a vector principle which produces a

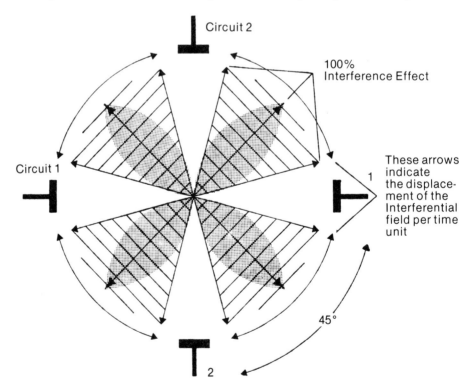

The Interferential Rotating Vector System

scanning movement of the interferential field similar to that of a radar beam, so that all parts of the tissue are subject to the maximum interference effect. The interference field is rotated to an angle of 45° in each direction. The push button for the vector system in the Nemectrodyn displaces the static interferential field and generates a dynamic interferential field covering the whole area.

However, because the interferential field is scanning the tissues, only part of the treatment time will be spent treating the lesion. Therefore the vector system should only be selected if the site of the lesion cannot be accurately localised.

Electrokinesy. The Endomed has a further variation termed electrokinesy, where the interferential current is generated inside the unit before it is applied to the patient. The actual current applied to the patient is 4000 Hz but carrying a low frequency modulation. The modulation is set at 50 Hz. The current is applied via a glove electrode worn by the therapist.

Surged current. The Endomed has an arrangement whereby the current produced in the electrokinesy mode is further surged. The number of surges may be varied from 2 to 12 per minute.

Interferential current with galvanism (DC). In the Endomed it is possible to give interferential therapy combined with direct current and also to select a suitable pole for the tissues.

Stereodynamic Interferential currents. These currents have recently been developed to attempt to overcome the problem that conventional interferential tends to be basically two-dimensional, whereas the body tissues are three-dimensional. Three pairs of electrodes are used, commonly the star electrode shown below.

The stereodynamic interferential waveform exhibits an additional modulation which is said to be a more effective current as there is likely to be less adaptation and habituation to it.

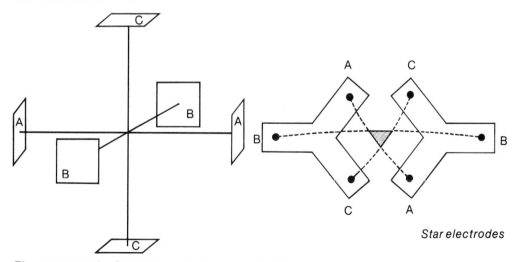

Star electrodes

The concept of a Stereodynamic Interferential Current
A diagrammatic representation of the concept of a three dimensional interferential field. Also shown are the 'star' electrodes used to deliver the current to the patient.

Calibration of circuits. Each apparatus has a calibration mode which ensures that the intensity in both circuits is balanced and the ground frequencies of both circuits are equalised.

The Nemectrodyn 5 and 8 and the Bosch have an automatic calibration unit. The old Electrodyn and the Endomed have control knobs which permit calibration. It is important to calibrate carefully before turning up the intensity. Calibration in the Endomed takes practice, and it is important for the therapist to become familiar with this operation before turning up the intensity. All apparatus generally has an indicator which shows when the optimum level of calibration has been reached.

Oscilloscopes. Some brands of equipment have an oscilloscope which displays the interference mode being applied to the patient.

PHYSIOLOGICAL EFFECTS OF INTERFERENTIAL THERAPY

The physiological effects on the tissues depend on the following factors:
frequency range selected;
the use of rhythmic or constant frequency swings;
intensity of current used;
accuracy in electrode placement with good calibration and no skin currents;
accurate localisation of the lesion;
patency of circulation and neurological function;
underlying pathophysiology in relation to the desired effect.

100 Hz constant. These currents cause oscillations which have marked amplitude and cause fine vibration of ions without producing heat. The fine vibrations act on the sensory nerve endings, producing an analgesic effect. This may occur via Sweet and Wall's theory of large fibre stimulation. Here minimal stimulation of large diameter fibres causes a mild tingling sensation and interferes with the perception of pain. A 10 to 15 minute stimulation can produce relief of pain lasting for over an hour.

Lim has stated that pain receptor sites are anionic or rich in electrons, while analgesic agents such as plasma peptides are cationic or deficient in electrons. It is possible that the interferential current could alter the distribution of the ions locally. The refractory period of nerve is 1 ms. As medium frequency currents are 4000 Hz or thereabouts, repeated stimuli come within the refractory period and thus cause no further excitation. Consequently the use of higher frequencies leads to rapid fatigue of the pain receptors of the skin.

Direct stimulation by the interference current at a constant 100 Hz produces inhibition of the sympathetic system. The passage of interference currents through the stellate ganglion will relieve causalgia or pain seen in patients with reflex sympathetic dystrophy, such as the shoulder-hand syndrome. Skin temperature changes can be noted if the interference current is given to the cervical sympathetic ganglion.

Increased vasodilatation is seen following the use of interference currents on the sympathetic ganglion. This could also help to relieve pain by removing the pain metabolites, and mobilising exudate if present.

1 to 10 Hz constant. This module has a more specific effect on motor nerves and causes muscle contraction, including mobilisation of tissue ions. The sensation of muscle contraction produced by interferential currents is different from that produced by faradic-type currents. There is less sensory stimulus, a greater depth of contraction and it is quite pleasant to feel. *It will stimulate only normal innervated muscles.*

1 to 100 Hz rhythmic. The use of the rhythmic modulations of the interferential current produces more stimulating fine vibrations of the ions, and further facilitates ion movement in the cells. There is alternate rhythmic excitation and relaxation of the tissues, producing more active hyperaemia and increased cellular activity. There is some alteration of the permeability of the cell membrane, which aids ion movement to and from the cells.

There is also an increase in venous and lymphatic flow, and an increase in the tone of tissues and vessels which aid in the relief of oedema and in facilitating the healing process.

90 to 100 Hz rhythmic. This is an automatic frequency change from 90 to 100 to 90 Hz in a 15-second cadence. The basic effect of this interference mode is analgesic, and it also has a vasodilatory effect on the tissues. It is particularly useful for neuralgic types of pain like migraine and brachial neuralgia. There is much less adaptation and habituation than with 100 Hz constant.

1 to 10 Hz rhythmic. This has a stimulating effect on motor nerves and tissues. It has increased vasodilatory effects and, if applied over exudate which is tenacious and gross, it will have a vigorous pumping effect which will help to start the physiological mechanisms for the absorption of the exudate.

Electrokinesy (50 Hz with a 4000 Hz current). This mode of interference is used with glove electrodes worn by the therapist. It is useful for patients with pain and muscle spasm. 'Deblocking' the spasm is brought about by giving strong contractions to the muscle in spasm for 2 to 3 minutes. It breaks the cycle causing over-activity of the muscle spindle. A strong *surged* electrokinesy current can be used as it is comfortable for the patient.

Impulse current. This is a rectified medium frequency DC current, surged at 50 Hz. The frequency is 4000 Hz with a pulse duration of 0.1 ms. It produces a strong sustained analgesic effect and can be applied by a bipolar technique.

INDICATIONS

Pain. The treatment of pain with interferential therapy is best effected by treating both the cause and the referred pain pathway directly. Selection of 100 Hz constant or 90 to 100 Hz rhythmic has marked analgesic effects for pain which is of sympathetic origin, such as causalgia, reflex sympathetic dystrophy, migraine, and neuralgia. Pain caused by stump complications, herpes zoster, and vascular insufficiencies without any skin breakdown are also effectively treated. For herpes zoster it is best to give as maximal a current as the patient can bear.

Interferential therapy is not effective in post-traumatic pain in the acute stages, but is effective in cases of chronic pain with or without swelling, particularly after prolonged immobilisation in plaster of Paris. It is more effective than ice packs.

Muscle spasm. Electrokinesy currents have been used by some therapists to give strong contractions to muscle spasm, to interrupt the cycle of pain metabolites triggering impulses to the antagonistic muscles, which then go into a protective spasm.

Oedema. Rhythmic frequencies from 1 to 100 Hz or 1 to 10 Hz have been found to be useful for aiding the absorption of exudate.

Haematoma. During the first 24 hours, 100 Hz constant, together with ice packs, is useful for the resolution of haematoma. If pain persists in the chronic stages, then interferential therapy and ultrasound are useful.

Chronic ligamentous lesions. Interferential therapy is useful for the relief of pain, if done in conjunction with ultrasound and mobilisation techniques. The interferential is given if other measures such as ultrasound or ice packs are not giving sufficient relief of pain, but are only useful for mobilising the tissues.

Trigger spots in myofascial syndromes. The use of constant 100 Hz and rhythmic 1 to 100 Hz is useful to relieve pain and mobilise the trigger spot.

Stress incontinence. Weakness of voluntary and involuntary muscles controlling the openings of the urethra, vagina, and rectum in the pelvic floor is effectively treated by the use of vacuum electrodes placed around the orifices. The dosage used is either 1 to 10 Hz rhythmic or 1 to 100 Hz rhythmic for 15 minutes. Stronger and more effective contractions are obtained with this method in comparison with those obtained with faradic pulses. The patient is able to take more current intensity with comfort. Results have been encouraging. The patient lies in the half-lying position, and electrodes are positioned on the lower abdomen just above the pubis, and on the inside of the thigh on the upper postero-medial side, using suction electrodes.

Delayed union and Sudek's atrophy. Nikolova has, since 1968, advocated the use of interferential treatment for delayed union. He used the constant 100 Hz with a moderately strong dosage for 15 to 20 minutes for 2 to 3 weeks daily. Results were said to be encouraging.

CONTRAINDICATIONS

Arterial disease is a contraindication as the stimulatory effect of the current could produce emboli.

Deep vein thrombosis or thrombo-phlebitis in the acute stage should not be treated as it would be possible to dislodge the thrombi or increase the inflammation of the phlebitis.

Infective conditions could well have the infection spread or exacerbated by the stimulatory effect of the currents.

Pregnant uterus. It is not safe to give it directly over the pregnant uterus, but cases of sacro-iliac strain during pregnancy can be effectively treated for pain with interferential therapy provided the field is superficially placed over the sacro-iliac ligaments.

Danger of haemorrhage. The stimulating effects of the interferential can cause further bleeding.

Malignant tumors. Direct stimulation of a tumor is contra-indicated, but referred pain from cancer or metastasis can be treated.

Artificial pacemakers. Generally a fixed rate pulse generator is immune to most electrical devices, but a demand unit must sense the electrical activity of the heart. It is safer not to treat anybody with a pacemaker.

During menstruation. It is contra-indicated over the abdomen only.

Febile conditions. These may be exacerbated by interferential.

Large open wounds. These will cause concentration of the current and distortion of the interferential field.

Unreliable patients. Patients who are unable to understand the warnings and instructions, for example very young or very old patients.

Dermatological conditions. Interferential may exacerbate any dermatological conditions in the area being treated.

DOSAGE

Intensity. The current level is adapted to suit the subjective sensitivity of the patient. He should feel a definite but pleasant tingling sensation. Higher frequencies are less sensitive than lower frequencies. Unpleasant sensation should be avoided. The current intensity is dependent on the size of the electrodes. The smaller the electrode, the greater the concentration of current density on the electrode. It is expected that the sensation reduces after a few minutes. The current intensity can be increased further, but after this it is best to leave it at the dosage selected.

The following differentiation may be used:

low doses	— not noticeable by the patient;
medium doses	— just noticeable;
high doses	— clearly experienced by patient as a vigorous, pleasant sensation;
very high doses	— strong, vigorous, almost unpleasant sensation.

The meter does not register the exact amount of current passing through the patient, it merely helps the therapist to find the optimum dosage in relation to the patient's reaction.

Frequency and duration

Analgesia

For acute pain, 90 to 100 Hz rhythmic, medium dosage, 10 minutes.
For chronic pain, 100 Hz constant, medium dosage, 10 minutes.
1 to 100 Hz rhythmic, medium dosage, 10 minutes.

Oedema

100 Hz constant, medium dosage, 10 minutes (if painful).
1 to 100 Hz rhythmic, medium dosage, 15 minutes.

Tenacious exudate

1 to 100 Hz rhythmic, high dosage, 10 minutes.
1 to 10 Hz rhythmic, high dosage, 10 minutes.

Pain due to sympathetic dysfunction
100 Hz constant, medium dosage, 10 minutes.
90 to 100 Hz rhythmic, medium dosage, 10 minutes.
For acute cases, 90 to 100 Hz, low dosage, 5 minutes.

Stimulation of weak muscles with normal innervation
1 to 10 Hz rhythmic, high dosage, 5 to 10 minutes, slowly increasing to 15 minutes if necessary.

Posterior root ganglion irritation
For patients with herpes zoster, 100 Hz constant, a very high dose, for 5 to 10 minutes. The patient must be warned about the discomfort.

Paraesthesia
90 to 100 Hz rhythmic, low dosage, 10 to 15 minutes.

Migraine
90 to 100 Hz rhythmic or 100 Hz constant, medium dosage, 10 minutes,

Parametritis (pelvic inflammation)
100 Hz constant, 15 minutes, medium dosage.
1 to 100 Hz rhythmic, 10 minutes, medium dosage.

Stellate ganglion block
Use equal double electrode pads. Place one electrode on the stellate ganglion and the other on C7 and C8.

Phantom pain
100 Hz constant or 90 to 100 Hz rhythmic, moderate dosage, 10 minutes.

METHODS OF APPLICATION

A. Metal Plate Electrodes and Pads
The electrodes are available in a variety of sizes and are usually encased in a sponge or felt envelope which is first moistened with water.

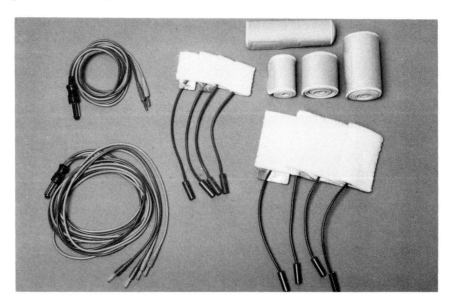

B. Quadripolar Plate Electrodes

These are an alternative to the standard plate electrodes. The electrodes are covered with a sponge material which must be moistened, and are embedded in a non-conducting rubber pad.

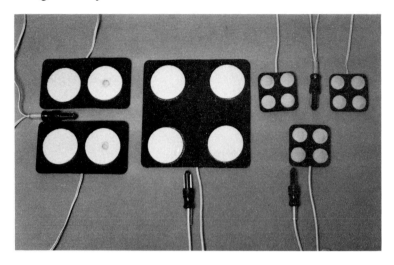

C. Suction Cup Electrodes

These are available in various sizes. The electrodes are applied to the patient through the suction cups which have a sponge pad and electrode incorporated inside the cup to carry the medium frequency currents. The suction force and speed can be regulated. Suction pads massage the area while the current is passing through the tissues, which causes further breakdown of any skin resistance by the propulsion of the electronic ions through the skin. There is an increased vasodilatory effect on all blood vessels, causing further suffusion of ions through the tissues. It will also help to speed the removal of mobilised exudate in the region.

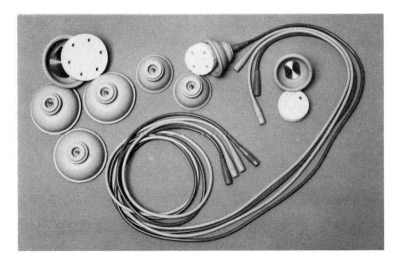

D. Quadripolar Suction Cup Electrodes

These are available in a variety of sizes as an alternative to the quadripolar plate electrodes. There is only one suction line, which is connected to any one of the four suction outlets. The other outlet for this circuit is left open, while the outlets for the second circuit are bridged by a short tube.

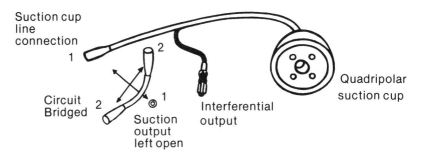

E. Quadripolar Probe Electrode

This is useful when it is difficult to locate the exact area of the patient's problem. There are four minute electrodes embedded in the end of a short tube. The end of the tube is moistened and, usually with the machine set on a frequency of 1–10 Hz rhythmic, the intensity is turned up to a medium sensation on an area of skin on an adjacent unaffected area. The probe is then moved over the affected area, and the site of the problem will be located as trigger points where the sensation becomes greatly increased, often painful.

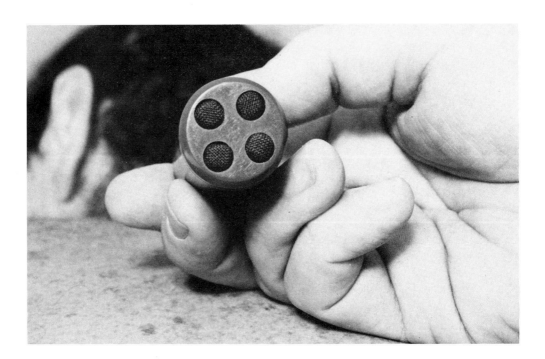

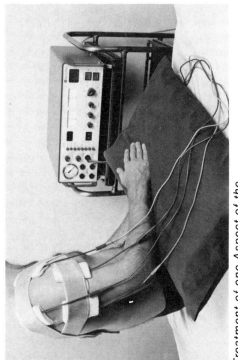

Treatment of one Aspect of the
Shoulder Region using Four Plate Electrodes and Pads

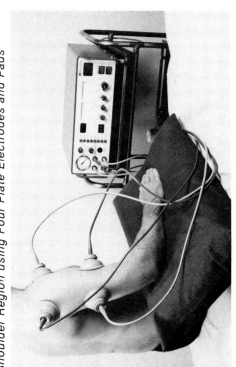

Treatment of the shoulder region using four suction electrodes

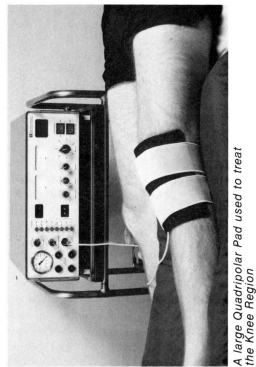

A large Quadripolar Pad used to treat
the Knee Region

Treatment of the Lateral Elbow Region
using a 60 mm Quadripolar Suction Cup
Electrode (in this case a 'tennis elbow')

TECHNIQUE OF APPLICATION

Equipment required
interferential unit
electrodes to fit the size of the lesion
pads — sponge or Wettex, 10 mm thick when compressed
velcro straps
plastic
sheets
vaseline

Position the patient comfortably with the area to be treated adequately supported, exposed, relaxed and elevated.

Inform the patient about the rationale for treatment and the sensation to be experienced — a vigorous or mild prickling sensation which is pleasant and will reduce within a few minutes.

Check that there are no contra-indications to treatment with interferential currents.

Inspect the part for any cuts, abrasions, excessive swelling, temperature or infection, and any raised edges or skin conditions. Insulate any skin lesions with vaseline.

Accurately locate the site of the lesion to be treated and mark out the position of the electrode placement, to ensure that the crossed field is on the lesion.

Skin test over the entire area to ensure intact pain sensation.

Wash the part to be treated to remove all grease, dirt, liniments (if any), dry scales and any cream if rubbed in prior to treatment.

Connect the electrodes to the machine through the quadripolar lead unit.

Soak the pads in a 1% saline solution, or in water.

Select the required frequency, constant or rhythmic.

Place your forearm on all 4 electrodes with leads of the same color diagonally opposite one another.

Ensure that the intensity is at zero.

Push in the mains button.

Slowly turn up the intensity dial and ensure that you feel the current. Watch the meter dial going up slowly.

Tell the patient what you are feeling.

Apply the electrodes firmly to the patient, ensuring that they are positioned so that the two circuits will cross at the site of the patient's problem.

Make sure that the electrodes are in the middle of the pads.

The pads must be evenly moist and not dripping wet.

Position the electrodes so that the red and white leads are diagonally across and, where the leads are close together, they are of the same polarity. This means that the knobs are of the same color.

Warn the patient that there should be:
(a) no increase of the presenting symptoms of pain or tenderness;
(b) no feeling of heat or a burning sensation;
(c) no intense, uncomfortable prickling sensation;
(d) if using vacuum electrodes, no discomfort or pinching sensation from the suction cups;

(*e*)   no movement to disturb the electrode placements.

Turn on the mains power control.

Slowly turn up the intensity control, asking the patient to tell you what he feels.

Be guided by the patient's subjective feelings and the meter dial to obtain a moderately strong prickling sensation which is pleasant. Make sure the meter dial does not reach its end limits.

Ask the patient if the prickling sensation is occurring at the site of the lesion. If not, it will be necessary to turn the intensity off and adjust the electrode position.

It may be necessary after 3 or 4 minutes to give the patient a little more intensity. Warn the patient again of the dangers, and remind him that the prickling will die down.

Turn down the intensity.

Switch off the machine at the mains.

Remove the electrodes and pads.

Inspect the part for redness.

Assess the part for swelling and pain.

DANGERS

Burns

Burns may be caused by:

(*a*)   bare metal electrode against the skin;

(*b*)   skin currents if the electrodes that lie close together are of the opposite polarity;

(*c*)   increased intensity with skin currents;

(*d*)   insufficient moisture in the pads.

Haematoma

The vacuum pump tends to produce a haematoma if the pressure is high and the speed is too fast.

Poor results

Poor results may be due to:

(*a*)   faulty positioning of the electrodes;

(*b*)   poor balancing of the circuits if the calibration dials are not properly positioned;

(*c*)   incorrect choice of frequencies.

ADVANTAGES

(*a*)   Large doses of interferential current can be given without the fear of producing a chemical burn. Any dosage at a pre-selected depth can be given within the body without surface discomfort and the danger of a burn.
Chemical burns can occur where a DC component is superimposed on the medium frequency current and great care should be taken in regard to the dampness and firmness of the pads. A slow increase and decrease in intensity must be used.

(*b*)   Decreased skin sensation is not a contra-indication to treatment, as the patient's deep sensation and the meter on the unit are satisfactory guides, but care should be taken if a large intensity is given over small trophic areas as changes in the skin may cause a slight blister.

(c) The current can be localised more effectively in a specific area by careful positioning of the electrodes. Lesions at any depth and in an extensive area can be treated.

(d) Metal is not a contra-indication as it is with so many other physiotherapy treatments normally used to help pain. There are a number of problems of pain and swelling in patients with metal implants which can be eased effectively by interferential currents.

(e) Provided the interferential therapy is not applied directly over a malignant tumor, referred pain can be effectively treated in some cancer patients.

9.2 Transcutaneous Nerve Stimulators

ELECTROANALGESIA AND TRANSCUTANEOUS NERVE STIMULATION

Local electroanalgesia has been done by the use of sinusoidal currents, cathodal galvanism or the interferential currents. After the publication of the Gate theory of Melzack in 1965, the use of electrical stimulation for pain relief gathered momentum once again. C. N. Shealy, a neurosurgeon, translated the Gate control theory into a neurosurgical tool, the dorsal column stimulator (DSC).

Shealy implants tiny wires into the dorsal column of the spinal cord and attaches them to an electronic receiver implanted in the skin of the back. A control unit is worn by the patient on his belt or shirt pocket so that he can turn up the current when needed. The device produces a vibrating sensation which tones down the pain and alters pain perception, thus allowing the patient with chronic intractable pain to carry out normal activities.

The basic assumptions underlying TCS are that nerves can transmit currents and that large nerve fibres can be selectively stimulated by adjusting the pulse amplitude, pulse width and repetition rate of specially selected wave forms. Large fibres have a lower threshold and faster conduction velocity than small fibres, and if they are recruited they can set a gating mechanism in motion to block small fibre activity and stop the pain signals going through.

The ascending and descending portion of the pulsed current depolarises nerve endings and produces a nerve impulse pattern which interferes with the ability of the central nervous system to perceive and interpret the messages. It also arrests synchronous firing in reverberatory circuits and produces some biochemical changes at the spinal cord level of the neurological imbalance. Both acute and chronic pain are effectively treated with TCS or DCS.

INDICATIONS

Post-traumatic and post-surgical pain, acute and chronic.
Phantom pain.
Causalgia (nerve pain).
Pain of arthritis.
Low back pain.
Neck pain.
Post-herpetic pain.

COMPLICATIONS AND CONTRA-INDICATIONS

Skin irritation: Due to electrolyte or long usage at high output voltage. Treatment is to remove the cause, or move the electrode temporarily.

Unpleasant sensation: A very few patients find stimulation unpleasant enough to preclude further use of this treatment.

Influence on cardiac pacemakers: Inhibits the output of some pacemakers. Stimulation is not recommended in patients with pacemakers.

Stimulation of sensitive carotid sinus nerves: May be risky in some patients when the electrodes are placed on the neck.

Alteration of sensation: TCS should be discontinued if the patient reports increased pain or has decreased sensation.

Spasm of laryngeal and pharyngeal muscles: May close off the airways when electrodes are placed on the neck or in the mouth.

Removal of protective influence of pain.

Neurotic addiction to stimulation: behavior modification.

Distraction of operators of dangerous machines when the intensity of stimulation is changed suddenly.

Safety in pregnancy has not been proved for nerve stimulation.

PRECAUTIONS

Diagnosis should be made before treating the pain.

Sometimes undiagnosed pain must be treated.

Pain of malignant or psychogenic origin does not respond well.

If there is an area of sensory loss, stimulate proximally and distally to the affected area within the painful region.

Contact dermatitis may occur after prolonged use. Careful cleansing of the skin and the use of different sites for the electrodes help to avoid this.

EQUIPMENT

Cutaneous stimulators consist of battery powered pulse generators with two carbonised rubber electrodes. Two circuits will have four rubber electrodes, on some equipment.

Output	— 0 to 100 mA
Voltage	— up to 150 volts
Frequencies	— 10 and 300 pulses per second
Pulse duration	— 50 to 500 microseconds

The pulses are half-wave rectified direct currents which are also depolarised. Their intensity is too small to stimulate motor nerves. Their prime action is on the sensory nerves. Models like the Stim-Tech and Neuromod have durations and frequencies that are adjustable. The cheaper models (Painblock, Biostim) have only the intensity adjustable. Adjustability in frequency is important to produce better coupling with the large fibres. Herman suggests the following points be kept in mind when selecting pulses:

Wider pulse widths may cause coupling to small fibres, lower perception thresholds, increased pain after stimulation despite pain relief during treatment, and cardiac fibrillation. High frequencies require greater stimulus amplitudes to produce depolarisation of larger fibres.

The electrodes make contact with the skin through electric gel or saline solution. They are held by tapes or rubber straps and can even be incorporated into prosthetic sockets. They usually measure 10 to 20 cm^2.

METHOD

The nerve supplying the painful area is stimulated preferably by placing the two electrodes over it. More than one pair of electrodes may be used at the same time to stimulate several nerves. The skin is cleaned and electrical contact is secured between it and the electrodes. The proximal electrode (anode) is placed over the nerve root close to the vertebral column to stimulate the posterior primary rami of the recurrent meningeal nerve and the site of autonomic or somatic convergence. The cathode is placed over one of the following:

(a)   the nerve trunk, for example, greater sciatic foramen for sciatic pain;
(b)   a trigger zone, a point of increased sensitivity when activated by pressure;
(c)   an area where the peripheral nerve lies most superficially in its course (often coinciding with a motor point);
(d)   an acupuncture point designated for the same pain pattern

Alternative methods may be used for the treatment of two painful sites within the same dermatome. Bilateral vertebral placement of the electrodes may be used for back pain. If pain does not follow a dermatome, the electrodes are positioned along a linear pathway. If the pain pathway is long, it is treated in two sections.

The intensity is turned up slowly until a tingling sensation occurs. This should not be unpleasant and no muscle twitching should occur. If it does, it means that the intensity is too high.

The most effective pulse width is selected by trial and error. The frequency is usually set at 100 pulses per second, but can be modified after the intensity and pulse width have been selected.

Maximal pain relief occurs after 20 minutes.

Stimulation is given for 1 hour, 3 to 4 times per day, although at times it may have to be continuous.

The patient learns from the beginning to adjust the parameters. Initially it takes up to 1 hour to identify the effective pulse and sites of treatment.

9.3   Summary of Medium Frequency Currents

Medium frequency currents, from 3900 Hz to 5000 Hz, are used for the relief of pain and the control of swelling. These currents are capable of gaining entry into the body without meeting a high resistance from the skin and causing discomfort. They can also stimulate deep-seated lesions. Low frequency currents such as the sinusoidal current and the faradic-type current have the disadvantage of skin resistance with high intensities and cannot be effectively localised to deeper tissues.

Other uses of medium frequency currents are as pain block stimulators, where the output ranges from 0 to 100 mA with a voltage of up to 150 volts and frequencies of between 10 and 300 pulses, per second, and a pulse duration of from 50 to 500 ms. Small pulse widths are used to effect a better coupling of the large A fibres and produce relief of pain (after the Gate theory of pain).

References

De Domenico, G, 1981, Basic guidelines for interferential therapy, Theramed Books, Sydney.

Frampton, V M, 1982, Pain control with the aid of transcutaneous nerve stimulation, *Physiotherapy*, 68, 3, 77-81.

Ganne, J M, 1976, Interferential therapy, *Aust J Physio, 22*, 63, September.

Gersch, Meryl Roth et al, 1980, Evaluation of transcutaneous electrical nerve stimulation for pain relief in peripheral neuropathy, *Physical Therapy*, 60, 1, 48-52.

Hansjurgens, A, Dynamic interference current therapy, *Phys Med und Rehab*, 311, Uelzen 1.

Heintz, N, 1975, The treatment of lumbar neuralgia, *Lecture SICOT International Congress*.

Herman, 1977, Transcutaneous nerve stimulation, *Physio Can, 29*, No 2.

Janko, Martin et al, 1980, Transcutaneous electrical nerve stimulation: A microneurographic and perceptual study, *Pain*, 9, 219-230.

McCloskey, D I et al, 1981, Excitation and inhibition of cardiac vagal motoneurones by electrical stimulation of the carotid sinus nerve, *J Physiol*, 316, 163-175.

Melzack, R et al, 1980, Ice massage and transcutaneous electrical nerve stimulation: comparison of treatment for low-back pain, *Pain*, 9, 209-217.

Nikolova-Troeva, L, Jan 1967, Interference current therapy in distortions, contusions and luxations of the joints, *Munch Med Woche, 109:11*, 579-582.

Schuster, G D et al, 1980, Pain relief after low back surgery: the efficacy of transcutaneous electrical nerve stimulation, *Pain*, 8, 299-302.

Shealy, C N, Taslitz, N, Mortimer, J T and Becker, D P, 1967, Electrical inhibition of pain-experimental evaluation, *Anes Anal Curr Res, 46*, 299-304.

Shealy, C N, Mortimer, J T and Hagfors, N R, 1970, Dorsal column electroanalgesia, *J Neurosurg, 32*, 560-564.

Shealy, C N, 1971, *Proc Internat Headache Symposium, Elsinore, Denmark*.

Shealy, C N, 1972, Transcutaneous electroanalgesia, *Surg Forum, 23*, 419.

Wilkie, C D, 1969, Interferential therapy, *Physiother, 55*, 12.

10 Electrodiagnosis

Some Key Points in this Unit

Accommodation is the property of tissue to adapt itself to slowly increasing stimulation intensities. This delays the build-up of the critical excitatory level for excitation of an impulse. It is lost when a muscle is completely denervated.

Refractory period is the time in which a tissue excited by means of a stimulus does not react to a second stimulus. Full recovery takes 10 to 15 milliseconds, but the first millisecond is the absolute refractory period.

Rheobase is the minimal voltage with a prolonged pulse duration necessary to excite a muscle causing a minimal perceptible and palpable contraction. Normal rheobase is from 5 to 35 volts.

Chronaxie is the minimum time required to excite tissue for a stimulus which is twice the strength of the rheobase. Normal chronaxie is 0.05 to 0.5 ms.

Strength-duration curve or intensity/time curve is a curve obtained by joining points that graphically represent the threshold values along the ordinate for various durations of stimulus displayed along the abscissa. The normal curve has a characteristic shape.

Erb's point is where stimulation of the brachial plexus at a point lying in the lower inner angle of the supraclavicular fossa can be produced, causing simultaneous contractions of the deltoid, biceps, brachialis, and brachioradialis muscles.

Reaction of degeneration describes a failure of muscle to respond to the tetanic currents (faradic-type currents), thus denoting denervation.

Neuropraxia is the physiological interruption of nerve conductivity due to pressure or ischaemia. Recovery is generally expected.

Axonostenosis is localised compression of the axon which is prolonged and severe — axon continuity is present, but excitability and conduction velocity are reduced over the affected length. It responds to a 100 ms rectangular current.

Axonotmesis is axon discontinuity with Wallerian degeneration, and only long duration pulses will stimulate the muscle. The neurolemma sheath is intact. It responds to long duration exponential progressive currents.

Neurotmesis is discontinuity of the whole nerve following complete section. There is no stimulation response. Wallerian degeneration is complete and only realignment by surgery will ensure recovery.

Nerve conduction test. When a nerve is stimulated in a suitably superficial position by pulses of short duration, visible responses can be obtained from all muscles supplied by the nerve.

10.1   Introduction to Electrodiagnostic Procedures

Electrodiagnosis is concerned with the study of electrical activity in motor units when stimulated by electrical pulses. It also considers the normal and abnormal behavior of the response of a motor unit when stimulated, and of the interpretation of its results for diagnosis and prognosis in disorders of the neuromuscular complex of the locomotor system.

Over a hundred years ago, Erb (1868) made his classical observation on the *reaction of degeneration* in muscles deprived of their nerve supply. He observed that a few days after nerve injury, muscles could not be excited by faradic shocks, but they still responded to galvanic currents (long duration pulses), and the sensitivity to galvanism increased, reaching a maximum one month after denervation. In 1872 Duchenne introduced electrical testing in patients suffering from Bell's palsy to distinguish between the excitation of a nerve and a muscle. In 1917 Adrian applied Keith Lucas's (1907) intensity/time curve for the investigation of human nerve injuries. He used rectangular pulses of varying durations provided by a pendulum driven stimulator and plotted it against the intensities needed to produce a twitch. Adrian noted that the responses of denervated muscles, when plotted, showed a pattern different from that produced by a normal muscle.

Hill, Katz, and Solandt (1936) were the first to describe the use of strength-frequency curves in the diagnosis of lower motor neuron lesions. Intensities required to produce a twitch were plotted against varying frequencies, but Ritchie found deficiencies in this method and the strength-duration curves were the main ones used for diagnosis. In 1944 Bauwens and Ritchie constructed an electronic stimulator producing rectangular pulses, and refined the method of strength-duration curves (SDC).

PHYSIOLOGICAL BASIS OF ELECTRODIAGNOSIS

The physiological basis of electrodiagnosis is the mechanism underlying normal electrical activity of muscle and nerve when stimulated by electrical impulses.

Stimulation of nerve fibre. In the resting state a neuron is a charged cell not conducting a nerve impulse. The difference in electrical potential of 90 mV between the tissue fluid outside and the intracellular fluid inside the neuron maintains the dynamic equilibrium of the resting neuron, and underlies the generation and propagation of the nerve impulse. If a brief minimal duration impulse between 0.02 ms and 1 ms is sent to the nerve, it will be sufficiently long to stimulate the nerve, and cause depolarisation followed by muscle contraction. Nervous tissue demonstrates the *phenomenon of accommodation*, by which the threshold of stimulation increases as the stimulus develops. If the rate of the stimulus is slow, as in triangular or saw-tooth pulses, it will fail to overtake the increasing threshold and excitation does not take place. So a slow rising pulse with the same intensity as a sharply rising long duration pulse will fail to excite a nerve.

Stimulation of the biceps muscle at its motor point (minimal contractions)

PULSE DURATION	SHAPE OF PULSE	INTENSITIES
1 ms	rectangular	30 volts
0.02 ms	rectangular	55 volts
100 ms	rectangular	30 volts
1000 ms	rectangular	30 volts
1000 ms	triangular	55 volts

Generally the intensity needed to produce a minimal perceptible contraction is always less than 2.2 times that needed to produce a contraction with a 100 ms pulse duration. If ever it is greater than 2.2 times the rheobase value at 100 ms, then it denotes denervation. Tetanic-like contractions at 100 ms need an intensity of twice the rheobase generally. If it is less than twice the rheobase, this denotes denervation.

Stimulation of muscle fibre. Like nerve fibre, muscle is bounded by a cell membrane which has a potential difference of 70 mV. It has a highly specialised neuromuscular junction where the nerve enters the muscle. It is possible to excite the muscle directly, and produce depolarisation of the muscle membrane, causing excitation of the muscle using pulses of varying duration.

Muscle has a much smaller accommodation property and thus will respond better to slow rising long duration pulses. This is particularly seen in denervated muscles, where a good response is obtained from a slow rising triangular pulse with a duration of 1000 ms. It is difficult to obtain a contraction with shorter rectangular pulses if the muscle is denervated.

The electrical properties of nerve and muscle must be considered in electro-diagnosis.

Electrical excitability is characterised by three factors:
　　intensity of current;
　　duration of current flow;
　　speed at which peak intensity is reached.
In cases of partial or complete denervation electrical excitability is altered specifically.

Refractory period is the time in which a tissue excited by means of a stimulus does not respond to a second stimulus. In denervated muscles the refractory period is longer.

Accommodation is the property of a tissue to adapt itself to slowly increasing stimulation intensities. If a muscle is denervated it has lost most of its power of accommodation, and only those pulses with a long duration and a slow rise in peak intensity will be able to produce a brisk contraction.

Action potential is the ability of nerve and muscle membrane to develop transient changes in potential which can be transmitted from one point to another, and which confers upon nerve and muscle the special property of excitability. The propagated change of membrane potential is the *action potential* or impulse.

Reaction of degeneration (RD). In 1868 Erb made his classical observation on the reaction of degeneration in muscles deprived of their nerve supply. Since then much progress has been made in the use of this observation for diagnosis. The term used today in the same context is *denervation*.

Reaction of degeneration describes the failure of muscle to contract when stimulated by a tetanising current. The tetanising current may be an interrupted current or a rapid sinusoidal current. It is generally of 1 ms pulse duration, and the muscle is stimulated through its motor point. A bipolar technique could be used for testing purposes also. The presence of RD means the muscle is denervated. The absence of RD means that the muscle is normally innervated.

Partial reaction of degeneration (PRD). If trauma, disease, or other factors have produced a partial lesion of the motor unit there will be an obvious diminution in the contractile response when a tetanising current is applied to such a muscle. This response is called *partial reaction of degeneration*. If, with the progress of time, PRD is less apparent, then the prognosis is good. Today it is also termed *partial denervation*, which means some of the muscle fibres have conducting nerves while in other muscle fibres the conducting nerves have been damaged.

Complete reaction of degeneration (CRD). If the lesion totally obstructs the activity of the motor unit, there will be no response when a tetanising current is applied to the affected muscles. Depending on the extent of the lesion, the muscle will respond to long duration rectangular pulses or slow rising saw-tooth or triangular pulses. If the denervation is more profound, pulses of 1000 ms with a trapezoidal or saw-tooth shape will be the most effective. This is also termed *complete denervation*.

Absolute reaction of degeneration (ARD). When denervation with marked degeneration has been present for over a year, muscle atrophy with replacement of muscle fibres by fibrous tissue takes place and there will be no response to any electrical stimulus. Occasionally a long duration pulse of 2000 ms, triangular in shape, may produce a sluggish reaction. This is termed absolute reaction of degeneration.

Occasionally denervated muscles that have been exposed to the cold and are poorly nourished may, within a year from onset, show no response to electrical stimulation. In such cases it is necessary to assess the extent of damage with an EMG report and bear in mind the history of the lesion. Here the lack of response is due to high resistance from the skin and superficial tissues, and poor nourishment. DO NOT MISDIAGNOSE.

Polarity reversal. When obtaining the threshold values of stimulations with long or short duration pulses, differences in the amount of intensity needed are noted when the cathode is replaced by the anode as the active electrode.

Normally, the cathode is positioned as the active electrode and takes less current than if the anode is positioned as the active electrode. (This is the cathode closing contraction.)

In partial and complete denervation, the cathode closing contraction is more effective.

In degeneration with atrophy, the anode is positioned as the active electrode and takes less current.

There is generally a sluggish reaction even to triangular long duration pulses.

This is a very crude test and is not reliable. Sometimes in cases of complete and partial denervation, the reverse may occur. It is always best to try both the cathode and the anode as the active electrodes before recording any values.

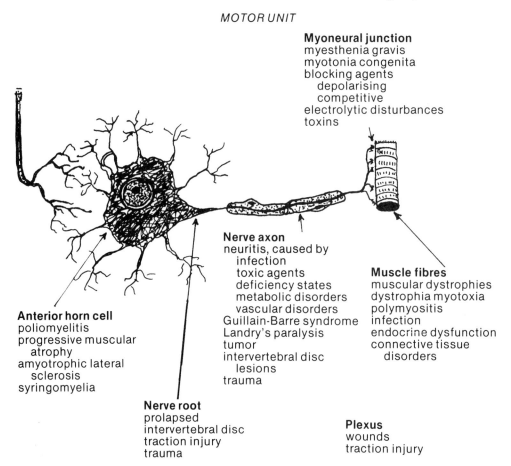

MOTOR UNIT

Myoneural junction
myesthenia gravis
myotonia congenita
blocking agents
  depolarising
  competitive
electrolytic disturbances
toxins

Nerve axon
neuritis, caused by
  infection
  toxic agents
  deficiency states
  metabolic disorders
  vascular disorders
Guillain-Barre syndrome
Landry's paralysis
tumor
intervertebral disc
  lesions
trauma

Muscle fibres
muscular dystrophies
dystrophia myotoxia
polymyositis
infection
endocrine dysfunction
connective tissue
  disorders

Anterior horn cell
poliomyelitis
progressive muscular
  atrophy
amyotrophic lateral
  sclerosis
syringomyelia

Nerve root
prolapsed
intervertebral disc
traction injury
trauma

Plexus
wounds
traction injury

CLINICAL APPLICATIONS; Routine electrodiagnosis is done for disorders of the motor unit, as indicated above.

10.2 Methods of Electrodiagnosis

RHEOBASE AND CHRONAXIE

Rheobase is the intensity of current required to produce a minimal perceptible and palpable contraction, using a pulse of infinite duration. Generally pulses of 100 or 300 ms duration are used to record rheobase. The shape of the pulse is always rectangular. It is measured in milliamperes or volts, depending upon whether it is a constant current or constant voltage machine.

Rheobase is measured using the cathode on the motor point of the nerve or by using a bipolar technique. Normal values of rheobase are 2 to 18 mA or 5 to 35 volts.

Some examples of the normal rheobase values (mean values) of different muscles are:

deltoid:	14 volts, 5 mA
triceps:	18 volts, 5 mA
abductor digiti minimi:	30 volts, 8 mA
frontalis:	14 volts, 4 mA

See the table at the end of this section for rheobase values of other muscles.

The actual value obtained in a rheobase test is often variable and is dependent on many factors such as:

Resistance of skin and subcutaneous tissues. Generally the palm of the hand and the skin over the lower leg, which are exposed to the environment, have high skin resistance and need higher intensities (14 to 50 V). Following denervation trophic changes occur in the skin due to the loss of the sympathetic nerve supply, and the skin becomes dry and scaly. This will alter the rheobase value.

Oedema and inflammation will make it difficult for the impulse to reach the muscle membrane. The excessive fluid will dissipate the current, and high intensities too uncomfortable to bear would be needed to obtain a contraction.

Ischaemia and underlying pain will make it difficult for the patient to tolerate any intensity at all.

Temperature variations will alter rheobase values. Heat lowers the rheobase value and cold raises it.

The value of the rheobase depends on the *position of the stimulating electrodes*. Minimal values are found if the cathode is placed on the motor point, or if the cathode is placed on the distal end of the muscle in a bipolar technique.

The amount of subcutaneous tissue between electrode and muscle will distort rheobase values.

In clinical studies, the following deductions can be made from a diagnostic point of view:

Degeneration. For about 10 to 15 days after a nerve lesion, the rheobase is increased.

Denervation lowers the rheobase value to about 59% of its normal value. Often it will be found that rheobase values are high, but this is due to the many factors that alter rheobase. It can fall below normal 10 to 20 days after denervation and remain low. This is not a uniform finding.

Partial denervation generally produces no change in rheobase.

Re-innervation can show a sharp rise in rheobase which heralds clinical recovery. Values rise to 5 to 6 times normal, then slowly fall. After nerve repair the threshold increases abruptly when nerve fibres have reached the muscle, and then returns to normal.

For some time it was thought that the phenomenon of low threshold during denervation, with increase of values on neurotisation, would be adequate to determine the state of neurotisation, but as so many variable factors affect the value of the rheobase, it is not possible to make a positive diagnosis or prognosis.

Chronaxie is an index of excitability and is the time, in milliseconds, necessary to induce minimal visible contractions with a stimulus of twice the strength of the rheobase. Any measurement of the chronaxie must include the rheobase.

Normal values of chronaxie are less than 1 ms (0.05 to 0.5 ms). There are variations depending on whether a constant current machine or a constant voltage machine is used.

Some mean values for chronaxie

MUSCLE	CONSTANT VOLTAGE	CONSTANT CURRENT
deltoid	0.01 ms	0.1 ms
abductor digiti minimi	0.04 ms	0.2 ms
tibialis anterior	0.04 ms	0.1 ms

At birth, chronaxie is 10 times higher than normal. At the 3rd month the values are lower, but are still high. By the 18th to 20th month the chronaxie falls to normal values.

Chronaxie values of proximal muscles are higher than those of distal muscles. Chronaxie values of the facial muscles are small.

Several variables affect the value of chronaxie, including:

Texture of skin — a dry skin will alter chronaxie values or make it difficult to obtain a value.

Ischaemia raises threshold values and decreases muscle excitability. Chronaxie rises by 100% under ischaemic conditions.

Oedema causes difficulty in obtaining chronaxie values.

Fatigue — if the muscle is tired, the chronaxie is increased to double, but then reverts back to the former value.

Position of stimulating electrode — if the stimulating electrode is not positioned on the motor point of the nerve, then the value of the chronaxie is that of the muscle, which is generally at least 10 times greater than the chronaxie at the motor point; in small muscles particularly, incorrect positioning greatly alters the chronaxie values.

In clinical studies, the following deductions can be made from a diagnostic point of view:

Denervation causes a rise in chronaxie if the whole muscle is affected. The rise is 50 to 200 times the normal value, going up to 25 ms. It then drops down to about 15 ms by the 30th or 40th day after denervation.

Partial denervation — this depends on the extent of the lesion; if part of the nerve is intact following the lesion or in a slow progressive lesion, there is little change.

Re-innervation — a progressive fall of chronaxie values occurs with neurotisation; it does not precede clinical recovery and gives no indication of recovery. *Chronaxie is the last criterion to reach normal.* Voluntary movement precedes normal chronaxie levels.

Nerve root lesions — there is evidence of raised chronaxie levels in the muscles supplied by the affected nerve root; for example, in a root lesion of the fifth lumbar and first sacral nerve roots, the chronaxie of gastrocnemius is high. The method could be used if there is difficulty with manual procedures of assessment to locate the lesion.

Peripheral neuropathies that are caused by infective, industrial, and toxic substances produce increased excitability of the nerve followed by lowered levels of excitability. It was found that in industrial lead workers there was hyperexcitability of extensor digitorum showing reduced chronaxie levels before clinical evidence of toxicity.

Myopathies — there is no significant change.

Rheobase and chronaxie measurement
Equipment required
low frequency generator with varying pulses from 0.02 to 1000 ms
moist saline pads
electrodes
leads
bandages
plastic protectors

The patient is positioned with the affected muscle placed in a supported and relaxed position. The muscle is maintained in the neutral resting position. The area to be treated is warmed for 10 to 15 minutes after all dry skin has been removed and the part washed. A large dispersive electrode is positioned at a convenient position away from the affected muscles and the course of the nerve. The active electrode (cathode) is positioned over the motor point of the muscle. The dials of the machine are positioned at 100 ms or 300 ms pulse duration and a suitable frequency (if needed). The current intensity is turned up until a good brisk contraction is obtained. This is performed 8 or 10 times, then the intensity is turned down until a minimal perceptible and palpable contraction is obtained and the rheobase value determined.

The next step is to raise the intensity of the current to twice the rheobase. At this intensity varying pulse durations are selected starting from 300 ms to 0.02 ms to search for the duration which will give a minimal perceptible and palpable contraction. *The time of this pulse duration represents the chronaxie* value for the muscle. There are generators available which specialise in the readings of chronaxies and are termed chronaxiemeters. They are not used much in

Rheobase and chronaxie values as found with voltage-stabilised and current-stabilised stimulators

	MUSCLE	RHEOBASE Volts Mean	Volts Range	Milliamperes Mean	Milliamperes Range	CHRONAXIE IN MILLISECONDS Voltage stabilised Mean	Voltage stabilised Range	Current stabilised Mean	Current stabilised Range
UPPER LIMB proximal	deltoid	14	10-22	5	3- 7	0.010	0.008-0.013	0.11	0.06-0.20
	pect. major	12	4-20	7	4-11	0.011	0.008-0.015	0.08	0.04-0.12
	biceps	8	4-13	4	2- 6	0.009	0.007-0.010	0.11	0.08-0.20
	triceps	18	13-24	5	2- 8	0.023	0.010-0.050	0.14	0.05-0.30
distal	flex. dig. subl.	13	3-20	4	2- 6	0.014	0.008-0.020	0.13	0.08-0.30
	flex. carp. rad.	13	5-20	6	4- 8	0.011	0.007-0.020	0.09	0.07-0.10
	ext. dig. comm.	18	9-25	7	3- 8	0.040	0.015-0.100	0.18	0.09-0.30
	ext. carp. rad. long.	18	10-28	6	3- 9	0.030	0.010-0.070	0.19	0.07-0.40
	dorsal inter. (1)	35	20-50	6	5- 9	0.050	0.010-0.100	0.11	0.50-0.20
	abd. dig. quinti	30	15-53	5	2- 7	0.040	0.010-0.080	0.22	0.10-0.40
LOWER LIMB proximal	rectus femoris	17	9-22	9	5-14	0.026	0.010-0.050	0.07	0.06-0.09
	vastus medialis	18	12-26	8	4-12	0.020	0.010-0.050	0.08	0.07-0.10
	biceps femoris	22	13-29	12	6-18	0.085	0.018-0.200	0.15	0.02-0.30
distal	gastrocnemius	18	14-20	6	3- 9	0.066	0.050-0.100	0.12	0.10-0.17
	tibialis anterior	19	14-22	5	2- 9	0.042	0.010-0.080	0.10	0.02-0.15
	peron. longus	19	13-24	5	4- 7	0.082	0.020-0.170	0.25	0.06-0.50
	ext. dig. longus	21	18-23	10	8-11	0.068	0.025-0.100	0.13	0.08-0.22
FACIAL	frontalis	14	8-24	4	3- 6	0.070	0.020-0.200	0.18	0.08-0.30
	orbicularis oculi	10	6-18	3	2- 5	0.110	0.040-0.300	0.18	0.10-0.25
	mentalis	18	7-25	4	2- 6	0.076	0.020-0.100	0.16	0.10-0.30

Australia. In practice each pulse duration should be tried 5 to 8 times before making any judgment. It is important to keep the electrodes on the motor point with uniform pressure, and to soak the pad in 1% saline solution constantly. Make sure the water does not drip over the patient.

First the normal side is tested and then the affected side.

Determination of accommodation. *Accommodation* is the property of nerve or muscle membrane to react less strongly to a slowly increasing current intensity by accommodating the electrical impulse. Each time the speed of rise of current intensity is slowed, an increase of intensity will result in a renewal of the current's ability to cause a contraction. The measure of the constant of accommodation is *lamda*.

Lamda or accommodation ratios are calculated from the ratio of the rectangular wave rheobase and the value for the progressive current rheobase, using a 1000 ms pulse duration. If the ratio is in the neighborhood of 3 to 6:1, it means that the progressive current impulse is 3 to 6 times greater than the rectangular pulse. Ratios of 1.5 to 1.0 : 1 indicate denervation. With a quotient of 1, accommodation ceases entirely.

$$\text{accommodability (lamda)} = \frac{\text{triangular impulse threshold in milliamperes or volts}}{\text{rectangular impulse threshold in milliamperes or volts}}$$

            normal —3 to 6
            denervated —below 3
            no accommodation —1 and below

The test will give some indication of the presence and extent of the lesion. It should be done in conjunction with the strength-duration curve, and great care taken in reading the threshold values of the various pulse durations. It is valid only if meticulous care with threshold value testing is exercised.

PULSE RATIO

Pulse ratio is the ratio of the intensity of the current needed to produce a muscle contraction with 1 ms duration to that required if the duration of the pulse is 100 ms. The strength of contraction is standardised. With innervated muscle which has been stimulated at the motor point there is little or no difference. If it is stimulated via the muscle membrane it can be a little higher, but nevertheless the values are always less than 2.2 : 1. Denervated muscles need much higher intensities at 1 ms, so the ratios are usually greater than 2.5 : 1. In complete degeneration there is no response to 1 ms.

It is a crude test, which has the same variables as the rheobase, and can be used as a guide for the progress of the lesion, if therapeutic use of low frequencies is made. The extent of partial denervation cannot be assessed from the test.

NERVE EXCITABILITY TEST

Nerve excitability is an electrical test which uses a short duration pulsed low frequency current to determine the state of excitability and conduction of a nerve trunk. When a normal nerve trunk is stimulated in a suitably superficial position by short duration pulses, visible responses are obtained in all the muscles supplied by the nerve as soon as the stimulus reaches the requisite intensity.

In this test of nerve excitability a rectangular pulse of either 0.1 or 1 ms pulse duration repeated once per second, is applied over the facial nerve trunk in front of the tragus. The threshold value needed to produce a minimal perceptible contraction is determined and recorded either in volts or milliamperes. This value is compared with values obtained on the opposite side. Bauwen advocates the obtaining of both minimal and maximal contraction values, as the obtaining of a pulse ratio will give further evidence for assessment. The normal values are:

facial nerve	2 – 16 mA, average 6.5 mA
	8 – 25 volts, average 12 volts
radial nerve	0.9 – 2.7 mA
median nerve	0.3 – 1.5 mA
ulnar nerve	0.2 – 0.55 mA
tibial nerve	0.28 – 0.5 mA

In assessing the facial nerve it has been found that there could be a variation from 2 to 6 mA or 4 to 8 volts between the right and left side. The right is generally a higher value than the left, but this is a variable factor. It is also essential to check the excitability of the three main nerve branches of the nerve trunk near the tragus.

Factors affecting nerve excitability tests include:

Temperature. Heat lowers, and cold raises threshold values.

Thickness of soft tissues. An increase of resistance to the pathway of the current by the interposition of any thickness of connective tissue will raise threshold values.

Position of electrode. The electrode must be accurately placed on the nerve trunk, which must also be superficially placed, anatomically.

Movement and tension of muscles. In cases of partial denervation, threshold values can be altered by movement and tension of muscles, particularly when assessing the facial nerve.

Daily assessment should be made, starting from the 3rd day after onset and continuing until the 10th day. If changes are noticed, continue until the 14th day.

When assessing the excitability of a superficially placed nerve trunk, it is important to assess both sides and note the difference between the two sides. A difference of 3 mA or more, or 8 V or more, will indicate denervation. It is not the value that matters, but the difference between the two sides.

The findings may be interpreted as follows:

neuropraxia	normal values of 1 to 2 mA or 2 to 4 V
denervation or *axonostenosis*	3 to 4 mA above normal
	8 to 12 V above normal
denervation or *axonotmesis*	5 to 7 mA above normal
	12 to 18 V above normal
neurotmesis or *severe axonotmesis*	nil

If there are changes in the values showing a progressive increase in the first 6 days, this will indicate an increase of swelling around the nerve, and calls for decompression by surgery or the use of steroids. It must be brought to the attention of the attending physician.

The tests of nerve excitability are of use early in the disease process to detect the presence and extent of denervation. If carried out carefully, there is sufficient evidence that the results are reasonably reliable. Wester states that in her studies about 10% of patients erroneously indicated a complete lesion, when it was incomplete. Yet it gives a fairly valid indication of the prognosis of the patient, particularly for cases of Bell's palsy.

Nerve excitability tests today are only carried out on the facial nerve for purposes of early diagnosis, as most of the large peripheral nerve trunks are inaccessible, inasmuch as they are not near enough to the surface to obtain accurate results. The facial nerve, the ulnar nerve as it lies near the medial epicondyle, the deep peroneal nerve as it lies around the neck of the fibula, are the only nerve trunks that could be satisfactorily stimulated.

Stimulation points of nerve trunks

Facial nerve: The three main branches of the facial nerve are separately stimulated immediately in front of the tragus or anterior to mastoid process where the nerve emerges out of the stylomastoid foramen.
ACTION. Contraction of the muscles supplied by the specific branch of the facial nerve or, if stimulated behind the ear, by all branches of the facial nerve.

Erb's point: Lower inner angle of the supraclavicular fossa.
ACTION. Simultaneous contraction of deltoid, biceps, brachialis and brachioradialis.

Ulnar nerve: Upper point — just above the medial epicondyle of the elbow.
ACTION. Strong wrist flexion and ulnar deviation and flexion of the lateral fingers.
Lower point — just above the wrist near the ulnar border.
ACTION. Adducts thumb and flexes the fingers at the metacarpal joints.

Radial nerve: Halfway down the arm posteriorly. The electrode has to be pressed fairly deeply against the arm.
ACTION. Extension of the wrist and fingers, and some radial deviation.

Tibial nerve: Slightly above the center of the popliteal crease.
ACTION. Plantar flexion of foot and toes.

Common peroneal nerve: Medial to biceps femoris tendon at the popliteal crease.

Deep peroneal nerve: Just behind head of fibula.
ACTION. Dorsiflexion of foot.

Superficial peroneal nerve: One centimetre below the deep peroneal nerve.
ACTION. Eversion of foot.

Nerve excitability testing for Bell's palsy. The presence of nerve excitability, the extent of the lesion if nerve excitability is lost and the level of the lesion can be determined by the performance of an accurate nerve excitability test.

Equipment required
low frequency stimulator producing rectangular pulses from 0.02 ms to 200 ms or

2000 ms; the pulses used are 0.1 ms and 1 ms, rectangular, with a frequency of 1 stimulus every second.

2 electrodes (indifferent approximately 150 mm × 80 mm placed centrally at the back of the neck, or on the upper arm on the same side of the lesion; the active a small single button electrode large enough to cover the nerve trunk; or 2 button electrodes joined together as a caliper which can be positioned over the nerve) leads

moist pads 170 mm × 100 mm, 10 mm thick when compressed (lint, sponge, Wettex)

piece of plastic to cover the pad

small basins of water

towels

soap

vaseline

spatula

cotton wool

The patient is positioned comfortably in lying with one pillow under the head. Half-lying can be chosen if the patient cannot lie down flat.

Place a plastic sheet and towel on the pillow.

Wash the patient's face in the region in front of the ear and behind the ear, on both sides.

Remove all dry scales. Check that there are no abrasions, raised edges, scars, acne or other skin lesions.

Check for integrity of sharp and blunt sensation.

Explain to the patient the need for the test and the sensation to be experienced, a mild prickling sensation which will be followed by the muscles of the face contracting. (If the patient notices any metallic taste in the mouth or flashing lights in the eyes, it would probably be due to the fillings in the teeth. To avoid this, use the indifferent on the same arm as the lesion or a bipolar button electrode technique.) Tell the patient he may feel a metallic taste in the mouth, and if it is too uncomfortable to let you know.

Warn the patient to inform you if there is pain, discomfort or a burning sensation under the electrode. Ask the patient not to move or touch any of the electrodes or the machine.

The operator should be sitting comfortably with the forearm holding the electrode supported. The operator should be able to reach the controls of the machine and see the patient's face.

Test the machine on yourself, setting the dials at 0.1 ms and 1 ms pulse duration with frequency at 1.5 Hz if the machine has a frequency control. The surge is switched OFF.

Now set the machine first at 1 ms rectangular pulse with NO SURGE. Check that the output dial is at zero. Place the indifferent electrode either at the back of the neck or on the upper arm of the same side as the lesion. Position the pad and plastic and bandage firmly. Check the polarity reversal switch. Check the mains control. Place the button electrode on the common motor point where the main nerve lies in front of the tragus on the normal side first. This is done as it gives a value for comparison with the affected side, locates the best stimulating points and shows which muscles are innervated by the particular branch at that level.

Switch on the machine and slowly increase the current intensity until the patient can feel some sensation. Let him get used to this sensation. Now increase the current until you obtain a reasonable contraction. Move the button around until you obtain a good brisk contraction of all muscles supplied by the facial nerve. Once the best response is obtained you must keep the button electrode *still* with a firm, but not too strong, pressure evenly distributed. Give 8 to 10 contractions on this spot involving all the muscles supplied by the nerve stimulated.

Reduce the intensity until one or more muscles just stop contracting. Increase the intensity until they are minimally contracting again. In practice it is best to locate a threshold value for the muscle furthest away from the nerve (any muscles in the midline of the face). You will find that at this value the strength of contraction of the various muscles will be slightly different. This is normal. Record this value.

Now turn the polarity reversal switch to the anode and obtain a threshold value. Turn the pulse duration dial to 0.1 ms and obtain a threshold value. This is done to make sure that it is the nerve that is being excited, as some neurologists have found more accuracy when using the 0.1 ms duration than the 1 ms duration, which could stimulate muscle fibre. Again in cases of marked denervation the anode may give the lower values. Now obtain a value for the upper, middle and lower branches of the facial nerve.

Having obtained all these values proceed to the affected side and obtain values for the following:

main nerve	—	cathode and anode	—	at 1 ms and 0.1 ms
upper branch	—	cathode	—	at 1 ms and 0.1 ms
middle branch	—	cathode	—	at 1 ms and 0.1 ms
lower branch	—	cathode	—	at 1 ms and 0.1 ms

The average threshold value at 0.1 is higher than at 1 ms, but it is the difference between the normal and the affected side that is important.

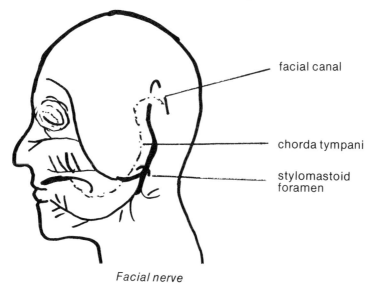

facial canal

chorda tympani

stylomastoid foramen

Facial nerve

STRENGTH-DURATION CURVES (SDC)

Synonyms: intensity/time curves; intensity/duration curves.

At the end of the first world war, Adrian (1919) applied the findings of Lucas (1907), who had experimented on the alpha and gamma excitabilities of muscle and nerve, to the investigation of human nerve injuries. In 1944 Bauwens and Ritchie produced an electronic stimulator to refine the earlier primitive equipment used for the production of a strength-duration curve, and since then many physicians such as Pollock, Wynn Parry, MacKenzie, and a host of others, have contributed much to its diagnostic value. Whilst it is not regarded today, by many neurologists, as a valid instrument, nevertheless it has many uses if employed correctly.

When nerve and muscle are stimulated by electric currents, they respond in a characteristic manner related to the strength of the exciting stimulus and its duration. A curve obtained by joining points that graphically represent the threshold values along the ordinate for various durations of stimulus displayed along the abscissa, is called the *strength-duration curve*.

The normal curve has a characteristic and constant shape. There are slight variations in the curve, depending on whether a constant current or a constant voltage stimulator is used, or if the values for the curve are found by stimulating the nerve at its motor point or on muscle membrane.

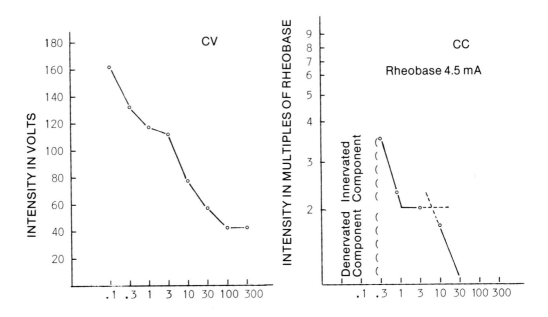

TIME IN MILLISECONDS

Intensity/duration curves from partially denervated muscle
CV, using constant voltage stimulator
CC, using constant current stimulator

Nature of stimulus. Any change in the environment of an irritable tissue is regarded as an electrical stimulus. If the stimulus fails to cause excitatory post-synaptic stimulation potential (EPSP), and produces a response, it is a *sub-minimal stimulus*. If it elicits a maximal response from the tissue, it is a *maximal stimulus*. Any greater stimulus is *supramaximal*. As electric currents are effective in producing a response from both nerve and muscle, and can be accurately measured and graded, they are the most suitable method of stimulation to produce contraction of a muscle for diagnostic purposes.

The factors influencing the effectiveness of the stimulus and the degree of response depend on the *strength of the excitation*, its *duration,* and the *rate of change*. The rate of change is important because of the phenomenon of accommodation. As nerve accommodates well, it may not be stimulated by a low intensity when the rate of change is low, as in a progressive pulse with a long duration. Muscle has very little power of accommodation and is not as easily affected by progressive pulses.

A strength-duration curve shows the relationship between the magnitude of the change of the stimulus and the duration of the stimulus. The curve provides valuable information on the state of excitability of nerve and muscle.

In normal muscle two components respond to electrical stimulation. These are (*a*) the intramuscular nerve fibres, and (*b*) the muscle fibres. Because nerve fibres respond to currents of shorter duration, and muscle fibre responds better to longer duration pulses, the typical curve of a normal muscle depicts the short time constant characteristic of nerve fibres. If a muscle is partly or completely denervated it will depict the longer time constant characteristic of muscle fibres.

An electrical impulse, starting with a long pulse duration of 1000 ms (or the longest pulse duration offered by the low frequency stimulator), is applied to the muscle being investigated, and the amount of intensity needed to produce a minimal perceptible contraction is noted and expressed in milliamperes or volts. The duration of the impulse is progressively shortened from 1000 ms to 0.02 ms. The possible range of impulses in low frequency stimulators is 2000 ms, 1000 ms, 600 ms, 200 ms, 100 ms, 30 ms, 10 ms, 1.5 ms, 1 ms, 0.5 ms and 0.2 ms. A choice

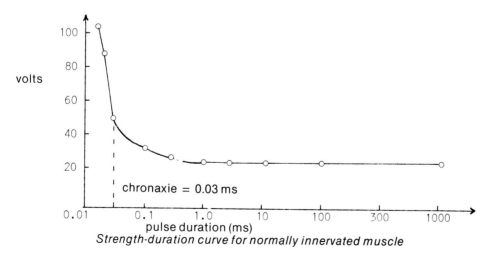

Strength-duration curve for normally innervated muscle

of at least 6 pulses to a maximum of 10 pulses may be taken. The longest pulse duration must be at least 100 ms.

For each pulse duration the intensity of current needed to produce a minimal contraction is noted. With the pair of values found, a curve relating to the strength of current and the pulse duration can be drawn. It is a continuous flat curve with an upward trend in voltage or current at the extreme left of the curve when short duration stimuli are used. Generally the current intensity necessary for excitation rises steeply with pulses between 0.1 and 0.01 milliseconds. The impulses of longer duration produce a response with the same strength of stimulus irrespective of their duration. This is due to the difference of critical excitatory levels and the accommodation powers of nerve and muscle as discussed earlier.

Several factors affect the validity and reliability of strength-duration curves, including:

Skin temperature alters the value of rheobase. An increase in temperature lowers values, while a decrease in temperature will raise the rheobase. It is important to ensure a consistent temperature of the skin prior to testing.

Humidity of the environment will alter the value of rheobase.

Deeply placed muscles cannot be accurately located and therefore can give invalid results.

Oedema will cause difficulty in obtaining a value.

Ischaemia will cause a rise in the threshold values of the curve and may even cause great discomfort and pain to the patient, as high intensities will have to be used.

Any quantity of *superficial tissue and fat* lying over the muscle will add resistance to the pathway of the current.

Large muscles like the deltoid and the quadriceps group must be assessed in sections. Only small muscles can be assessed wholly.

Position of the stimulating electrodes. Anatomical accuracy is essential in the positioning of the electrodes in both the monopolar and bipolar techniques. Care must be taken that adjacent or deeper muscle fibres are not inadvertently stimulated.

Pressure variations of the hand-held electrodes during the entire testing procedure will give faulty values.

Determination of the *rheobase* without any operator bias is essential. It must relate information to the muscle being tested. Use of an assistant can eliminate operator bias.

It is important that all factors which would alter the strength-duration curve are carefully eliminated, and the technique of doing a SDC is meticulously followed. Whenever it is difficult to obtain an electromyogram for a patient, the next alternative electrodiagnostic technique would be the SDC. Often there is difficulty in taking a patient to the electromyography clinic because the patient may be immobilised in the ward or there is a shortage of personnel operating the clinic, and thus it is left to the physiotherapist to assess the lesion. There should be no doubt as to the reliability of the technique if all care is taken to standardise the conditions that would otherwise alter the curve. It is the most reliable of all the techniques that the physiotherapist can perform.

Strength-duration determinations require a rigorous standardised testing procedure done with extreme care in a laboratory atmosphere.

Optimum timing for strength-duration curves

Patients with peripheral nerve injuries can have the strength-duration curve done 10 to 14 days after the onset of the lesion, when the motor end plate is no longer functioning and Wallerian degeneration, if present, would have occurred. For other lesions of the motor unit, if there is paralysis or paresis present following acute onset or a slow, insidious onset then, after considering the relevant pathology for prognosis, the strength-duration curve may be utilised to assess the extent of the lesion, and to monitor progress. It is best done weekly under the same conditions, until there is recovery or a decision has been reached on the eventual final state of the muscle. Once recovery takes place there will be changes expected in the curve every fortnight or so.

Practical uses of the strength-duration curve in diagnosis:

(a) to detect the *presence or absence of excitable nerve fibres* in the muscle; if a muscle is completely or partly denervated, the shape of the curve will denote the extent and size of the lesion, so it is also used to assess the *extent of denervation*.

(b) It will detect *signs of re-innervation* in a muscle; in most cases the onset of regeneration is evident well in advance of the clinical return of voluntary contractions.

(c) the *value of chronaxie* can be measured from the strength-duration curve; the value of twice the rheobase is noted and a horizontal line drawn from this point until it intersects the curve; a vertical line is dropped down to meet the time on the ordinate and this time value will indicate the chronaxie.

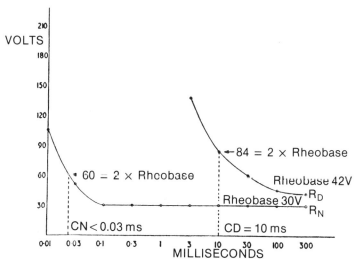

Left hand curve, normal innervation; right hand, denervated. This shows derivation of chronaxie values from the S-D curve.

(*d*) it will *monitor progress of the lesion* and denote whether the lesion is recovering or regressing.

(*e*) it will permit *identification of utilisation time*, which is the point at which the curve begins to flatten horizontally; this point is taken vertically down to the ordinate line; the pulse duration noted will signify the probable pulse duration which will be suitable for stimulation if the muscle is to be treated therapeutically with low frequency currents.

In clinical studies the following deductions can be made from a diagnostic point of view:

In completely denervated muscles, the strength-duration curve shows only the responses of the muscle fibres, which are less excitable than nerve fibres. So it is only the long duration pulses which will elicit a response from the muscle, and there will be a need to increase the current intensity from about the 10 ms pulse duration. The curve is no longer horizontal on the right hand side, but is converted into a distinctive steeply rising parabola which is displaced towards the right (that is, towards the long duration pulses). As atrophy advances, there will be no response with short duration pulses, practically no horizontal part, and a curve which slopes upward sharply within the range of the longer duration pulses from 1000 ms to 30 ms.

Partial denervation may occur from the onset, or if there is a slow process of degeneration of nerve fibres. Here the rapid nerve fibre response is partially lost or declining. According to the dominance of one or other component the strength-duration curve will reveal, by the form of curve discontinuities, whether there are more denervated fibres than innervated fibres.

The partial loss of nerve fibres or the reduction in excitability is reflected in the normal strength-duration curve in the form of discontinuities or kinks which usually appear in the curve between the 3 and 10 ms pulse durations. The kinks divide the curve into two parts, one which denotes the rapid nerve component with a short time constant, with a curve characteristic of impaired nerve fibres, and the other curve denotes the long time constant of the growing muscle fibre response which masks the nerve fibre decline.

The appearance of a kink or discontinuity in a curve is a reliable early sign of denervation, and in cases of progressive involvement of nerve lesions it provides slightly later evidence of denervation than electromyography. The extent of denervation can be picked up by the shape of the curves and the kinks. If a large part of the muscle is denervated, the greater part of the curve resembles that of the denervated curve with the kink, but if only part of the fibres is denervated and the majority innervated, then the curve resembles that of a normal curve with a kink in it.

Re-innervation characteristics in a curve were first described by Adrian in 1916. The first sign of recovery is the appearance of a kink or discontinuity in the denervated strength-duration curve. The kink first appears between the 3 ms and 10 ms pulse durations, and next appears between 30 ms and 10 ms or between 1 ms and 3 ms. Sometimes there is an appearance of a kink between 1 ms and 3 ms right from the beginning. The appearance of a kink generally heralds clinical recovery by 6 weeks. At times it can appear even 3 to 4 months before the return of voluntary activity.

The figure illustrates the variations which occur in strength-duration curves performed on normally innervated muscles, and on partially and totally denervated muscles. Movement of the kink towards the 30 ms level indicates progressive recovery.

Advantages

Strength-duration curves have many advantages as a percutaneous testing procedure.

The procedure provides a *more comprehensive picture* than other methods of electrodiagnosis.

When taken serially it plots the neurotisation progress, or lack of it, with minimal discomfort.

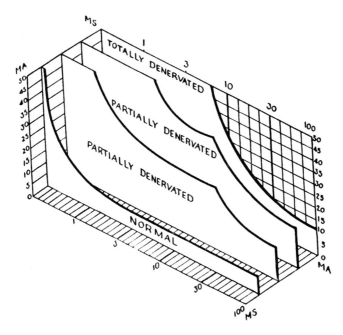

Comparison of strength duration curves showing a normal nerve, partial and complete denervation

It provides a *sensitive test* for the presence or absence of denervated fibres, particularly when using exponential progressive pulses for the SDC.

With the use of progressive pulses it can *obtain a discrimination of 10 to 20 times* in favor of denervated fibres against nerve or normal fibres.

It is useful in cases of *mild neuropraxia* where most of the fibres are intact and when the EMG may record normal conduction times.

In cases of *nerve block*, stimulation of the nerve trunk below the lesion with or without simultaneous electromyography may reveal the presence of surviving direct axons, but only a specific test by direct stimulation of the muscle can reveal the number, presence and state of progress of the denervated fibres.

In all these cases the use of triangular pulses or any of the other exponential pulses is important to obtain these advantages. The triangular pulse SDC gives the best results.

Strength-duration curves can be reproduced with a sufficient degree of reliability. Variations of rheobase chronaxie and current intensity at the selected points can be eliminated if the hand-held electrode is carefully attached to the skin without producing skin irritation, and eliminating all other factors that invalidate the SDC, as discussed earlier. The time taken to perform a SDC is minimal when the procedure has been mastered.

It causes the least discomfort to the patient of all the electrodiagnostic procedures.

Disadvantages
It can accurately assess only the superficial muscles. With great care some of the deeper muscles can be assessed.

The establishment of a detailed protocol in the administering of a SDC is not always possible in a busy department.

The use of progressive currents for electrodiagnosis
Progressive currents are pulses which reach their maximal intensity slowly. By the use of progressive currents such as triangular, trapezoidal, or saw-tooth pulses, the factor of accommodation of nerve and muscle to electrical stimuli can be utilised. The pulses ensure the stimulation of denervated fibres only, particularly when long duration pulses are used. The provision of pulses up to 1000 ms duration enables the physiotherapist to detect accurately the presence and quantity of denervated fibres, and assess the extent of the lesion. In cases of denervation with atrophy the long duration progressive currents, such as 1000 ms triangular pulses, will be the best stimuli to cause a brisk contraction with minimal intensity.

Strength-duration curves with progressive currents
An intensity/duration curve is plotted using pulses which range from 1000 ms to 0.2 ms duration with a triangular pulse shape, where the magnitude of the rate of rise and decay are the same. The current interruption is not too abrupt, and prevents unwanted break excitation. The curve obtained on the left hand side where shorter duration pulses are being used coincides with the rectangular pulsed curve at short durations.

This is to be expected from the fact that at short durations the quantity of electricity required for stimulation is constant regardless of the shape or duration of the pulse. At a duration longer than chronaxie, the triangular pulse curve levels off and reaches a minimum 10 to 20% higher than the rectangular pulse. At longer pulse durations the curve starts to rise again as accommodation begins. The shape of the curve and its lateral position are controlled entirely by the changes in chronaxie and accommodation time constant.

The curve for motor nerve is almost flat between 1 and 10 ms, with a broad minimum in the region of 5 ms. The curve rises steeply from 30 ms onwards.

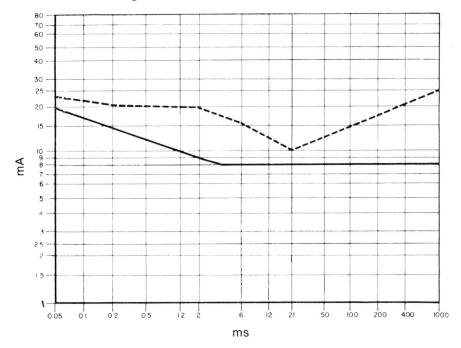

ms

Normal curves. The broken line indicates the progressive current curve; the solid line, strength-duration curve. Note the dip in progressive current curve at 21 ms; this is utilisation time.

The curve for normal muscle fibres shows a sharply defined minimum in the region of 30 to 50 ms. The threshold tends to be higher than that of the motor nerve.

Denervation curves. The threshold drops after 14 to 21 days following denervation, and the accommodation time constant increases. Once there is denervation and progressive atrophy, the threshold value rises. The drop in the threshold value in the first 30 days is generally 5 to 10 times lower than normal. In complete denervation the shape of the curve is similar to the rectangular pulse denervated curve, where the whole curve is displaced to the right and upwards (that is, the excitability has decreased).

Partial denervation or the intermediate stages of degeneration and regeneration show a shift of utilisation time to the right and some kinks or discontinuities, as seen with rectangular pulsed curves.

Advantages of the use of progressive currents for SDC
It is a very sensitive test for the presence or absence of denervated fibres in a muscle.

It can obtain a discrimination of 10 to 20 times in favor of denervated fibres against nerve or normal fibres.

In cases of mild neuropraxia it can detect or confirm the presence of denervated fibres when EMG has failed to detect it.

It is more comfortable to the patient.

It can be used for the more accurate identification of utilisation time.

Strength-duration curve technique

The excitability characteristics of muscle or nerve fibre can be expressed as a curve obtained by joining points that represent the threshold values along the ordinate for various durations of stimulus displayed along the abscissa.

Equipment required

low frequency electronic stimulator producing square wave or progressive wave pulses from 0.05 ms to 1000 ms

leads

disc electrode

suitably sized electrode to fit the muscle belly

piece of plastic to cover pads

moist pad, 10 mm thick (lint, sponge or Wettex)

small basins of water

spotlight

towel

soap

insulating cream

spatula

graph paper to draw curve

Position the patient comfortably with the desired muscle groups relaxed, supported and adequately exposed.

Place a plastic sheet and towel on the pillow supporting the affected area.

Explain to the patient the need for the test, the sensation to be experienced (a prickling sensation with long duration pulses followed by muscle contraction, a variable sensation with short duration pulses which varies with extent of denervation, or painful if denervated).

Check that there are no contra-indications to the use of low frequency currents.

Examine the area to be treated for cuts, scars, skin lesions, oedema, dry skin, and pain. Insulate all cuts, abrasions and raised areas. Check for integrity of sharp and blunt sensations (thermal sensation should be tested if sensory impairment is marked).

Soak the area to be treated in a bath of warm water or cover the area with a moist warm towel to reduce skin resistance.

Soak the pads in warm water.

Check that all controls are in the zero position. Plug in to the mains supply, having checked the plug integrity. Connect the leads firmly to the machine and the electrodes, having checked the leads for breaks. Select the settings for the pulse duration, frequency, shunt, and polarity (frequency 1.5 Hz, 120 shunt, polarity normal, pulse duration to be started with 200 ms).

Cover the metal electrodes with the pads and test the machine on yourself. Test on all pulse durations. Describe to the patient the sensation felt and demonstrate the contraction produced.

Remove the hot soak and insulate any breaks or raised areas on the skin.

Moisten the skin lightly where both electrodes are to be placed.

Position the electrodes on the muscle at each end of its belly. Use a bipolar technique. If the muscle is small, use a monopolar technique. If diagnosing a nerve, place the disc electrode on a motor point and the indifferent on a proximal, superficial nerve trunk.

Two bipolar electrodes are soaked in 1% saline solution and positioned longitudinally along the long axis of the muscle. The electrodes must be lightly placed on the muscle belly, as too firm a pressure might conceal a minimal contraction. The electrodes are placed on each end of the muscle belly. The distance apart would depend on the size of the muscle. The longitudinal muscle shows more accurate readings, as with monopolar techniques there is spread to other muscles, or in the partially innervated fibres, only some fibres will be picked up depending on the current pulse used.

Warn the patient to inform you if the area stimulated is painful or produces a burning sensation. Ask the patient not to move or touch any of the equipment.

The operator must have the machine on one side and the patient on the other, so that he can operate the machine with one hand while holding the electrodes with the other hand. The light must be correctly directed on the muscle. The operator's eyes must be above the muscle level.

Check that all controls are at zero.

The pulse duration selector switch is set at the longest duration pulse, the frequency to 1.5 (one every two seconds), and the apparatus checked to ensure accurate calibration. The output is then gradually increased until a good contraction of muscle is observed and the quality of contraction (sluggish or brisk) is noted. About 6 to 8 strong contractions are produced, as this is a final precaution in lowering skin resistance, and ensuring the same rheobase.

The output is then gradually lowered until the contraction disappears. The output is increased until the bare minimal perceptible contraction is produced,

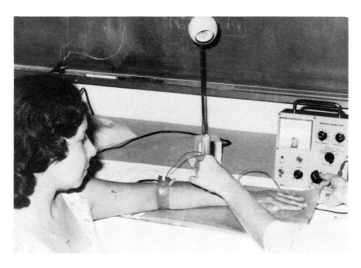

Technique of application of strength-duration curve. The lighting in the area must be directed on the part to ensure that a true minimal visible contraction is obtained.

and the output is read and recorded off the dial. The pulse duration is switched to the next pulse without moving the position of the electrodes, and the same procedure done, for all the remaining pulses. A curve is now drawn relating duration with amount of current, noting the rheobase and the chronaxie values.

If the muscles have an easily palpable tendon, one finger may be on the tendon to feel activity. On completion of the test return all dials to zero. First the output dial is returned to 0 before returning the pulse duration switch back to the longest duration.

Changes in electrical reactions to be noted
Quantitative changes — brisk/sluggish
Hyperexcitability or hypoexcitability
Pain

Interpretation
Sluggish contraction at the anode — poor prognosis.
Persistent contraction — may be indicative of spasm.
Contraction quickly ceases — may be due to fatigue.
No response to short duration pulses and sluggish response to long duration pulse — prognosis is poor.

As well as recording the results on the graph, it is essential to record full details of the technique used, to ensure that it can be exactly reproduced for future testing. For example, the sizes of the electrodes used, the length and temperature of the hot soak, the anatomical positioning of the electrodes, are all variables which must be accurately recorded.

THE GALVANIC-FARADIC EXCITABILITY TEST

This is a crude test which is considered to have little value as a diagnostic procedure. A denervated muscle is stimulated with varying pulses and the following responses obtained. Factors such as temperature, swelling, dry skin, pain, and infection may inhibit excitation.

Detection of reaction of degeneration

PULSE	RESPONSES	DIAGNOSIS
1 ms rectangular pulse	brisk	no RD
1 ms rectangular pulse	nil	presence of RD
100 ms rectangular pulse	brisk (no response to 1 ms)	RD
1000 ms triangular pulse	brisk (poor response to 100 ms) (no response to 1 ms)	CRD

GALVANIC TETANUS RATIO

Galvanic tetanus ratio is the relationship between the current strength required for a minimal visible and palpable contraction and the current strength required for a sustained tetanic contraction with a 100 ms pulse duration. It can be done with the muscle in a neutral position or stretched with resistance.

However, this test is no longer commonly used as there are now more accurate methods of electrodiagnosis available. Some patients may find the high intensities required very uncomfortable and this may result in inaccuracies in the results.

The ratio measures the difference in accommodation between nerve and muscle tissue. The old theory was that muscle contracts only on 'make' and 'break' of current.

Pollock and his colleagues called attention to the fact that either normal or denervated muscle may remain in sustained contraction, or tetanus, throughout duration of the current flow (galvanotonus). With this current the strength necessary to obtain tetanic contraction in denervated muscle is much lower than in normal muscle as there is less accommodation.

The following figures indicate the presence or absence of nerve fibres:

Normal — 3.5 to 6 : 1.

In degeneration, immediately after section of a nerve, the tetanus ratio may increase for 30 days to as high as 10 : 1, then it becomes progressively lower until it reaches unity.

In denervation, the ratio is 1.5 to 1 : 1. Approximately the same amount of current strength that causes minimal visible contraction in a denervated muscle also causes tetanus. Contraction described as 'worm-like' is probably incomplete tetanus.

In regeneration, the ratio increases to as high as 20 : 1. Then as regeneration progresses, it decreases to normal limits again. Voluntary contraction is usually present before the ratio reaches normal limits.

Tetanus ratio is relatively uninfluenced by local factors such as oedema. The time since the injury must always be considered in interpreting the significance of the tetanus ratio. Examples:

ratio 1.5 : 1 with the distal segment 250 mm, 100 days since injury
(continued denervation with unfavorable prognosis)
ratio 10 : 1 with the distal segment 250 mm, 100 days after injury
(nerve fibres have reached the muscle)
ratio 8 : 1 with the distal segment 250 mm, 20 days since the injury
(degenerating).

The following precautions in interpretation must be observed:

(a) tetanus ratio may be high indicating regeneration when the nerve fibres reaching the muscle are too few for functional recovery; rambling nerve fibres may bridge the gap of the divided nerve; branches from another nerve may innervate the muscle.

(b) do not expect neurotisation when there has not been time for regrowth of fibres; successful regeneration may be taking place although fibres have not yet reached the muscle.

(c) do not rely on a tetanus ratio based on one examination unless there is evidence of complete denervation.

Analysis of nerve injures

	NEUROTMESIS	AXONOTMESIS	NEUROPRAXIA
CAUSES	cuts and lacerations missiles fractures traction injections operation ischaemia	missiles fractures traction compression: prolonged friction (a combination of traction and compression) injections freezing operation ischaemia	missiles traction compression: momentary freezing operation ischaemia
Pathological anatomical continuity essential damage	may be lost complete disorganisation	preserved nerve fibres interrupted Schwann sheaths preserved	preserved selective demyelination of larger fibres: no degeneration of axons
Clinical motor paralysis muscle atrophy sensory autonomic	complete progressive complete complete	complete progressive complete complete	complete very little usually very little usually very little
Electrical phenomena reaction of degeneration nerve conduction distal to the lesion motor unit action potentials fibrillation	present absent absent present	present absent absent present	absent preserved absent occasionally detectable
Nerve excitability strength-duration curve	nil shows CRD	nil shows CRD or PRD	normal or 2 to 3 mA above normal normal

Recovery
surgical repair
rate of recovery
 	
march of recovery
 	
quality
	essential
	1 to 2 mm a day after
	  repair
	
	according to order of
	  innervation
	always imperfect
		not necessary
		1 to 2 mm a day
		
		according to order of
		  innervation
		perfect
			not necessary
			rapid; days or weeks;
			2 to 52 weeks, depending
			on extent of block
			duration
			
			no order
			
			perfect

Results of testing patients with suspected neuropathy or peripheral nerve injury affecting various nerves, at various stages after the onset of symptoms

DIAGNOSIS	SDC (RECTANGULAR PULSES)	CHRONAXIE	ACCOMMODATION	UTILISATION TIME	PROGRESSIVE CURRENT CURVE
radial nerve injury following fracture (40 days)	severe partial denervation	7 ms	1.5	500 ms	severe partial denervation
contusion of common peroneal nerve (28 days)	partial denervation (mild)	1 ms	5	50 ms	mild partial denervation
alcoholic peroneal neuropathy (60 days)	partial denervation	4.5 ms	4	100 ms	mild partial denervation
axillary nerve contusion following dis- located shoulder (28 days)	normal	normal	4	10 ms	partial denervation
Bell's Palsy (21 days)	denervated	20 ms	2	1000 ms	partial denervation (severe)

10.3 Bell's Palsy — Some Aspects of Facial Nerve Paralysis

In 1821 Sir Charles Bell demonstrated that the facial nerve was the motor nerve of the face. Paralysis of the facial nerve can cause a great deal of anxiety and discomfort to the patient, as it is intimately involved in emotional expression. There is considerable disability involving eating, drinking and speech. There are many known causes of facial paralysis. A lesion anywhere on its entire course can be pinpointed and the clinical features exhibited will depend on the site of the lesion, and the cause of the lesion. One of the common causes (75% of all cases) of facial paralysis is idiopathic in origin and is called Bell's Palsy. It can occur at any age, but is most common between the ages of 20 and 55.

Definition: Bell's palsy is a spontaneous paralysis of the face due to a lesion of the seventh cranial nerve. It is generally due to ischaemia of the facial nerve. Its cause is unknown and more than half of the patients suffer a simple block of conduction from which they recover. Triggering factors are exposure to draughts, hypertension, diabetes, pregnancy, and middle ear infection.

Criteria for the diagnosis of Bell's palsy
Sudden onset of complete or partial paralysis of the muscles supplied by the seventh cranial nerve.

Absence of other signs of central nervous system disease.

Absence of disease of the middle ear or posterior fossa.

Absence of herpes zoster.

Pathological changes following Bell's palsy show oedema, dilated capillaries, and degeneration of the medullary sheaths and axis cylinders of the facial nerve. In severe cases there is later degeneration of the Schwann sheaths and finally fibrosis of the nerve. The most important factor is the absence of inflammatory cells. It has been shown that two arteries supply the vertical part of the facial nerve, and they give off branches which enter the nerve perpendicularly. The veins do not enter perpendicularly and any minor swelling can compress the veins and deprive the nerves of their blood supply.

The initial change following the onset of the lesion is an interstitial oedema of the nerve. A conduction block occurs because of demyelination in the region of the histological damage. The fast conducting fibres are the first to be affected. Matthews points out that degeneration is not an all-or-none phenomenon. Some nerve fibres may degenerate, and others remain intact or in a state of reversible block. Such a reversible block may persist for as long as 6 to 12 months after the onset of facial paralysis. Electrodiagnostic tests can show the presence and extent of the lesion fairly accurately. Study of the response to electrical stimulation from the onset of the lesion has shown fairly consistent results.

Clinical features exhibited will depend on the extent of the lesion of the facial nerve as it travels through the posterior cranial fossa, the facial canal and then emerges to the face through the stylomastoid foramen.

Location of the lesion in peripheral facial paralysis: The length of the facial nerve (i) in the posterior cranial fossa is 23 to 24 mm; (ii) in the internal auditory meatus, 7 to 8 mm; (iii) in the facial canal the labyrinthine segment is 3 to 4 mm, the tympanic segment 12 to 13 mm, and the mastoid segment is 15 to 20 mm.

If the lesion is outside the stylomastoid foramen the signs are on the affected side. The mouth droops and may draw to the other side. Food collects between the cheeks and gums, and deep facial sensation is lost. The patient cannot whistle, wink or close his eye, or wrinkle his forehead. Tears are shed if the eye is unprotected. Paralysis is of the flaccid lower motor neuron type. The reaction of degeneration appears in 10 to 14 days, depending upon the extent of damage. Superficial sensation to the face is supplied by the trigeminal nerve, and so is not lost.

The degree of paralysis is assessed by examining tone, deformity, functional activities, loss of taste in the anterior two-thirds of the tongue, and tinnitus. Wrinkling the forehead will test the highest branch. Closing the eyes is a protective reflex. Blinking aids the lachrymal system. Wrinkling the nose tests the midface. Grinning, whistling, and blowing out the cheek test for the lower branches. Depressing the lower lip depends on an intact mandibular branch. Testing the platysma measures the integrity of the cervical branch of the facial nerve.

If the lesion is in the facial canal and involving the chorda tympani nerve, all of the above signs are present, as well as loss of taste in the anterior two-thirds of the tongue and reduced salivation of the affected side. The chorda tympani nerve contains taste fibres, preganglionic secretory fibres to the submaxillary and sublingual salivary glands, and fibres for common sensation at the intra-oral part of the 'geniculate zone'. These sensory fibres were postulated by Hunt, and later confirmed by Costen and Bishop as originating in the geniculate ganglion.

Lesions higher up in the facial canal will involve the stapedius muscle and add the sign of tinnitus or hyperacusis because of the paralysis of the stapedius muscle.

Lesions higher up outside the canal may involve the geniculate ganglion.

ELECTRICAL TESTS

The four electrodiagnostic tests used in the assessment of Bell's palsy are:

(*a*)   measurement of nerve excitability; this is done in the first 10 days following onset of the lesion.

(*b*)   measurement of nerve conduction (latency); this is also done in the first 10 days following onset.

(*c*)   the strength-duration curve; this is the graph of the excitability of nerve, muscle or both; this is done 10 to 14 days after onset when the motor end plate excitability is lost if the lesion is marked.

(*d*)   electromyography; this will detect action potentials elicited by nerve stimulation when the muscle contraction is too weak to be observed with the unaided eye; with denervation, fibrillation potentials will appear.

Electromyography and nerve conduction latency tests are the most valid data found today, but nevertheless, as stated earlier, there have been fairly consistent

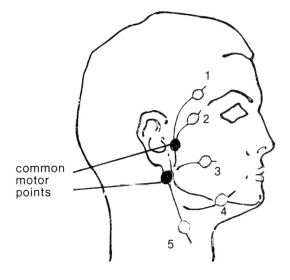

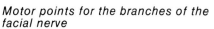

Motor points for the branches of the facial nerve

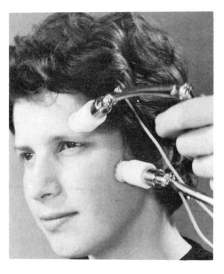

Use of caliper electrodes to stimulate the facial nerve

findings with the nerve excitability tests provided they are done carefully. The SDC can also be reasonably valid if meticulously done, and provides useful information to the physiotherapist. It is necessary to confirm your findings with nerve conduction latency tests or EMG if possible. Do not divulge information obtained by the nerve excitability test to the patient unless confirmed by other data.

Synkinesis is aberrant innervation. In most patients with recovered Bell's palsy, some degree of synkinesis can be detected. A common form is that of retraction of the angle of the mouth when the eye is closed. This can be demonstrated by the use of a 3-channel EMG. Occasionally even the mildest cases of Bell's palsy may show synkinesis. With denervation there is axon degeneration and regrowth. The profuse pattern of axonal regrowth may lead to the fibres intended for one muscle going over to another group.

Nerve excitability tests should be performed daily from the 3rd to the 10th day. If changes are noticed, continue daily until 14th day.

Changes shown from the 3rd to 4th day after onset include:

Neuropraxia	normal values
Physiological block and denervation	2 to 3 mA above normal (or 6 to 10 V)
Denervation	not excitable
Neurotmesis	not excitable

Slowly increasing changes seen in the first 6 days indicate compression and call

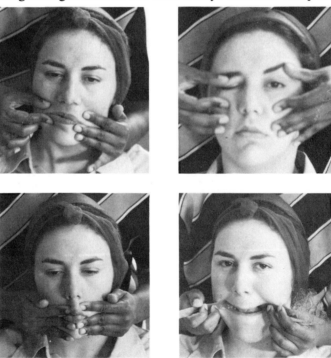

Facilitation techniques for the facial muscles.

for decompression or steroids. Today the use of steroids in the early stages is proving beneficial, and decompression is rarely done.

Detection of disease process in the early days of the disease and establishment of a prognosis must be confirmed with nerve conduction latency tests.

Measurement of nerve conduction (latency) is a measurement of the response to electrical stimulation of the myelinated motor nerves. The time taken for an impulse to spread from site of stimulation at nerve trunk to a terminal muscle is known as nerve conduction latency measurement. A concentric needle is placed into frontalis-orbicularis oculis or orbicularis oris. The nerve is stimulated and the appearance of the evoked muscle action potential is measured in milliseconds and reflects the rate of conduction of the facial nerve.

Bell's Palsy — Natural history and nerve excitability studies

DIAGNOSIS	NERVE EXCITABILITY TESTS	PROGNOSIS
neuropraxia (58%)	difference of 2.3 to 3.5 mA, 6 to 10 V mean 3.3 mA, 8V	recovery within 12 weeks
denervation — axonostenosis (18%)	difference of 5 to 7 mA, 14 to 20 V mean 6 mA, 16 V	recovery within 6 months
denervation — axonotmesis (14%)	difference of 7 to 10 mA, 18 to 26 V mean 8 mA, 20 V	incomplete but satisfactory recovery within 8 to 13 months
neurotmesis — complete degeneration (10%)	no response with maximal stimulation	poor and unsatis- factory recovery

The normal latency for frontalis, 100 mm from the point of stimulation is 3 ms, and for orbicularis oris at 80 mm is 4 ms.

Bell's Palsy — Latency measurements and natural history (orbicularis oris)

DIAGNOSIS	LATENCY	OUTCOME
neuropraxia	4 ms (mean)	complete recovery within 12 weeks
denervation — axonostenosis	6 ms	complete recovery within 6 months
denervation — axonotmesis	7 ms (mean)	incomplete but satisfactory, recovery within 1 year
neurotmesis — degeneration	no response	poor and unsatis- factory recovery

Strength-duration curves

The distal portion of the nerve will remain excitable for as long as 5 days. Excitability at the motor end plate will remain normal for about 10 days. It then declines and only muscle tissue remains excitable. The strength-duration curve will remain normal for the first 10 days, and then the following changes may occur:

Neuropraxia	normal SDC
Physiological block and denervation	swings upwards and to the right; larger intensities for 30, 10 and 1 ms
Degeneration	no response with pulses after 30 ms; swings upwards

This method of electrodiagnosis will differentiate the extent of the lesion.

10.4   Electromyography

Written by Dr. J. C. Walsh, Royal Prince Alfred Hospital, Sydney.

INTRODUCTION

Nerve and muscle differ from all other tissues in the body in that their functioning is associated with the generation of electrical signals. These electrical signals result from the rapid exchange of sodium and potassium ions across the surface of the muscle and nerve cell membranes. It is not possible to obtain any feeling for electromyography and nerve conduction methods unless there is some basic understanding of the anatomy and physiology of normal nerve and muscle tissue. The smallest functioning unit in the normal peripheral nervous system is the motor unit, and it is essential to understand the structure and functioning of this unit.

THE MOTOR UNIT

A motor unit is defined as one anterior horn cell lying in the anterior grey matter of the spinal cord, its single axon, the terminal branches of the axon and the muscle fibres that each branch innervates. There are many thousands of anterior horn cells along the length of the spinal cord and the cells are often referred to as the final pathway for information from the central nervous system to the muscles. There are many different kinds of nerve endings in contact with the anterior horn cells; some have a stimulating and others have an inhibitory effect so that the membrane potential of the anterior horn cell is constantly fluctuating.

When the excitation threshold is reached the anterior horn cell fires once and then is immediately switched off by the action of the Renshaw cell. The upper motor neuron is the major stimulating fibre from the motor cortex acting upon the anterior horn cell, but there are many other imputs to the anterior horn cells such as the vestibulospinal, rubrospinal, and reticulospinal pathways. It is the combination of these many negative and positive instructions to the anterior horn cells which causes the cell to fire off or not to fire off.

Each motor nerve fibre extends from the anterior horn cell in the spinal cord to the muscle it supplies, passing through the relevant motor roots, plexus and peripheral nerves on the way. These nerve fibres are all myelinated fibres permitting rapid nerve conduction. The fibres range in size from 3 to 18 μm in diameter, and if one considers the motor fibres from the lumbosacral cord to the small muscles of the feet, the nerve fibres may be up to 1 metre in length.

It is helpful to consider an example to illustrate the way in which motor units are arranged. Consider the lateral head of the triceps muscle; the innervation of the triceps depends upon about 5000 anterior horn cells which lie in the cervical spinal cord between the C7 and C8 levels on the same side as this muscle. The anterior horn cells are not grouped but are mingled with the anterior horn cells which innervate other muscles at the same segmental level.

The microscopic fibres come out of the side of the spinal cord in bundles forming the central nerve roots and these enter the axilla where they fuse with other motor and sensory roots from C5 to T1 to form the brachial plexus. Out of the plexus emerge the three major nerves to the upper limbs, the radial, median and ulnar nerves. The fibres under consideration that are destined for the triceps muscle pass in the radial nerve. On reaching the muscle each of the 5000 or so fibres divides into about 150 fine branches. Each of these fine axonal branches is attached to one muscle fibre so that each one of the 5000 anterior horn cells innervates approximately 150 muscle fibres.

If a particular anterior horn cell fires once then all of the muscle fibres that it supplies will also fire once. The triceps muscle itself is anchored to the bone at each end by a tendon but the muscle consists of long thin cells in parallel that run all the way along it and some of them are up to 250 mm in length, but are only 30 to 90 μm in diameter.

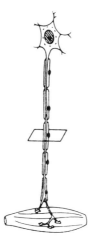

Myelinated motor neuron

The muscle contains about 750 000 muscle fibres and as has already been mentioned each fibre is innervated by one fine filament derived from a motor axon. Therefore in the triceps muscle there are about 5000 motor units, each one of which is made up of 150 single muscle fibres.

Let us return then to the anterior horn cell which in firing off once results in the generation of a nerve action potential along that motor fibre and along each of the branches to the 150 muscle fibres of the motor unit. At the junction between nerve and muscle there is a chemical reaction leading to the generation of a muscle fibre action potential in each of the muscle fibres. The single muscle fibre action potential is the potential on which all EMG studies are based.

The shape and size of the potential is the same from every muscle fibre; the duration of a single muscle fibre action potential is about 1 ms or less and the amplitude of the potential depends upon how far away the recording electrode is from the surface of the muscle fibre. If the recording electrode is within the muscle fibre, a potential change across the membrane of 70 mV is recorded, but if the electrode is 1 mm away from the muscle fibre a potential change of only a fraction of a millivolt will be recorded because the exchange of sodium and potassium is only local at the surface of the membrane, and is small in amount.

However, in normal muscle we never see the electrical activity of a single muscle fibre because normal muscle functions in terms of motor units, and if one anterior horn cell only fires off, we record from the muscle a summation of the muscle fibre potentials from the 150 or so muscle fibres making up that motor unit. They fire off at slightly different times because of the variation in the lengths of the fine axonal sprouts at the end of the nerve fibre. The muscle fibres of a particular motor unit are not necessarily together; it is usual for the muscle fibres of different motor units to be intermingled with one another, and this is one of the several mechanisms responsible for the smoothness of muscle contraction.

THE PERIPHERAL NERVES

The peripheral nerves contain the motor and sensory axons, which are the extensions of the nerve cell bodies. The cell bodies of the motor nerve fibres are the anterior horn cells which lie in the grey matter of the spinal cord; the cell bodies of the sensory fibres lie in the dorsal root ganglia. The longest axons extend from the sacral cord through the sciatic nerve to the small muscles of the feet and are almost one metre in length. All of the nerve fibres in a peripheral nerve are associated with Schwann cells.

There are two vastly different ways in which the axons are related to these supportive cells and this association is the basis of a morphological classification of nerve fibre type there is a series of Schwann cells wrapped around the axon and are associated with that axon alone.

The lipid membrane of the cell is wound around and around the axon like the layers of an onion skin, effectively insulating the axon membrane from the interstitial fluid at all points except where there is a junction of one Schwann cell with another. The area where the nerve axon is exposed to the interstitial fluid is known as the node of Ranvier. These nerve fibres are the fast conducting fibres and the diameter of the myelin sheath and axon ranges from 1 to 18 μm.

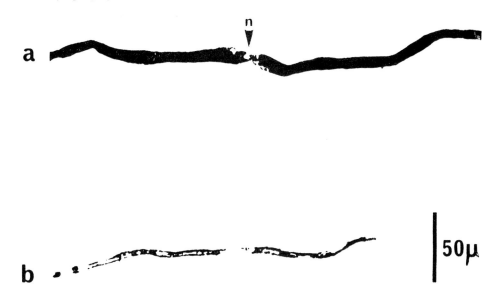

A normal large myelinated fibre (a), *and small myelinated fibre* (b). *The nodal area* (n) *is where the axon is in contact with the interstitial fluid.*

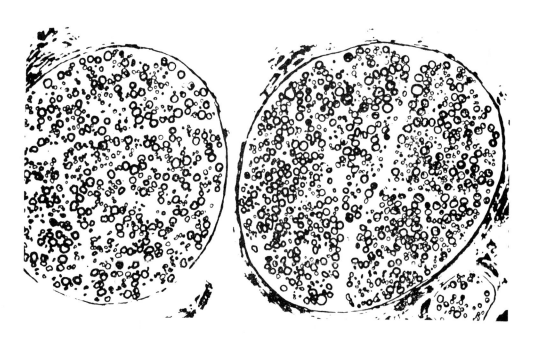

The transverse section of a normal sural nerve stained for myelin. In each of the two large fascicles there are several hundred myelinated nerve fibres. The myelin sheath is seen as a black ring and the axon as the non-staining central portion.

In a transverse section of a peripheral nerve the myelin layer around each of the fibres is easily visible in lipid stained sections as a dark ring and there are 5000 to 10 000 myelinated fibres for each square millimetre of nerve area. Motor fibres are composed of this as are the sensory afferent fibres responsible for position sense and light touch. There are almost four times as many unmyelinated fibres; these fibres have a diameter of from 0.2 to 2.6 μm and have a different relation to the Schwann cell. One finds that there are several small axons associated with one Schwann cell, each of them lying in a gutter in the cell surface and they are not effectively insulated from the interstitial fluid. For this reason the fibres conduct relatively slowly. The fibres are responsible for some aspects of pain appreciation and also for efferent sympathetic activity.

THE CONDUCTION OF THE NERVE IMPULSE

A great deal of knowledge about the nerve impulse mechanisms has been derived from experimental studies on the large axons of the squid for the simple reason that they have a diameter of 500 μm and are easy to handle and study in experimental circumstances. However, since the early studies much of the information has been supported by studies on man and other animals.

If one considers motor conduction we have to look at myelinated fibres and realise that the presence of long segments of insulating myelin gives the fibres a remarkable property. The electrical events which occur to produce the nerve action potential develop only at the uninsulated areas of the node of Ranvier and hence jump from node to node. The phenomenon results in rapid conduction along the length of the fibre.

If one measures the potential difference across the axon membrane at a node of Ranvier the inside is at –70 mV to the outside. The measured value is not rock steady as there are slight fluctuations up and down depending upon the leakage of sodium and potassium ions and other substances across the membrane. If an external electrical stimulus is applied at the nodal region and the potential difference rises from –70 mV to –60 mV, a small potential change at a small distance within the fibre occurs, but is not propagated because the internal resistance of the axon to electrical conduction is high.

However, there is a level at about –40 mV at which an uncontrollable event occurs because of a structural change in the axon membrane. This voltage level is known as the threshold, and when that point is reached, sodium rushes into the axon and within –0.5 ms the inside of the axon at that point is at +40 mV, that is, a change of 100 mV or so. As this occurs, potassium is also leaking out of the fibre, probably through separate holes in the membrane. When the rate of potassium loss equals the rate of sodium influx the potential swing reverses, and the membrane reverts to its original structure and the holes are closed.

This recorded event is known as the spike potential and the energy for this is derived from the local concentration gradient of sodium and potassium ions across the membrane at the node of Ranvier. The overall exchange of sodium and potassium is very small, and is about 50 picamoles per square centimetre of squid axon. In other words 5000 or so nerve action potentials have to occur before a readily measurable change of concentration of sodium or potassium occurs in the interstitial fluid.

Now this has happened at a node of Ranvier near the applied electrical stimulus. When the potential inside the fibre swings to $+40$ mV, it is a sufficient change for current to flow internally through the axon to the next node, which is at -70 mV, and raise the potential at the next node to threshold, producing a second nerve spike potential at the adjacent node of Ranvier. In this manner the nerve impulse is propagated from node to node along the length of the fibre.

It is often thought that the active transport of sodium across the membrane is an integral part of the nerve action potential generation but this is not the case. The active transport pumping of sodium out from the inside of the fibre is a slow process and will switch on after 100 or so exchanges have occurred. This is a mechanism to slowly repair the deficit in electrolyte levels at a leisurely speed following a series of nerve discharges.

Many factors affect the behavior of the cell membrane; for example, the calcium ion has a role in the structural side of the axon behavior, and if the level is lowered, as in a person who has hypocalcemia, the membrane becomes more sensitive and spontaneous nerve firing occurs leading to 'tetany'. The velocity of conduction of the nerve spike from node to node along the fibre depends upon several factors including the temperature, the diameter of the axon, the internodal length (that is, how far apart the nodes are), and finally upon the width of the nodal gap.

The largest fibres of about 18 μm conduct at a velocity of 100 m/s or more but as a rule there are only one or two such fibres in every square millimetre of nerve. There are a large number of fibres in the range of 10 to 15 μm and these conduct at a velocity of 50 to 70 m/s. These larger fibres are more sensitive to external depolarisation by a stimulus than are the smaller ones. The larger fibres are used in the procedure of estimating nerve conduction velocities.

The generation and propagation of a nerve action potential does not depend upon the metabolic function of the axon but depends upon structural features of the cell membrane. This is illustrated by experimental studies on the squid axon, in which all of the contents of the axon may be extruded and the internal space filled with a solution containing potassium ions and other substances. The semi-artificial structure will function normally for many hours and produce thousands of completely normal nerve action potentials propagated from one end to the other.

The unmyelinated fibres conduct very slowly by comparison with the myelinated fibres. Velocities are usually in the range of 0.5 to 1.5 m/s. Once the external stimulus has generated a nerve action potential at a point on the surface of an unmyelinated nerve fibre membrane, the internal positivity produces a change in the adjacent membrane and not in a part of the membrane at a distance, as in the case of a myelinated fibre. For this reason the change in membrane potential spreads much more slowly along the entire length of the membrane from one end to the other.

THE PATHOLOGY OF THE PERIPHERAL NERVE AND ITS RELATION TO CONDUCTION STUDIES

In spite of the large variety of injuries, disease and afflictions that may befall the peripheral nervous system there are only a limited number of pathological reactions that occur. One of the commonest problems results from concussion, contusion, traction, or compression of a peripheral nerve or nerve plexus. The exact nature of the pathological changes has now been clearly worked out. It forms a basis for understanding the abnormalities which occur in electrical studies, and in assessing the prognosis for these patients.

If we consider a compressive lesion of the ulnar nerve sustained in an intoxicated individual as a result of his arm hanging over the edge of a table, the pathological changes depend on the force of compression and the duration for which it is applied, and occur at the edges of the compressive band or edge where a *gradient* of pressure occurs. The mildest abnormality is the displacement of the myelin sheath from areas of high pressure to areas that are not compressed. The effect is to remove the myelin from a length of axon with little damage to the underlying nerve fibre. When this happens there is associated local oedema around the bare axons and it has been postulated that the oedema fluid is rich in potassium.

The two factors act to produce a conduction block at the site of myelin displacement, known as neuropraxia. The affected axons will not conduct through the blocked region. Therefore the more axons that are affected, the more motor and sensory loss will be demonstrable on clinical examination. If an electrical stimulus is applied to the nerve distal to the block, there will be a normal contraction of the supplied muscles and the conduction velocity in the distal segment will be normal. However, when the stimulus is moved to the proximal side of the block there will be a failure of conduction as the nerve action potential cannot pass through the blocked region.

Electromyographic studies of the muscles in such a situation will reveal no evidence of denervation. There will be no spontaneous fibrillation but the interference pattern is reduced or absent depending upon the number of fibres that have been blocked. This type of lesion has an excellent prognosis for recovery which may be expected to occur within days or weeks at the most.

Now imagine that the pressure is more severe or prolonged; in addition to the pathology already described, axonal interruption will occur in some of the fibres. Once this happens to motor fibres there will be spontaneous fibrillation in muscle fibres that have been denervated. For these fibres to recover, the motor axons have to regrow at a rate of about 1 mm per day from the site of compression to the muscle. Degenerated axons will be electrically inexcitable after 3 to 4 days.

So the points that emerge are as follows:
The problem of assessment of the degree of nerve injury and the outlook for recovery hinges upon deciding how much of the lesion is the result of local loss of the myelin, and how much of the lesion is the result of axonal interruption. The more spontaneous fibrillation and the less the excitability to external electrical stimulation of the nerve trunk distal to the lesion, the worse is the prognosis for recovery. The two types of pathology that may occur in the acute nerve lesions also occur with chronic local nerve injury, such as lesions of the ulnar nerve at the elbow, or the median nerve at the wrist.

The commonest peripheral nerve entrapment is that of the median nerve in the carpal tunnel. Narrowing of the canal through which the nerve moves backwards and forwards every time the person flexes and extends the wrist is a common complement of aging but it may also occur in young people. Here again the milder type of pathology is that of segmental loss of myelin from the axons leading to slow conduction through the carpal tunnel areas as measured by the electrical tests. If untreated, however, progressive axonal degeneration will occur with gradual loss of more and more fibres.

Diffuse metabolic disturbances of the peripheral nerves usually produce mainly one or other type of pathological abnormality, for example the peripheral neuropathy associated with nutritional deficiency, alcoholism, diabetes, and the side effect of drugs, results mainly from axonal degeneration of the distal ends of the longest fibres. This probably arises because the cell bodies malfunction and are unable to transport nutrients to the distal end of the fibres. Obviously the longest ones will be the more affected and this is the reason that sensory and motor disability is most marked in the feet and legs in this type of patient.

By contrast the peripheral neuropathy associated with the Guillain-Barre Syndrome and many of the congenital neuropathies such as Charcot-Marie Tooth Disease is predominantly a disorder of the Schwann cell leading to extensive segmental loss of myelin. This has a different pathological appearance in nerve biopsy and produces marked slowing of conduction.

NEUROMUSCULAR TRANSMISSION

The conduction of the nerve impulse is fundamentally an electrical event and the contraction of the muscle fibre is associated initially with an electrical event which spreads through the fibre and is linked to mechanical contraction. However, the transmission of the nerve impulse from the nerve membrane to the muscle membrane depends upon a chemical reaction. The terminal filaments of a motor nerve fibre lie in a shallow gutter on the muscle fibre surface and are separated from the muscle by a gap of 0.1 μm.

The amount of current flow resulting from arrival of the spike potential is too small (2.3×10^{-8} A) to affect the resting membrane potential by any more than a fraction of a microvolt. However, it is now established that the arrival of the nerve potential at the end of the fibre leads to the release of a substance called acetylcholine, which is manufactured within the nerve fibre and is stored in tiny vesicles at the nerve terminal. At rest these vesicles rupture spontaneously into the gap between nerve and muscle at a rate of 1 every 4 to 5 seconds.

Acetylcholine diffuses across the gap and leads to a slight depolarisation of the muscle membrane, resulting in a small potential change of about 1 mV. The phenomenon can be recorded and is called the 'miniature end plate potential'. The short-lived action of the released acetylcholine is the result of the action of an enzyme called cholinesterase, active on the surface of the muscle membrane. The enzyme rapidly destroys the substance soon after its release.

However, when a nerve impulse penetrates the region, many thousands of vesicles are released simultaneously; the amount of acetylcholine flooding the muscle membrane is sufficient to allow the depolarisation to reach the threshold level and a muscle action potential is generated which spreads at about 5 m/s along and through the muscle fibre leading to contraction of that fibre. The chemical event which occurs at the neuromuscular junction results in a delay in transmission of about 0.7 to 1 ms.

The number of vesicles released is reduced if the serum calcium falls, if the magnesium rises, and by the action of neomycin, and is completely abolished by the presence of the toxin of botulinus infection. The sensitivity of the receptors is increased by the veratrum alkaloids and this has been used as a theoretical basis for increasing the strength of the muscles in a person with myasthenia gravis. In this condition it is thought that the amount of acetylcholine in each vesicle is reduced, leading to a reduction in size of the miniature end plate potentials, and in a failure of the production of acetylcholine to keep up with the demand of repetitive muscle contraction. The sensitivity of the receptors on the muscle membrane is reduced by atropine and curare which are very effective muscle relaxants used in anaesthesia. Muscle relaxants such as scoline act by depolarising the muscle cell membrane so that potential changes cannot occur.

Electrophysiological methods may be used to assess the status of neuromuscular transmission. They include repetitive supramaximal stimulation of a motor nerve and the recording of the force of contraction of a supplied muscle together with a recording of the amplitude of evoked muscle action potential. A defect in neuromuscular function will be shown by a fall in the amplitude of the evoked response with successive stimuli, which results from the inability of the production of acetylcholine to keep up with the demand.

Another method is the recording of single muscle fibre potentials from muscle fibres that are members of the same motor unit. This is done by using a small recording electrode with a small surface area; the patient makes a slight effort and the muscle is explored until two muscle fibre potentials that belong to the same motor unit are obtained. If the neuromuscular transmission is normal, then the potentials will have almost the same interval between them every time the motor unit fires off.

If one or other neuromuscular junction fatigues however, on some occasions there will be a longer interval between the fibre discharges. On other occasions one or other muscle fibre will not fire at all. This is probably one of the most sensitive means available to assess the adequacy or otherwise of neuromuscular function.

THE RECORDING AND DISPLAY OF ELECTRICAL ACTIVITY FROM MUSCLE

The electrical activity of the motor units in a muscle is easily examined using modern equipment. Before outlining the various means of recording the electrical signals, let us consider the apparatus used to display the information. The electrical activity recorded from a muscle may vary in amplitude from 50 μV to 15 mV or so. The signals are led from the patient through wires attached to the recording electrodes and are amplified electronically.

The amplified signals may be handled in various ways; it is common to display them on a cathode ray oscilloscope and to display simultaneously a calibration signal of known amplitude so that the size of the potentials can be measured accurately. A time scale is also displayed. With a photographic system attached to the oscilloscope, a permanent record can be made. A tape recorder may be used to store EMG information so that it may be redisplayed at will. Since the frequencies in an EMG signal lie in the audible range, it is convenient to listen to

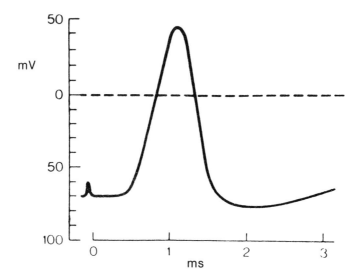

The change in potential across the surface of a nerve cell membrane as the permeability change passes through the area.

the EMG signal on a loudspeaker, and it is often easier to detect subtle abnormalities in the EMG from the sound than from the visual display. Steps have to be taken to prevent electrical interference by earthing the patient, and by the use of an electrically screened room for the examination area.

RECORDING ELECTRODES

Surface recording electrodes made of silver, covered with material and moistened with a suitable conducting medium may be strapped to the skin over the surface of the muscle. If a person is thin and can contract one or two superficial motor units, it may be possible to get some idea of the size, shape and duration of the potentials. In practice this is unsatisfactory because of the insulating layers between the recording electrodes and the muscle. Surface recording is however useful for other applications such as to determine how much of a muscle is contracting in response to a voluntary effort, or in response to electrical stimulation of the nerve supply.

To obtain a good look at the motor unit action potentials, we have to get close to them. The only means of achieving this is to use a needle recording electrode. The commonest recording electrode in use is known as the Concentric Needle Electrode. It consists of an insulated wire contained within a hypodermic needle. The cut surface of the wire at the end of the needle forms one electrode and the shaft of the needle forms the other. It may be introduced into a muscle with almost no discomfort at all and an accurate recording can be obtained for a distance of up to 7 mm from the needle tip.

Motor unit potentials have been studied for many years now and there is a considerable fund of knowledge as to what is normal and what is not. If a person makes a slight effort then it is fairly simple to activate only one motor unit in the recording field of an electrode like this. It is found that a motor unit potential usually has an amplitude from 0.5 to 3 mV and a duration of up to 9 ms. There are usually three to four phases. There is considerable variation in the size, shape and number of phases of normal motor units in normal muscles. It has to be remembered that the motor unit potential is made up, for example in the triceps, by the summation of about 150 single muscle fibre potentials which fire off at slightly varying times. For this reason the amplitude and shape of any particular motor unit potential depends upon the number of muscle fibres in the motor unit, how far away the fibres are from the recording electrode, the size of the recording electrode, the resistance of the recording electrode, and the orientation of the recording surface of the central electrode to the muscle fibres that form the motor unit.

In addition there is considerable variation from muscle to muscle; motor units in the quadriceps contain approximately 800 muscle fibres, in the biceps approximately 160 muscle fibres, and in the external ocular muscles only 8 to 9 muscle fibres. It is obvious therefore that considerable experience is needed to interpret the significance of changes of the size, shape and duration of motor unit potentials.

THE PERFORMANCE OF ELECTROMYOGRAPHY

With the needle electrode introduced, observations are made of the oscilloscope screen which displays electrical activity in the recording field of the electrode (namely in a hemisphere around the angled tip of the needle with a radius of about 7 mm); the sound of the electrical activity is audible over the loudspeaker.

Normal muscle

Needle insertion into a normal relaxed muscle is accompanied by one or two seconds of muscle fibre potential discharges which are of small amplitude and last 1 ms or less. They are produced by the mechanical irritation of the needle passing through and between the muscle fibres ('insertion activity') and ceases immediately the needle is at rest in the muscle. A normal muscle is electrically silent at rest; no motor unit activity is recorded; nothing is seen on the oscilloscope nor heard over the loudspeaker.

If the subject is now instructed to make a slight contraction there will be one or two motor units only firing under voluntary control in the recording field of the electrode. The amplitude of the motor unit potentials will vary from 0.1 to 3 mV and depends upon several factors, including how far away the motor unit is from the needle tip, the surface area of the recording electrode and its orientation in relation to where the motor unit is, and the number of muscle fibres in that motor unit. There may be from two to four phases in normal motor units, but 2 to 3% of motor units in control subjects are polyphasic.

The duration of the motor unit potential will not usually exceed 9 or 10 ms, with a mean duration of about 4 ms. It is noted that the firing rate is regular and that with slight effort the discharge frequency varies from 1 to 5 per second. Therefore it is possible to examine the size, shape and duration of motor unit potentials and by moving the electrode to various sites in the muscle to fairly rapidly assess the features of several motor units.

As the patient increases the force of contraction more and more motor units begin firing in the vicinity of the needle electrode so that by the time that maximum effort is produced there may be 15 or 16 motor units being recorded; because they fire asynchronously the action potentials overlap one another so that it is not possible to distinguish the shape and form of individual potentials. For this reason the pattern is known as an 'interference' pattern because the features of individual potentials are lost. There is a characteristic rumbling sound on the loudspeaker, somewhat like the sound of distant thunder.

Abnormalities may be revealed at electromyography either in the resting muscle or during effort.

ABNORMALITIES AT REST

Spontaneous fibrillation. Normal muscle is electrically silent at rest. Spontaneous fibrillation is an abnormality which occurs in resting muscle and is characterised by the presence of spontaneous single muscle fibre activity. Because they are potentials from single muscle fibres they are of small amplitude with a conventional recording electrode and usually never exceed 300 μV; the duration of single muscle fibre potentials is 1 ms. The commonest cause of spontaneous fibrillation is interruption of the axon responsible for the innervation of these muscle fibres.

When the nerve supply to a muscle fibre is interrupted, the fibre becomes hypersensitive to the small amounts of acetylcholine normally circulating in the interstitial fluid. Because of the hypersensitivity, the muscle fibres fire regularly and repetitively. The finding of spontaneous fibrillation is a sign of acute denervation and the amount is proportional to the extent of axonal interruption. Therefore it is a good measure of the severity of an acute nerve injury.

Spontaneous fibrillation may not appear for up to 18 days after injury so that its absence during the early interval does not exclude the possibility of axonal damage. Spontaneous fibrillation potentials have a characteristic appearance on the oscilloscope and have a crackling sound over the loudspeaker. Small amounts of spontaneous fibrillation may be found occasionally in muscles with myositis, and occurs as a result of necrosis of a portion of a muscle fibre which effectively separates part of it from the neuromuscular junction. The effect is the same as an interruption of the nerve supply.

Fasciculation. Fasciculations are the spontaneous discharge of motor units. They are clinically visible as a flickering of the muscle under the skin if they affect motor units near the surface of a muscle. The features of fasciculations are that they are involuntary, the repetition rate is irregular and the amplitude and duration of fasciculating potentials is similar to that of normal motor unit potentials, but may be up to 9 or 10 mV in amplitude in patients with chronic denervation and re-innervation. Fasciculations are most commonly seen with chronic diseases affecting the anterior horn cell or motor root, such as motor neuron disease and cervical or lumbar spondylosis. Occasional fasciculations are seen in subjects who have peripheral neuropathy and it is not uncommon for normal people to have fasciculations occur occasionally in one particular muscle; if they are confined to the calf muscles, the phenomenon is usually of no pathological significance.

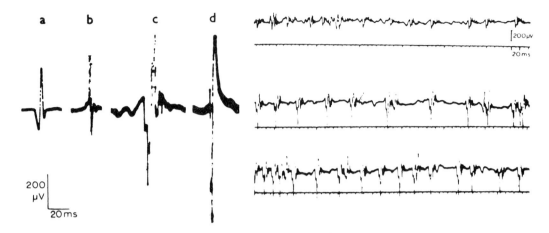

Four motor unit potentials recorded
from the biceps muscle

The interference pattern on slight (upper
trace), moderate (middle trace), and full
(lower trace) voluntary effort illustrating
motor units firing in isolation as a result
of partial denervation

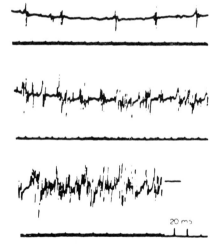

The interference pattern on slight (upper
trace), moderate (middle trace), and full
(lower trace) voluntary effort in a muscle
of a patient with muscular dystrophy
illustrating the increased number of
small multiphase motor unit potentials

Myotonia. These are high frequency spontaneous discharges of muscle fibres or groups of muscle fibres, initiated by touching or moving the muscle or by voluntary contraction. Following initiation of the myotonic response, there is a gradual fall in frequency and amplitude, giving a characteristic sound on the loudspeaker something like a motor cycle engine. The spontaneous discharge is usually accompanied by the clinical symptoms of muscular stiffness, or slowness of relaxation and is a feature of some inherited diseases of muscles such as dystrophi myotonica, Thomsen's disease, and other diseases in which there are disturbances of potassium metabolism.

High frequency discharges. Sometimes in a muscle that is either denervated or has a compressive lesion of its nerve supply, motor unit potentials will suddenly fire rapidly at high rates at rest. As a rule there is no clinical disability associated with this phenomenon, and it is observed only at electromyography. The potentials do not have the waxing and waning sound of myotonia and are abolished if the nerve supply to the muscle is blocked using a local anaesthetic.

Positive sharp waves are monophasic positive potentials recorded in a muscle the nerve supply of which has been acutely interrupted. They are a sign of denervation. The signals are regular and have a long duration, up to 80 ms.

Abnormalities of the EMG on voluntary effort. In the presence of a neurogenic lesion with complete interruption of the nerve supply to the muscle, there will obviously be no motor units firing in response to attempted voluntary effort. If there is a partial lesion of the nerve supply to the muscle there will be less motor units than normal firing on voluntary effort. This EMG pattern is another means of assessing the degree of severity of a nerve injury.

On full voluntary effort it is not possible to determine the shape or size of individual motor unit potentials because there are enough of them in the recording field of the electrode to overlap each other. If, however, there is a reduced number of motor units functioning as a result of interrupted nerve supply, then on full effort one will be able to see the remaining motor units firing at high rates of 30 per second or more. The form of the surviving motor unit potentials will obviously be within normal limits if it is an acute lesion. Certain abnormalities of the motor units will be found in the presence of subacute or chronic lesions.

If there is a chronic disease leading to denervation of some motor units then the denervated muscle fibres will be re-innervated by axonal branching from the nerve fibres of surviving normal motor units. In other words, the territory of the motor units will become larger than normal. An axon in the triceps innervating 160 muscle fibres may extend branches to some components of adjacent denervated units, and may then innervate over 500 muscle fibres. Hence that motor unit potential will be larger than normal, exceeding 9 or 10 mV, and it will have a longer duration because the conduction is slower through the axonal branches to the new components.

Thus the finding of motor units that are larger than normal, have more phases, and are of longer duration than normal is evidence of long-standing denervation with re-innervation. The common causes are motor neuron disease and injuries of the spinal nerve roots. Nascent motor units are motor units that are forming following interruption of a nerve supply to a muscle. The new motor units often contain a small number of muscle fibres, hence the amplitude of the motor unit is low and it is composed of small clusters of single muscle fibre spike potentials. They have a characteristic crackling sound in the loudspeaker.

By contrast there is a different type of alteration to the motor unit potentials in the muscles of subjects who have muscle disease. There are many different conditions responsible for primary disease of the muscles and the commonest are the congenital muscular dystrophies and polymyositis, which is an inflammatory condition affecting mainly the proximal muscles. In these conditions there is a random loss of muscle fibres from individual motor units.

The result is motor unit potentials of reduced amplitude and composed of many small spike components. In the loudspeaker they have a characteristic sound with a large number of high frequency crackling components. On full effort, the overall amplitude of the interference pattern is reduced and the crackling nature of the discharge intensifies in the loudspeaker, different from the dull rumbling sound of the normal interference pattern.

By studying the EMG of selected muscles at rest and during various degrees of voluntary effort it is therefore often possible to determine whether the particular muscle is normal or if there has been denervation, re-innervation, chronic denervation, or if the muscle is the site of a primary disease affecting muscle. Obviously there may be difficulty with very mild abnormalities and it is sometimes necessary to perform measurements of some of the features of the motor units to allow accurate comparisons with control data.

One approach is to photograph single motor unit potentials and to measure their amplitudes, and compare with studies on normal individuals. Another method is to feed the EMG signal into a computer which will automatically analyse the number of spikes occurring at a particular contraction load, and compare with values from normal muscles. It is possible to detect minor abnormalities in the EMG on effort, and is particularly useful in the early diagnosis of patients who have muscle disease.

NERVE CONDUCTION STUDIES

We have outlined the information obtained by electromyography from muscles at rest, and contracting in response to voluntary effort. The third phase of the examination is the study of the response to electrical stimulation of the motor nerve supply. The peripheral nerves contain a mixture of myelinated and unmyelinated nerve fibres. The radial nerve contains several thousand myelinated fibres which are a mixture of motor efferent and sensory afferent fibres, and of unmyelinated sensory fibres.

All fibres in a nerve are capable of artificial stimulation by applying an electric shock to the nerve trunk. The fibres most easily stimulated are the myelinated fibres of large diameter, and those less easily stimulated are the small unmyelinated fibres. The motor fibres are all myelinated, and if an electric shock is applied to a normal nerve trunk via the skin it is possible to simultaneously activate all the motor fibres in that nerve using a stimulus that is bearable for the patient. The technique is the basis of assessing motor nerve conduction.

Muscle responses may be recorded with a concentric needle electrode within the muscle or with a surface recording electrode strapped to the skin over the muscle. The former method allows a slightly more accurate measurement of the onset of the response, which is not attenuated by the insulating properties of the overlying skin and adipose tissue. By contrast, the latter method using surface recording electrodes provides additional information in that the amplitude of the evoked response is a measure of the amount of the responsive muscle tissue that is present.

It is helpful to refer to the following diagram of recordings obtained during a study on a median nerve using surface recording electrodes.

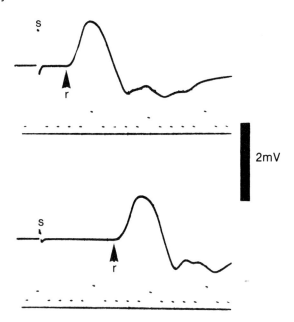

2mV

The evoked muscle potential recorded from the abductor pollicis brevis in response to stimulation of the median nerve at the wrist (upper trace) and at the elbow (lower trace). s = stimulus, r = the onset of the evoked response.

Two silver recording electrodes have been strapped over the thenar eminence so that the active electrode is over the belly of the abductor pollicis brevis muscle, and the reference electrode is over the metacarpophalangeal joint. A negative deflection at the muscle belly electrode produces an upward deflection on the oscilloscope screen. The stimulating electrode is now positioned over the median nerve at the wrist just proximal to the carpal tunnel. The cathode is placed distally (that is, nearer to the recording electrode) since the cathode is the more efficient of the two at producing depolarisation of the underlying nerve.

The amplitude of the stimulus is increased until a maximal response is obtained from the muscle. This ensures reproducibility of the results and allows comparison with control subjects. The duration of the stimuli is usually 0.2 ms, and the amplitude of the necessary stimulus depends to some extent upon skin resistance, but in control patients is usually no more than 150 volts. It is therefore possible from the photographic records to determine the latency of conduction through the carpal tunnel region to the muscle, the time elapsed from stimulus to the first response from the muscle. In other words, we are looking at the conduction in the fastest conducting fibres.

The amplitude of the response may also be measured. The site of application of the cathode is marked, and the median nerve is then stimulated at a proximal site in the ante-cubital fossa. The stimulus is increased again until a supramaximal response is recorded from the thenar eminence. It may be seen that the latency is considerably longer because the nerve impulses have to spread from the elbow to the muscle. The site of stimulation is now marked, and the distance measured from the elbow to wrist with a millimetre rule. It is now possible by simple proportion to determine the conduction velocity of the fastest fibres in the median nerve from the elbow to the wrist in metres per second.

The three measurements obtained in motor conduction velocity studies are thus:

(a) The terminal latency from the distal stimulation site to the muscle. The distal segment response cannot be expressed in terms of velocity. One has to take into account the delay at the neuromuscular junction, and the delay due to the spread of the electrical signal through the muscle membrane. In control subjects the upper limit of normal for adults in the median nerve is 5.0 ms, in the ulnar nerve 4.0 ms, and the lateral popliteal nerve 7.5 ms. The latency may be increased in one nerve only if there is a compressive lesion affecting that nerve, or it will be increased in all nerves if there is a diffuse disease affecting the motor fibres, such as peripheral neuropathy.

(b) The motor conduction velocity; the lower limit for control adults is 49 m/s in the upper limb and 40 m/s in the lower limb. The velocity will fall in one nerve if there is a disorder localised to that nerve, or it will be reduced in all nerves if there is a diffuse disturbance of the anterior horn cells or of the peripheral nerves. Several factors must be considered when making comparison between the same patient on different occasions, and between a patient and a group of control subjects. Both latency and motor conduction velocity are affected by age, temperature, and by the care taken to perform accurate measurements of distance on the skin, and of the photographs of the recorded responses. For example, velocity falls by 2.4 m/s per degree C lowering, in nerve temperature.

On some occasions a clue to the underlying pathology may be given by the finding of extremely slow conduction velocities such as 17 or 18 m/s, a feature of segmental demyelination, in which there is a specific disorder affecting the Schwann cell insulating layer on the myelinated fibres.

(c) The amplitude of the evoked muscle potential. The wide range of amplitudes for control patients partly depends on the resistance of the overlying skin to the passage of electrical signals. However, useful information may be obtained when one compares the amplitude of the response obtained from stimulating at different sites along the course of a nerve. For example, if a person has a peripheral neuropathy, and some of the motor fibres are conducting inefficiently, the amplitude of the response obtained from stimulating at a proximal site may be smaller and more dispersed than a response obtained by stimulating nearer to the recording electrode, because of dispersion of the descending volley of impulses in the motor nerve trunk as the result of the presence of 'sick' axons.

Another finding of importance is the marked reduction in amplitude of the response when there is a compressive lesion between the stimulus site and the recording electrode. A good example is ulnar nerve lesion at the elbow.

A recording made from the abductor digiti minimi on stimulating the ulnar nerve at the wrist gives a normal response. The stimulus is now moved to the elbow above the level of the medial epicondyle, the common site for compressive lesions of the ulnar nerve. The nerve impulses from the stimulus now have to pass through the region of abnormal nerve, and many of the impulses will be slowed.

There is a reduction in amplitude of the evoked response and in the appearance of late components related to the delay in transmission in some fibres across the abnormal area. The slowing up of the conduction in some fibres results from oedema and from loss of myelin at the site of compression.

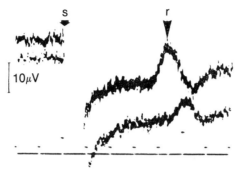

The superimposed responses recorded from a normal sural nerve (upper trace), and from a sural nerve (lower trace) from a patient with a neuropathy. The stimulus is applied at s, and the latency of the response is measured to the peak r.

SENSORY CONDUCTION STUDIES

Conduction in sensory nerve fibres is easy to assess in the upper limbs, since the interdigital nerves contain only sensory fibres. Ring electrodes may be attached to the index finger with the cathode nearer to the palm and stimuli applied. A response may be recorded from the median nerve at the wrist via surface electrodes strapped to the skin. The recording is of a sensory nerve action potential, and the amplitude in control patients is small and ranges from 9 to 40 μV. In a similar manner the little finger may be stimulated and a response recorded from the ulnar nerve. The sural nerve in the foot may also be studied.

The usual practice is to measure the latency of the sensory action potential to the peak of the response and to measure the amplitude of the response. Here again there are well defined values for control patients and the upper limit of peak latency for the median is 4.0 ms, for the ulnar nerve 3.5 ms, and for the sural nerve 4.5 ms. In healthy adults, the responses should be no smaller than 9 to 10 μV in amplitude.

The sensory action potentials are a sensitive measure of sensory nerve fibre function. They are lost completely early in the course of a neuropathy or compressive lesion and may be the only evidence of abnormality. For example, one only has to lose 4 or 5% of large myelinated fibres to completely lose the recordable sensory action potential, but one has to lose at least 30% of these fibres before there is demonstrable sensory loss on clinical examination.

PRACTICAL ASPECTS OF ELECTROMYOGRAPHY AND NERVE CONDUCTION STUDIES

The wide variety of patients referred for these investigations include patients with weakness localised to one or more muscles, or generalised in nature, patients suspected of having a peripheral neuropathy, root lesion or disease of the muscles, patients suspected, or known to have had an injury to a nerve, and patients who may have rather vague symptomatology and who are a problem in diagnosis.

The procedure can be carried out only by a neurologist, since the preamble to the examination involves taking neurological history and neurological examination of the patient to decide which procedures are most likely to yield useful information to the referring specialist. The one exception is the referral of patients with known nerve injury to a specialist in physical medicine who may perform electromyographic studies to determine the extent of the injury and prognosis for recovery. Electromyography may also be used in a research situation such as in the study of kinesiology.

Case 1. A seventeen year old man is referred with a four-week history of left-sided facial weakness. The illness began with aching in the ear about nine days after a viral illness. On examination, there is an almost complete lesion of the left facial nerve. No movement is noted of the angle of the mouth and the eye will not close.

The orbicularis oculi and orbicularis oris muscles are sampled with a concentric needle electrode. There are small numbers of spontaneous fibrillation potentials in the muscles, but on attempted voluntary effort numerous motor units respond. Electrical stimulation of the facial nerve at the angle of the jaw produces visible movement of the muscles and a response is recorded of latency 3.8 ms to the orbicularis oculi and 4.0 ms to the orbicularis oris.

Comment. Although there is little clinical evidence of function in the muscles supplied by the facial nerve, the small amount of spontaneous fibrillation on EMG, and the good response to electrical stimulation indicate that there is little axonal degeneration and that the face is paralysed because of a conduction block of the facial nerve, probably in the facial canal. This is a typical example of Bell's palsy.

The severity of the lesion is assessed by considering the amount of spontaneous fibrillation found in the muscles, the responsiveness of the muscles to voluntary effort and the responsiveness to electrical stimulation. With a complete lesion, there would be profuse spontaneous fibrillation and no units would respond either to voluntary effort or to electrical stimulation of the facial nerve. The prognosis in such a case would be poor.

Case 2. A girl of 19 is about to be married. There is a vague family history of some muscle disease, and she wishes to determine whether there is a risk of her having affected children.

The first step is to take a detailed family history, to determine as far as possible the features of the history that have raised the possibility of muscle disease and to examine as many members of the family as possible. The second step is to perform a careful neurological examination of the patient. She is found to have slight weakness of the facial and shoulder girdle muscles, although there is no wasting. A blood sample is taken to perform muscle enzyme estimations. Electromyography is performed on the right deltoid, lateral head of the triceps and supraspinatus muscles. Large areas of the muscles seem to be normal but others contain low amplitude multiphasic units consisting of small spike components.

Comment. There is clinical and electrical evidence of muscle disease and biopsy is arranged to be taken from a muscle on the side of the body opposite to the EMG to assist in establishing the nature of the pathology. This is essential to act as a guide for genetic counselling.

Case 3. A man of 51 has been referred because of dull aching in the right hand and inner aspect of the forearm for five months. On clinical examination there is a suggestion of wasting of the intrinsic muscles of the right hand but no other definite abnormality is demonstrable. The fingers are nicotine-stained. Electromyographic examination performed upon the deltoid, lateral head of the triceps, extensors of the forearm, biceps, abductor pollicis brevis, and abductor digiti minimi. The muscles of the arm and forearm are normal but the small muscles of the hand (which are supplied by T1) contain a markedly reduced interference pattern and motor units fire in isolation. Motor conduction velocities of the median and ulnar nerves are 51 and 53 m/s respectively and the latencies are normal. A normal median nerve sensory action potential of 18 μV is recorded but the ulnar nerve sensory action potential is only 3 μV.

Comment. The studies show partial denervation of the small muscles of the hand (T1) supplied by the median and ulnar nerves. However the median nerve sensory action potential is normal while the ulnar response is reduced. The ulnar sensory action potential is an assessment of the C8 fibres, and the combination of findings suggests a lesion that affects the C8 and T1 components of the brachial plexus, raising the possibility of a cervical rib or a lung cancer eroding the plexus. Pain in the hand either with or without wasting is a common symptom and there are often few if any clinical signs. The differential diagnosis includes conditions such as lesions of the median nerve of the wrist, lesions of the ulnar nerve at the elbow, cervical spondylosis, lesions of the brachial plexus, and psychogenic disturbances. The problem can be resolved only by the combination of neurological history, neurological examination and a carefully planned study including electromyography and assessment of motor and sensory nerve conduction.

Case 4. A 21 year old motor cycle rider is referred for the investigation of paralysis of the left arm following an accident; seven weeks have elapsed since the injury. There is slight contraction of the biceps, and good contraction of the deltoid supraspinatus and interspinatus but virtually no other motor power in the arm. On electromyography a relatively normal pattern is obtained from the deltoid biceps and supraspinatus muscles. The triceps, forearm extensors and flexors and the small muscles of the hand contain profuse spontaneous fibrillation, and no motor units appear on attempted voluntary effort or in response to electrical stimulation of their nerve supply. There is extensive sensory loss over the whole arm but in spite of this, normal sensory action potentials are recorded from the median and ulnar nerves at the wrist in response to stimulating the respective fingers.

Comment. The distribution of clinical weakness and the findings on electromyography indicate extensive involvement of the lower roots of the brachial plexus from C7 to T1. The preservation of the sensory action potentials in the median (C6) and ulnar (C8) nerves in spite of extensive sensory loss in these dermatomes indicates that the site of the lesions is on the proximal side of the dorsal root ganglion cells and that the nerve roots have been avulsed from the spinal cord. If confirmed by myelography, the outlook for recovery is hopeless. Fortunately, if muscles supplied by C5 and 6 are relatively intact, a useful artificial limb may be fitted.

Case 5. A 51 year old man is referred with a four month history of difficulty with swallowing; he has not noticed any weakness or sensory loss in any other areas of the body. On neurological examination, he has a spastic dysarthria and there is some wasting of the tongue muscle. The bulk of the limb musculature is good, but occasional fasciculations were noticed on examining the shoulder girdles, paraspinal muscles and the right quadriceps.

Electromyographic examination of the right deltoid, lateral head of triceps, abductor pollicis brevis, vastus medialis, and tibialis anterior reveals frequency fasciculation potentials and some spontaneous fibrillation is noted from the abductor pollicis brevis muscle. The interference pattern in the deltoid and tibialis anterior is within normal limits but in the other muscles there is reduced interference pattern and motor units are seen to fire in relative isolation on maximum effort; some of these motor unit potentials are over 15 mV amplitude. Motor conduction velocities are normal and the sensory action potentials are also normal.

Comment. The finding of fasciculations, spontaneous fibrillations and giant motor units in several muscles of both the upper and lower limb indicates a diffuse disorder affecting the anterior horn cells or roots; for example, motor neuron disease.

GLOSSARY OF ELECTROMYOGRAPHIC CHANGES

Normal motor unit

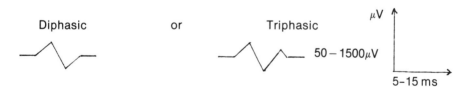

Fibrillation — muscle action potentials of short duration and caused by the firing of single muscle fibres spontaneously. It may be evoked by the mechanical irritation of the sarcolemminal membrane of a denervated muscle by needle protrusion or by mechanical stimuli such as needle movement or surface percussion of the muscle.

Fasciculation — involuntary contraction of the physiologic motor unit. It can be seen by the naked eye on the surface of skin and cannot be inhibited by voluntary relaxation. When seen in the absence of other signs of denervation, it is considered to be benign and of relatively unimportant clinical significance. It is irregular, from 1/min to 50/min, and is present when there is some voluntary element, and hence motor unit potential. It may occur in muscle cramps, benign myokymia anterior horn cell disease, and nerve root compression.

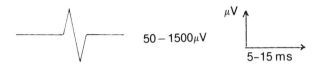

Positive sharp wave — spontaneous (positive deflection) potentials often seen in association with fibrillations, usually indicating denervation, but may appear days or weeks before the onset of fibrillation.

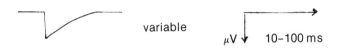

Polyphasic motor units — usually consist of four or more phases and two or more negative spikes.

    Polyphasic motor unit activity denotes that the nerve impulse travelling along the axon is slower than usual, and is usually the result of an alteration in the myelin sheath.

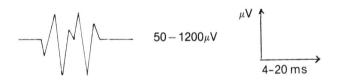

Insertion activity — A burst of action potentials ranging from fibrillation to positive wave forms. This may represent, in certain cases, the main EMG findings. It is more significant when the potentials occur in series.

Nerve potentials — Nerve potentials arise from the needle electrode contacting a nerve within the muscle substance. Amplitude: 20 to 250 μV. Duration: 1 to 4 ms. Wave form: diphasic. Frequency: 30 to 150/second. Sound: machine gun with a background of characteristic high pitched 'sea shell' murmur. Sometimes this action potential is referred to as pseudofibrillation.

Myopathic motor units — Tiny motor units recorded from diseased motor units, denoting that the muscular wasting is the result of disease of the muscle itself and rules out any alleged nerve pathology.

When accompanied by denervation activity, they are electrical manifestations of inflammatory polymyositis.

In the presence of atrophy, they can differentiate between atrophy of disuse or neurogenic atrophy.

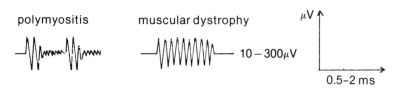

Myotonic waves — Denote the hyperexcitability of the muscle membrane and are usually recorded, on insertion, from persons suffering from myotonia congenita (with myopathic waves, indicates myotonia dystrophia). In muscle spasm, the presence of this activity establishes the diagnosis of myotonia congenita and eliminates all other conditions which cause muscle spasms.

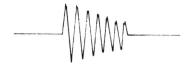

Bizarre high frequency discharges — usually recorded from muscles which have undergone neurogenic atrophy or in cases of polymyositis. They may be seen if the needle tip is in a muscle spindle.

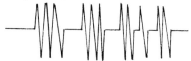

Giant motor unit — Usually seen in neuronopathy and indicates that the lesion is old. They develop over a period of months to years and are usually indicative of motor units which have branched to innervate fibres of an adjacent diseased motor unit.

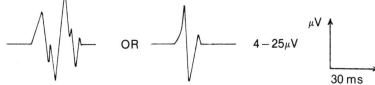

Negative nerve fibre activity — means that the needle tip has penetrated an intramuscular nerve fibre. They are of no clinical importance but can simulate fibrillation activity.

10.5 Summary of Electrodiagnosis

Low frequency currents are used effectively for electrodiagnosis. Standard methods used today are the strength-duration curves where the excitability characteristics of muscle or nerve fibre can be expressed as a curve obtained by joining points that graphically represent the threshold values of stimulation along the ordinate for various durations of stimulus displayed along the abscissa. Nerve excitability tests are done on the main nerve trunks, but the only such test done today which has any validity is that for lesions such as Bell's palsy. The validity and reliability of these tests have been queried by neurologists and hence it is important that meticulous laboratory-type care must be carried out when performing them to obtain accuracy. All the variables that could alter the findings must be considered if one is to make a valid diagnosis.

References

Adrian, E D, 1917, Physiological basis of electrical tests in peripheral nerve injury, *Arch Radiol and Electro, 21,* 379.

Alexander, Strength duration curves, *Arch Phys Med Rehabil, 55,* 74, February.

Bauwens, P, 1941, Electrodiagnosis and electrotherapy in peripheral nerve lesions, *Proc Roy Soc Med, 34,* 459.

Bickerstaff, E R, 1968, Neurological examination in clinical neurology, *Blackwell.*

Brown, E, The role of the physical therapist in EMG and nerve conduction studies, *JAPTA, 42,* No 1.

Brumuck, Joel, MD and Cohen, Hyman, MD, 1968, A manual of electroneuromyography, *Hoeker Medical Division, Harper and Row.*

Cawthorne, T, 1963, Indications for intratemporal facial nerve surgery, *Arch Otolar, 78,* 429.

Chusid, J, 1973, Correlative neuroanatomy, *California, Lange.*

Denham, K T, 1970, An introduction to electromyography, *NZ J Physio,* May.

di Benedetto, M, 1971, Electrodiagnosis: essentials for accurate neurological diagnosis, *Md State Med J, 20,* 89.

Goodgold, Joseph and Eberstein, Arthur, 1972, Electrodiagnosis of neuromuscular diseases, *Williams and Wilkins Co, Baltimore, Maryland.*

Hayden, J B, Evaluation of a peripheral nerve injury, *Phy Ther, 68,* 11.

Haymaker, Webb and Woodhall, Barnes, 1967, Peripheral nerve injuries, *W B Saunders Co, Phila.*

Hill, A V, 1936, Excitation and accommodation in nerve, *Proc Roy Soc, 119B,* 305.

Jantsch, H, 1952, The strength duration curve in the diagnosis of paralysis, *Brit J Phys Med, 15,* 252–253.

Jongkees, L B W, 1972, On peripheral facial nerve paralysis, *Arch Otolar, 95,* 317–323.

Joseph, J, 1960, Man's posture: electromyographic studies, *Springfield, Ill, Thomas.*

Lapicque, L, 1909, Definition experimentale de l'excitabilitie, *Compte Rendu Soc Biol, 67,* 280.

Licht, Sidney, Electrodiagnosis and electromyography, *Waverly Press Inc, Baltimore, Maryland.*

Lucas, K, 1907, The analysis of complex excitable tissues by their response to electric currents of short duration, *J Physiol, 35*, 310.

Marinacci, Alberto, 1968, Applied electromyography, *Lea and Febiger, Philadelphia*.

Norris, Forbes, 1963, The EMG, *Grune and Stratton, New York*.

Richardson, A T, Wynn Parry, C B, 1957, The theory and practice of electrodiagnosis, *Ann Phys Med, 4*, 1-2.

Ritchie, A E, 1944, The electrical diagnosis of peripheral nerve injury, *Brain, 67*, 314.

Spinner, M, 1972, Injuries of the major branches of peripheral nerves of the forearm, *Phila, Saunders*.

Stephens, W G S, 1971, A new technique for the assessment of muscle denervation using isosceles triangular pulse stimulation, *Proc Roy Soc Edin, B*, 71, 86.

Sunderland, S, 1968, Nerves and nerve injuries, *Edinburgh and London: Livingstone*.

Taverner, D, 1954, Cortisone treatment of Bell's Palsy, *Lancet, 2*, 1052-1054.

Taverner, D, 1954, Cortisone treatment of Bell's Palsy, *Lancet, 2*, 1052-1054.

Taverner, D, 1959, The prognosis and treatment of spontaneous facial palsy, *Proc Roy Soc Med, 52*, 1077-1080.

Taverner, D, 1965, Electrodiagnosis in facial palsy, *Arch Otolar, 81*, 470.

Taverner, D, 1968, The management of facial palsy, *Laryn Otolar, 82*, 585-590.

Wester, I, 1971, Bell's Palsy: The present state of electrodiagnosis and treatment, *J Can Physio Assoc, 23*, 5, 218-221.

Wester, I, 1974, Bell's Palsy: A review of the present status of electrodiagnosis and treatment, *Proc WCPT 1974 Congress*.

Yanagihara, N and Kishimoto, M, 1972, Electrodiagnosis in facial palsy, *Arch Otolar, 95*, 376-382.

11 The Fatal Current

11.1   Electric Shocks and Safety Factors

A seemingly harmless voltage of 20 millivolts can kill a patient under certain conditions. It could be generated by poorly designed or badly serviced electronic apparatus. Most apparatus used in physiotherapy departments is plugged into a mains supply of 240 V and frequency 50 Hz. Any apparatus plugged into the mains represents a hazard — the risk of electric shock. It would seem that a shock of 10 000 volts would be more deadly than 100 volts, but this is not so. Individuals have been electrocuted by appliances using as little as 40 volts direct current in industry, or by using household appliances. The measure of a shock intensity is the amount of current forced through the body. It is not the voltage, but the *amount of current* which does the damage.

After a person is knocked out by an electric shock it is important to give artificial respiration, since it is impossible to state how much current has passed through the vital organs of the body.

PHYSIOLOGICAL EFFECTS OF SHOCK

Up to 20 mA   —   labored breathing
                    breathing upset
                    painful
Up to 100 mA   —   cannot let go
                    muscular paralysis
                    ventricular fibrillation; at higher currents, the heart muscle
                    goes into spasm, which prevents fibrillation, and may even
                    improve the chances of survival
                    severe burns
100 to 200 mA —   unconsciousness
                    death
Above 200 mA   —   *death*

The skin resistance in a person can vary from 1000 ohms (Ω) in wet skin, to 500 000 Ω in dry skin. If a person contacts the mains supply, the body current can vary from 0.5 mA when the skin is dry to 240 mA when the skin is wet. The resistance of two electrodes placed on the skin can vary from 500 Ω to 0.5 MΩ, depending on moisture, dry skin and oils in the skin. If needle electrodes are placed into the body, the resistance of the body is zero. Under these circumstances a current as low as 20 mA will cause fibrillations. A voltage as low as 20 V can be fatal when there is faulty earthing of the machine.

HOW ELECTRIC SHOCKS OCCUR

In order to receive a shock, the person must become part of the electrical circuit by touching two terminals of a voltage source so that a shock current can flow. Two kinds of shock can occur: a macro-shock and a micro-shock.

A macro-shock. If the current flow is from the body surface through the skin into the body, a relatively large amount of current is needed to produce a harmful shock.

A micro-shock. If the current by-passes the surface of the body and enters the heart by way of a myocardial electrode or a transvenous catheter, a minute current can produce a fatal shock without the patient experiencing anything. For example, a therapist may be handling a patient with an electrical monitoring device on the heart. If at the same time he were to connect his hand to a faulty table lamp or some device with a broken ground connection, whilst palpating the patient's chest, then he could give the patient a micro-shock, and cause ventricular fibrillation.

A person can obtain a shock without touching the active wire of the power supply by the following mishaps:

(a)   Many electrical appliances have metal casings. An active voltage can be actually *shorted to the casing* because of dropping of the instrument, moisture, dust, deterioration of the equipment due to misuse or age. A person touching the casing could get a shock.

(b)   *The leakage current.* In all electrical equipment the intended current-carrying parts are separated from the rest of the equipment by insulators. With high quality insulation materials and good circuit designs there will be no problem with leakage currents, but with poor designs the leakage currents from the wires carrying the current will be hazardous.

(c)   *Two-pin connections.* It is important that all electrical equipment should have a three-pin connection with the earth connection, to avoid the leakage currents and hazards from metal casings. The three-pin system offers the protection of the fuse blowing if there is a leakage or a metal casing short-circuit. The three-pin system has the protective ground wire pin always longer than the others, to ensure that the ground connection is the first to be plugged in and the last to be unplugged. The building itself must carry a good grounding system for the power supply.

(d)   *Faulty components* in instrumentation and monitoring devices can cause a shock. Faulty transformers or leaky capacitors in the instrument's power supply can be hazardous.

ELECTRICAL BURNS

Electrical burns result in injury which varies depending on the physiological response of the tissues involved. Therefore therapy must be specific and individualised.

The main histological change in the tissues is coagulation necrosis. In blood vessels there is greater damage to the media layer since the bloodstream cools the intima. Delayed tissue death may be linked to necrosis of the media which results in progressive thrombosis within the blood vessels.

In the first 12 hours after electrical injury the skin is white surrounded by a line of hyperaemia. After this period, oedema and inflammation widen the demarcated area. In a few days the white skin turns black. Necrosis below the apparent skin damage may be extensive. Peripheral nerves fragment. Necrosis of fat, muscle and tendon occurs. Bone may be burned through.

Electrical burns on the mouth and lips should be treated conservatively to permit spontaneous sloughing, as early intervention may destroy important deep structures. Repair is delayed for at least one year. Burns of the skull are also treated conservatively. Extremities which are extensively and deeply burned and cannot be restored should be amputated early, since myoglobin released from extensively charred muscle may cause death from renal shut-down.

OTHER HAZARDOUS FACTORS

Short wave machines and microwave machines should not be placed close to an interferential machine as the latter will disrupt the frequencies, particularly of the short wave machine.

A microwave machine should not have its antenna in such a direction that it faces the open end of the room, as there is quite a leakage of radiation from the microwave circuits. Patient and therapists with metal rimmed spectacles can also have microwave reflected to their eyes, particularly when treating the neck or shoulder region.

Interferential, short wave, microwave and ultrasound should not be applied to any patient with a pacemaker as they will disrupt the operation of the pacemaker. In fact these machines have been shown to disrupt the operation of the pacemaker in a patient in the vicinity of the machine.

SAFETY FACTORS

The following safety precautions should be taken when using electrical equipment for therapeutic purposes.

Equipment use

All equipment which is enclosed with conductive materials must be connected to a three-pin supply plug.

The three-pin plug must be fitted into a power outlet. Do not use the same power outlet for two machines, by including an adapter.

Avoid the use of extension cords as they can increase leakage current flow to the ground, apart from the risk of somebody tripping over the cord.

Never pull the plug out of its socket by pulling on the wire.

Never drag short wave machines or microwave machines by the arms of the machine.

Be careful not to pull the cable connection of the movable angled ultrasound transducer heads.

Always check the power plugs and outlet for any loose connections.

Never disconnect a machine from the wall power outlet with the power turned up. This will cause arcing at the plug and receptacle, and heating and damage to the plug.

All equipment should be unplugged at the end of a day's work.

Always check the power controls and other monitoring devices for perfect working order before applying the modality to a patient. If any pilot light or control functions partially or sporadically, it must be repaired.

If water gets into any electrical equipment, it must be serviced before use.

Positioning of equipment

As all electrical equipment generates heat, the machine must be positioned so that there is ample ventilation space around it.

Ensure that the antenna of the microwave machine is directed against the wall so that any leakage of microwave will not come towards the operator.

Interferential machines must be placed 3 metres away from short wave and microwave machines, and 10 metres away from ECG machines and pacemakers.

Do not place electrical equipment next to radiator pipes or water pipes within the reach of the patient or the operator.

Treatment couches or chairs used for short wave or microwave treatments should be made of wood or plastic.

There should be no metal in the pathway of low, medium, or high frequency currents, fields or waves.

Patient precautions

The precautions, emphasised throughout the text, of checking for contra-indications to the use of a modality, skin testing for pain and/or thermal sensation as appropriate and warning the patient of the potential dangers of a modality must be strictly observed.

The following standard warnings for patients receiving heat or electrical treatments are recommended and must be given before *every* treatment, not only at the first treatment. In clinics where English is not the usual language of many patients, it is recommended that these warnings are translated into the appropriate languages and printed on cards so that the patients can read them. In addition, we recommend that large signs be displayed in the treatment areas giving the warnings in various languages as appropriate.

A STANDARD WARNING FOR PATIENTS ABOUT TO RECEIVE A HEAT TREATMENT

When receiving a heat treatment, all you should feel is a mild, comfortable warmth. If you feel anything hotter than this, or heat concentrated in one spot, *you could be in danger of being burned*. Call your physiotherapist immediately. Please do not move during your treatment, nor touch any of the equipment. Remember, if you have any doubts, ask your physiotherapist to assist, immediately. Do you understand?

A STANDARD WARNING FOR A PATIENT ABOUT TO RECEIVE AN ELECTRICAL TREATMENT

This is an electrical stimulation treatment. All you should feel is a "tingling" sensation in and around the area of the electrodes. This may be accompanied by a contraction of the muscles and you may see your limb moving. This is a perfectly safe treatment. Should you feel the sensation concentrating in any one spot, or becoming painful, you must call me immediately, *otherwise your tissues could be damaged*. Please do not move or touch any of the equipment. Do you understand?

An additional precaution, in the interests of patients with pacemakers — it is recommended that a sign be prominently displayed on the door of the treatment area, warning patients that machines are in use which may interfere with pacemaker function.

Machine servicing
Although we recommend that all machines are tested on the therapist before they are applied to the patient, it is also advisable to have all machines checked by a qualified service technician at least annually regardless of the amount of usage. In fact, lack of use can result in equipment malfunction in some instances.

Therapists should make themselves familiar with the recommendations of the Standards Association of Australia regarding Electrical Safety. The appropriate references are listed at the end of this unit.

11.2   Summary

All physiotherapists must be fully aware of the responsibility placed on them to be safe practitioners, capable of selecting a modality that will have no adverse effects on the patient, and administering the modality correctly and safely to obtain the desired effects. It is important that all hazards associated with electric current usage must be understood. The ways a current could become lethal to either the therapist or the patient must be known. It is not the sole responsibility of the designer and manufacturer of electrical equipment to produce safe instrumentation. The user should take proper care, arrange regular maintenance, and be alert to all hazards that could occur in the lifetime of a machine.

References

Cheng and Aston, 1976, Safe use of electromedical equipment, *Physio Can*, March, May.

Commonwealth Scientific and Industrial Research Organization, 1975, *Safety Booklet No. 1*, Electrical safety: A code of practice.

Conolly, C, 1976, The possibility of harmful effects in using ultrasound, *Biomed Eng*, March.

Flaws in medical design can kill, *Electronic Design*, September 1, 1967.

The fatal current, 1966, Clinical note, *Phys Ther, 46*.

Hollway, Hunter and Higgins, Report on radiations from microwave apparatus, New South Wales, Australia, *Nat Stand Lab, Chippendale*.

Mesley, J, 1975, Some therapy might be deadly, *Physio Can, 27*, 103.

Michels, E, 1975, Electrical hazards, *Phys Ther, 55*, 1139.

Standards Association of Australia, 1976, Report on effects of current passing through the human body, *Miscellaneous Publication MP30-1976*.

Standards Association of Australia, 1978a, Electrical installations in electromedical treatment areas, *Standard AS 3003-1976*.

Standards Association of Australia, 1978b, Electromedical equipment: general requirements, *Standard AS 3200-1978*.

Standards Association of Australia, 1980, Guide to the safe use and application of electrically operated equipment in patient care areas, *Draft Standard DR 80253*.

Standards Association of Australia, 1981a, Rules for the electrical equipment of buildings, structures and premises, *Standard AS 3000-1981*.

Standards Association of Australia, 1981b, Transformers in electromedical equipment, *Standard AS 3208-1981*.

Ward, A, 1980, Electricity, fields and waves in therapy, *Science Press*.

Ward, Alex, 1981, Electrical safety: an Australian perspective, *Aust J Physio*, 28, 1, 3-11.

12 The Selection of Physical Agents for the Management of Clinical Problems

Some of the common problems arising in the main pathological conditions that present for physiotherapy treatment are:

pain
pain and muscle spasm
muscle tension
oedema
effusion
contractures
adhesions
scars
inflammation
infection
indolent wounds and ulcers

The methods of treatment used today are largely empirical or selected randomly in terms of time available, access to the modality, and individual preferences. An attempt will be made to rationalise the selection of specific modalities for effective use in physiotherapy.

12.1 Classification of Physical Agents

The physical agents in use today can be classified according to their specific effects on biological tissues.

Classification of physical agents

EFFECTS	TYPE OF AGENT	MODALITIES
thermal	conductive heating agents heating by radiation	hot packs; paraffin wax; cryotherapy; peloids infrared
thermal and non-thermal	diathermy agents producing conversive heating and non-thermal effects	short wave diathermy; microwave diathermy; ultrasonic energy
stimulation of nerve and/or muscle	low frequency currents medium frequency currents	faradic-type currents; long duration pulsed currents; sinusoidal currents; direct current; interferential currents; didynamic currents; acupuncture; TNS
stimulation of circulatory mechanisms	compression units low frequency currents medium frequency currents	intermittent pressure cuffs with varying pressure and cycles faradic currents; sinusoidal currents interferential; didynamic currents
effects on skin and superficial tissue for infection and skin lesions	ultraviolet rays diathermy agents	mercury vapor lamps; fluorescent or 'black light' tubes; Kromayer or cold quartz lamps microwave; short wave diathermy; infrared radiation

12.2   Thermal and Non-Thermal Effects of Treatment

In the selection of physical agents for thermal effects one must consider the variables involved:
temperature
penetration depth
absorption
thermal conductivity of specific tissues
specific resistance of tissue
duration of temperature change
rate of temperature change
existing pathophysiology
patency of circulation
patency of sensation

contra-indications to heat or cold
size of lesion.

TEMPERATURE AND PENETRATION

Therapeutic ranges of temperature lie within 39° to 44°C for heat and 0° to 27°C for cold.

Conductive heating agents cause a *gradual rise* of temperature of from 2° to 5°C which fluctuates during the application. The depth of penetration is only to the level of the epidermis.

Conversive heating agents, such as short wave diathermy and microwave, cause a rise of temperature varying from 3° to 10°C.

Short wave diathermy using condenser electrodes produces an *immediate rise* of temperature of up to 5°C. The depth of penetration will depend on the arrangement of the rigid electrodes or space plates. The rise in temperature is maintained during the application. The use of the induction cable causes a rise in temperature of up to 7° to 8°C.

Microwave diathermy produces a temperature rise of 5° to 7°C and has an effective penetration of 30 mm, provided there is no large quantity of fat in the field. The rise in temperature is immediate and remains constant during the application.

Ultrasound produces a rise in temperature of up to 8°C in deeper structures, particularly around a joint or bone up to a depth of 100 mm, depending on the frequency of the machine. Frequencies of 0.75 MHz have a half-value penetration of 100 mm, while a 1 MHz frequency has a half-value penetration of 50 mm. The temperature rise in the muscles and superficial fascia is about 3° to 5°C.

Infrared rays produce a rise of up to 5° to 6°C in the superficial tissues only. The depth of penetration is to the level of the dermis. There is some rise in temperature of the superficially placed joints and muscles.

Conductive heating agents such as paraffin wax baths, hydrocollator packs, contrast baths and hot water baths are used for a gentle rise of temperature in the superficial tissues. The superficial tissues have an increase of 7° to 8°C, but this diminishes as the function of skin vasculature is heat regulation, and dissipation of heat rapidly occurs. Overall there is an effective rise of 2° to 5°C in the superficial tissues. A lowered temperature in the underlying joints may occur reflexly, and may account for pain relief in subacute cases of rheumatoid arthritis, which is characterised by raised temperatures of joints.

Conductive heating agents are characterised by the gentle moist heat which is markedly sedative for painful areas in a superficial region. They are easy to apply over larger muscle areas or, as with paraffin wax baths, the uneven surfaces of hands or feet may be heated evenly.

All forms of diathermy cause *a rapid rise in temperature*, with selective tissue heating occurring at the time of peak temperature (Lehmann, Abramson). Peaking occurs after 12 to 25 minutes. The increased tissue temperature remains for up to 30 to 45 minutes following removal of short wave, microwave or ultrasound.

It must be remembered that when heat is applied to an area the underlying joints receive the physiological effects of heat by reflex mechanisms. Any temperature rise in the skin is quickly dissipated because the function of skin circulation is to dissipate heat. The circulation in muscle is not increased by heat, but is only effectively increased by heat plus exercise.

Heat is used for its vasodilatation effect in the various tissues, for altering metabolic activities, accelerating the passage of sodium and potassium ions by altering cell permeability, and decreasing pain perception by blocking the pain pathways. Heat also affects the collagen content of tissues and accelerates extensibility and elasticity of soft tissue.

Cryotherapy will lower the temperature of the body, if required. The method of cryotherapy used determines the extent and the speed of temperature reduction.

Immersion icing produces the largest drop in temperature of 10° to 12°C. Sudden and large drops in temperature produce marked vasoconstriction followed by cyclic phases of vasoconstriction and vasodilatation for long periods of time even after the cessation of treatment. Ice packs produce a slow and smaller drop in temperature but, if maintained for a period of 15 to 20 minutes, produce effective analgesic and vasoconstrictive effects. After-effect vasodilatation is also seen. Cryotherapy is used for the blocking of fusimotor efferents to control spasticity. It is also used for its vasoconstriction and delayed vasodilatation effect. The vasoconstriction effect is useful for acute swelling. It is effective for reducing pain by blocking pain pathways. At specific temperatures, cold can improve isometric endurance, but generally it reduces muscle tone and elasticity of soft tissue.

If a temperature rise to 42° to 44°C is required for:

(*a*) Joints   —   use ultrasound for superficial or deep joints; depending on the depth required, use a 3 MHz, 1 MHz or 0.8 MHz frequency.

               —   use microwave for superficial joints with little fascia, fat or muscle covering the lesion and no subcutaneous bony prominences.

(b) Muscles   —   for superficial large muscles with little fat, use inductothermy, such as monode, minode or cable, or microwave.

               —   for deep muscles which are more than 50 mm deep, select ultrasound using 0.8 MHz frequency.

For a temperature of 39° to 40°C that is to be maintained for longer periods:

(*a*) Joints   —   select short wave diathermy using the condenser field technique.

(*b*) Muscles   —   select pulsed ultrasound in the ratio of 1 : 10 or 1 : 5.

For a gentle temperature rise of 2° to 3°C for:

(*a*) Superficial joints and muscles such as the hands and feet — use paraffin wax.
(*b*) Superficial muscles — use hot packs or infrared.

To reduce temperature by 10° to 18°C in superficial muscles, use immersion icing or ice cube massage.

To reduce temperature by 5° to 10°C in superficial muscles, use ice packs or iced towels.

ABSORPTION, THERMAL CONDUCTIVITY, AND SPECIFIC RESISTANCE

The absorption of short wave by the tissues of the body is dependent on fluid content. High fluid content tissues are muscle and vascular organs. Bone acts as an impedance in the field and causes displacement currents through it. Fat is easily heated up, even though it has a lower dielectric constant and thermal conductivity than muscle, because it has lymphatics and blood vessels in the areolar tissues which surround the fat cells, causing the greater heating. The vessels have high values of dielectric constant and conductivity and produce a high rate of heating.

Microwave is also absorbed well by tissues with high fluid content. The penetration and absorption of microwave is governed by the presence of bone and fat. If there is a moderate amount of fat between skin and muscle, there is reflection at the fat-muscle interface, causing more heating in the superficial fascia and very little penetration into muscle. With 2450 Hz microwave there is about 30 mm penetration into muscle if there is no fat or bone intervening. Microwave is also reflected at the muscle-bone boundary. Lower frequencies of microwave have better penetration and less reflection at fat-muscle or muscle-bone interfaces.

Ultrasonic energy is absorbed by tissues with a high protein content such as muscle, nerve, and bone. It is not absorbed by fat or fluids. It is reflected at the periosteum-bone interface and produces a high temperature rise in structures surrounding a joint. Absorption is frequency dependent. A frequency of 3 MHz has greater absorption properties but has only 30 mm half-value penetration. It is important to select a suitable frequency and dosage to gain maximum absorption (see Unit 5).

SIZE AND DEPTH OF LESION

Short wave diathermy and microwave can cover larger areas and produce a vigorous heating effect mainly in the superficial regions. Vigorous heating in large deep-seated lesions can be produced by short wave diathermy using the condenser electrode technique, but ultrasound produces the best rise in temperature in deeper areas without causing excessive heating in the superficial regions.

The microwave beam is more divergent than ultrasound and covers a larger area. There is a greater interference field in front of the ultrasound beam so that it is difficult to calculate the amount of absorption and heating that would occur. The heating effect from microwave is more predictable as long as the quantity of fat, fluid, and the bone-muscle interface is considered.

Hot packs produce a gentle, mild, moist heat to large areas and are useful for superficial large muscles. The gentle heat also produces reflexly a lower temperature at joints so that it is useful in cases of rheumatoid arthritis, where joint temperature is increased. The sedative action of moist, gentle heat is utilised here.

Infrared is useful for heating moderately large superficial areas such as the back, thigh, around the neck, shoulder and knees. It is sedative to superficial nerve endings and increases circulation to any superficially placed inflammation, thus aiding healing. Infrared reaches the dermis level so that some arterial circulation is increased.

Paraffin wax baths are useful for the extremities such as hands and feet, as the wax is moulded carefully around the joints. It produces a gentle rise in temperature which overall is no more than 2°C, even though temporarily there is a 7° to 8°C rise in the skin and fascia, but this is quickly dissipated.

Cryotherapy is used only for superficially placed muscles and soft tissue. There is some reflex effect of increased temperature in deeper structures.

EXISTING PATHOPHYSIOLOGY

It is generally accepted, according to Lehmann, Guy, and Griffin, that the following reactions to heat are desirable for therapeutic purposes;
the extensibility of collagen tissues is increased;
joint stiffness is decreased;
pain is decreased;
muscle spasm is reduced;
the resolution of chronic inflammatory processes is aided;
the absorption of acute and chronic traumatic exudate and oedema is accelerated
    by the diffusion of sodium and potassium ions in cells and tissue fluid;
    (reversal of the viscosity of intra- and extra-cellular colloidal substances).
Cold is desirable for the following effects:
the marked vasoconstriction effect which prevents formation of exudate in acute
    trauma;
decrease of pain;
decrease of muscle spasm and spasticity;
reflex stimulation of muscles with poor tone (with brief icing);
prolonged periods of vasodilatation which will enhance the desired effects of the
    vasodilatation.
Vigorous heating is useful for chronic states where there are contractures of joint capsule and other periarticular structures, and for lesions of tendons, muscles and ligaments around a joint. It is used for pain and swelling in an area, and for chronic inflammatory conditions such as pelvic inflammation and sinusitis. It is also used for the resolution of haematomas after injury or in surgical incisions. It is used for its metabolic effect, as when short wave diathermy is used to increase the activity of the uterine organs to aid conception.

Mild and moderate heating produces a gentle rise in temperature, which overall is no more than 2° or 3°C, even though initially the skin rises by 6° or 7°C. The temperature rise is effective only for short periods. Conversive diathermy agents can be used to produce minimal heating at deeper levels. Mild heating is used mainly for its sedative effects as it reduces pain perception. In the subacute phases it can gently accelerate the absorption of exudate. In any inflammatory conditions, heat generally aggravates the symptoms in the acute and subacute phases.

CONTRA-INDICATIONS

The contra-indications for each modality have been discussed in detail in the previous units and must be carefully excluded before proceeding with treatment.

NON-THERMAL EFFECTS

Non-thermal effects are the micromassage of ultrasound or the Krasny-Ergen effect, that is, the tendency of microscopic particles to rearrange under the influence of electrical fields. The Krasny-Ergen effect is yet unproved for microwave and short wave, but effects such as decrease in glycogen granules in muscle and liver, alteration of mitochrondria in liver, muscle, and kidney, destruction or increase of lysosomes, changes in transport across membranes, changes in electrophoretic mobility and ultrastructural changes in muscle, have been reported as not being due to heating or cavitation with ultrasound. These are still being investigated. For non-thermal effects of ultrasound, pulsed ultrasound in the ratio of 1:10 or 1:5 is used.

12.3 Stimulation of Nerve and Muscle

Low frequency currents are used today for diagnosis and for therapy. They have fallen into disrepute in many countries because over the years indiscriminate use has proved time-consuming and ineffective. It is important to evaluate the patient carefully, understand the physiological effects of these currents, and then make a selection.

STIMULATION OF NERVES

The currents are generally used for the following reasons:
(*a*) for the restoration of lowered muscle tone due to disuse atrophy or inhibition by pain from underlying pathological lesions such as injury to muscle or an underlying joint;
(*b*) for the hypertrophy of weak muscles.
The selection of faradic-type currents to achieve these objectives is made if therapeutic exercises are not being effective, or if the atrophy of muscle is marked and the patient has no memory of the pattern of movement. Even though the technique is time-consuming it is worthwhile as it has been proved that it reduces rehabilitation time. It is important to obtain good contractions and ensure that the patient participates actively in the treatment.

The currents used are:
(*a*) faradic-type currents — triangular or square wave pulses from 0.2 to 1 ms pulse duration with a frequency of 50 Hz and selectively surged;
(*b*) faradism, which is an uneven alternating surged current with a pulse duration of 1 ms at a frequency of 50 Hz, primarily followed by damped oscillation of 1000 Hz.

STIMULATION OF MUSCLES

According to Seddon, Sunderland and Guttman, it has been proved that the selective use of low frequency currents is valuable for the rehabilitation of patients with paralysed muscles. It is important that the most suitable pulses are used at the right time.

A prognosis of paralysis can generally be made by the current electrodiagnostic techniques available. In patients with neuropraxia, it has been found that use of 100 ms rectangular pulses given daily maintains the muscles in a good working order and reduces the rehabilitation time. In patients with denervation from axonotmesis, the use of long duration triangular, saw-tooth, or trapezoidal pulses on the smaller distal muscles is useful to prevent denervation atrophy, loss of extensibility and maintain the nutrition of the muscle. The treatment must be started as soon as possible after the onset of the lesion. There is no point in starting three months later. Good strong contractions given with the muscle stretched and resisted achieves the objectives mentioned earlier in Unit 8.

Currents used are triangular, square wave, trapezoidal, or saw-tooth slow rising pulses with pulse durations varying from 100 to 1000 ms with a frequency of 5 to 1.5 Hz.

12.4   Stimulation of Circulatory Mechanisms

OEDEMA

Oedema is the excessive accumulation of tissue fluid in the tissue spaces and serous sacs of the body, and is due to disturbance of the mechanisms governing fluid exchange. There are four mechanisms that govern fluid exchange:

(a)   osmotic pressure — decrease of osmotic pressure due to reduction of plasma proteins can cause oedema;

(b)   hydrostatic pressure — increase in hydrostatic pressure of the capillaries due to cardiac or renal failure upsets fluid exchange;

(c)   cell permeability — if increased permeability of the capillaries occurs from injury or inflammation, oedema ensues;

(d)   lymphatic obstruction — any damage to lymph nodes and lymph vessels will cause obstruction of fluid removal mechanisms and oedema.

The effects of oedema are:

(a)   disturbance of nutrition;

(b)   increase in spread of infection, if present;

(c)   loss of function of movement;

(d)   impairment of sensation;

(e)   if fibroblasts are present in the oedema fluid, it will become organised into fibrous tissue and the area will become hard and swollen; this is *woody oedema*, which is tenacious;

(f)   pain;

(g)   reduction of muscle tone resulting from inactivity, with possibility of contractures occurring.

Oedema may be general or local. General oedema may be:

(a)   *Cardiac oedema* — the two main factors are venous congestion and gravity (hydrostatic pressure seen in the feet and ankles first and gradually extending).

(b)   *Renal oedema* — the basis of renal oedema is the retention of fluid due to failure of damaged kidneys to eliminate enough water. The excess water is shunted into the interstitial spaces.

(c)   *Starvation oedema* — caused by imperfect nutrition, mainly protein insufficiency.

Patients suffering from general oedema due to renal or cardiac failure are not treated with physiotherapy. Any infective foci present in the oedema indicate that all physiotherapy measures are contra-indicated. Haemarthrosis is also a contra-indication.

Local oedema may be:

(a) *Traumatic oedema* — following injury to bone and/or soft tissues, there is possible damage to blood vessels and lymphatics, causing increased permeability of capillaries and extravasation of fluid into the tissue spaces.

(b) *Gravitational oedema* occurs if the main muscles responsible for pumping the circulation are impaired by lesions or immobilisation. This is seen when there is paralysis of the muscles, with circulatory problems or with prolonged immobilisation in plaster.

(c) *Obstructive oedema* is seen in patients who have had radical mastectomy for carcinoma of the breast and after a deep vein thrombosis. It also occurs with tight plaster and bandages.

EFFUSION

Effusion is the pouring out of fluid, which is either serous, purulent, or bloody, into tissue spaces or serous sacs. Effusion into a joint is called *synovitis* of a joint and is inflammation of the synovial membrane lining the capsule of the joint. *Bursitis* is inflammation of the bursa under areas of friction caused by tendons or muscles. Inflammation of the synovial sheath surrounding tendons is called *tenosynovitis*.

It is essential to determine the cause of the oedema or effusion, assess the quality and quantity of the swelling, and note any factors that may aggravate the condition.

Is the fluid watery, tenacious, purulent, bloody, or viscid?

Is it recent and acute, or is it chronic?

Is there any underlying rheumatology history, circulatory disturbance, inflammatory process, or infection?

RECENT ACUTE TRAUMATIC CONDITIONS

Treatment should commence within 48 hours of the injury.

If it is localised, immersion icing following by elevation and compression bandage is indicated.

If it is a large area, use ice packs and pulsed ultrasound, utilising a 3 MHz frequency with low dosage, followed by elevation with compression bandages.

Large areas can be treated with a cryogel pack and simultaneous use of the compression units. This is useful for injured muscles.

Ice produces a good vasoconstriction which prevents further bleeding and exudate formation. Pulsed ultrasound gently prevents the exudate from moving to a wider area.

Interferential therapy can be used 48 to 72 hours after the injury if the swelling is not reducing adequately. It also helps to relieve pain.

CHRONIC CONDITIONS

Chronic conditions occur when the oedema or the effusion becomes more organised and viscid. Continuous ultrasound is given to the exudate and the surrounds, plus short wave diathermy or microwave diathermy. If a muscle group is involved, treat with exercises in between the short wave and the ultrasound technique. Give exercises to the antagonistic group and exercise the muscle as a synergist or a fixator. Ultrasound produces a reversible decrease of viscosity of the intra- and extra-cellular colloidal substances.

If muscle spasm exists with the swelling, then continue to use ice packs for the whole muscle plus ultrasound.

If the pain and swelling are primary problems in the chronic stages, then use interferential therapy and ultrasound.

Compression units can be used after the ultrasound for widespread tenacious swelling. Firm bandaging, exercises, mobilisation for stiff joints, and counterbalance of gravity must always be used in association with the physical agents.

INFLAMMATORY CONDITIONS (NON-TRAUMATIC)

In conditions such as rheumatoid arthritis, ankylosing spondylitis, psoriatic arthritis, Reiter's syndrome, septic arthritis, gout, and systemic lupus erythematosus it is important to assess the inflammatory process and take all laboratory findings into consideration. These conditions are not generally treated with physical agents in the acute stages. In the subacute stages application of gentle heat such as hot packs or paraffin wax is used as it is thought that it lowers the temperature of the joints reflexly. Gentle heat will aid exudate absorption.

In the chronic stages, if the white cell count, synovial fluid analysis, ESR and other laboratory tests show control of the inflammation, then short wave, microwave and ultrasound can be used for the synovitis or oedema if present. The absorption of inflammatory products around the joint can be aided by the vasodilatatory effect which helps in the phagocytosis processes and the absorption of exudate. If heat aggravates the pain, then ice packs should be tried. Ultrasound will produce depolymerisation of the proteins and reverse the viscosity of the exudate.

In the acute stage of conditions such as tenosynovitis, bursitis, tendinitis, degenerative joint disease, osteochrondritis, and chondromalacia patellae, rest is important. Ice can be used to reduce swelling and pain. In the chronic stages, ultrasound and short wave are useful. Ultrasound will help absorption of the exudate and short wave will further aid in accelerating the healing processes.

THE CONTROL OF SWELLING

Today there are several modalities available for the control of swelling. There are three types of compression units:
(a)   total compression and relaxation of a limb either locally or for the whole limb; the machines have variable pressures and a specific rest phase.
(b)   as for (a), but with variable pressure and variable rest phase.
(c)   sectionalised compression units, where the cuffed limb units produce a sequential compression, starting distally, and proceeding proximally; it is like a milking action, on the lymphatics and other vessels.
Compression units are useful for large areas of swelling and also for tenacious exudate. Crushed hands and feet are treated with ice packs and compression units from the onset. 'Cork thighs' are treated in sports injury centers with cryogel

packs and compression units simultaneously.

Faradism under pressure has been the means of combating limb oedema for many years, but as it is a time-consuming treatment it has been superseded by the compression units. Nevertheless it can be the method of treatment for tenacious exudate which is not being sufficiently mobilised by the compression units and exercises. It has the advantage that it exercises the circulatory muscle pump and hence, with patients who have weak muscles, it could serve a dual purpose.

Interferential currents are the first choice for the treatment of localised swelling and oedema in the subacute and chronic stages. This has the advantage of selecting currents that would increase ionic movement in the tissue spaces as well as exercise the muscle pumps.

All these modalities are used in conjunction with exercise, elevation routines, and compression bandages.

12.5 Treatment of Skin and Superficial Tissue

Psoriasis may be treated effectively with ultraviolet rays, usually used in combination with other therapy, such as Leeds regime or the PUVA regime. Dosage levels have been discussed in Unit 6.

Acne. Occasionally severe and resistant cases of acne may present for treatment with ultraviolet rays. Medicated soaps, topical administration of antibiotics and other therapy must be continued in association with ultraviolet therapy. Suitable dosages are suggested in Unit 6.

Slow-healing wounds. Ultraviolet rays at an E_1 dosage level stimulate the growth of granulation tissue and epithelial cells and so assist in promoting the healing of wounds. In some cases the wound may be slow to heal because of lack of nutrients and oxygen in the area. Stimulation of the circulation by the vasodilatation effect of short wave diathermy, microwave, or infrared may promote healing in such cases.

Infected wounds. The effects of high doses of ultraviolet rays may be used to assist in the control of infection in wounds and ulcers. Low doses of ultraviolet rays may then stimulate healing once the wound or ulcer is clean. Suggested dosage levels have been discussed in Unit 6.

Carbuncles, boils and abscesses. Enclosed pockets of infected material (pus) may need drainage in order for the lesion to subside. Heating the superficial tissues using infrared, microwave or a co-planar application of short wave diathermy is often effective.

Plantar warts. Some cases of plantar warts have been successfully treated with ultrasound. Details of technique and dosage have been discussed in Unit 5.

Keloid scars are difficult to treat effectively, though a few successes have been reported by therapists using ultrasound.

Incipient pressure areas. When the circulation of the skin is interfered with due to prolonged pressure, particularly over bony prominences, as seen sometimes with prolonged bed rest, the skin may break down producing an open area prone to infection. If an incipient pressure area can be recognised, by redness of the skin, the breakdown can be prevented. The use of ultraviolet rays or stimulation of the circulation with infrared, in association with regular turning of the patient and positioning to prevent further pressure, have proved successful.

12.6   Pain

Language which is so expressive of all the sensations experienced in life has no words for the sufferer to describe a pain to his doctor — language at once runs dry. VIRGINIA WOOLF: On being ill.

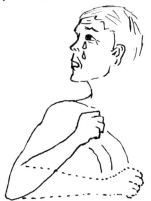

Pain is a perceptual state characterised by a highly complex interaction of various neural systems and psychological factors producing physiological, motivational, behavioral, cognitive, and psycho-dynamic mechanisms. The phenomenon of pain will be reviewed from the autonomic physiological and psychological aspects. It must be understood that pain still presents itself as a perplexing, poorly understood phenomenon that defies a precise definition.

DESCRIBING PAIN

Pain has been viewed through history in various ways. Aristotle equated pain with 'unpleasantness'. Spinosa thought of pain as 'focal sorrow'. Sherrington described it as a 'psychical adjunct of an imperative protective reflex'. Wolff defined pain as containing two parts: '(1) the awareness or perception of a stimulus that is potentially damaging to tissues; and (2) the association with a subjective feeling of discomfort or unpleasantness'.

Two definitions of pain point to its diversity:

(1)   Pain is an abstract concept which refers to (*a*) a personal, private sensation of hurt; (*b*) a harmful stimulus which signals current or impending tissue damage; and (*c*) a pattern of responses which operate to protect the organisms from harm. These responses can be described in terms which reflect certain concepts in neurological, physiological, behavioral and affective languages. (Sternbach, 1968.)

(2)   The word *pain* represents a category of experiences, signifying a multitude of different unique events having different causes and characterised by different qualities varying along a number of sensory and affective dimensions. (Melzack, 1973.)

NEUROPHYSIOLOGICAL ASPECTS OF PAIN

The concept of pain as an integrated experience can be considered as consisting of two components: *pain perception* and *pain reaction*.

Pain perception (localised in the thalamus) is the awareness of a painful sensation in response to afferent impulses from stimulated pain receptors. We must accept the fact that pain perception is purely subjective. It is a multidimensional experience which involves not only the capacity to identify the onset, duration, location and intensity of the physical characteristics of the stimulus, but it also *includes the motivative, affective, and cognitive functions leading to aversive behavior. It depends on such factors as experience, training, basic attitudes, culture and consciousness.*

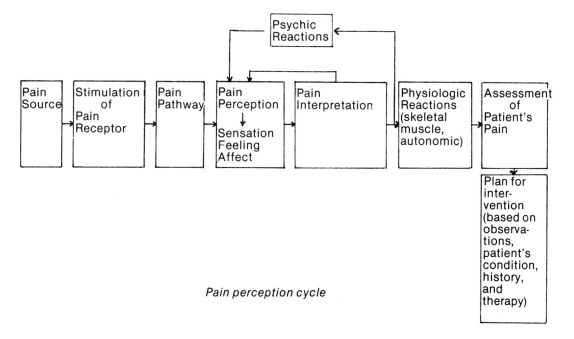

Pain perception cycle

Pain perception is a sensation, a feeling, an affect. It is a sensory discriminative component selected and modulated by the neospinothalamic tract.

Sensation gives us precise information about the site of the pain and the nature of the environment. It tells us where the pain is situated. It shows no tendency to irradiation.

Feeling — Sensation releases to a small extent the phenomena of summation, tracking, inhibition or change. Change inhibition or tracking is aroused by feeling.

Affect is the elementary or complicated defence reaction of the body to pain stimuli. It is coupled with movements of facial and bodily expression and emotion.

Pain reaction is affect. It includes all the psychological and physiologic responses of the body to painful stimuli.

Pain experience is not an isolated event, but is integrated with a person's previous pain experiences, cultural attitudes about pain, and pre-existing physiological and psychological states. Experience and training can reduce pain threshold. Consciousness, too, has an effect on pain reaction. When consciousness is limited, as in a state of intoxication or semi-consciousness, a pain stimulus can release a primitive reaction, an unrestrained emotional reaction, or in the opposite direction a person can become dull to the sensation of pain.

PATHOPHYSIOLOGY OF PAIN

The sense organs of pain are the nerve endings found in almost every tissue of the body. It has been proved experimentally that the free nerve endings which function as pain receptors also act as thermal receptors. In structure, there are thin myelinated and non-myelinated nerve endings. The difference is important for the speed of conduction.

Cutaneous receptors for pain are in the highest density, up to 200 pain receptor endings per square centimetre, in areas not exposed to tactile stimulation, such as the thigh, forearm, breast, back of the hand, and the forehead.

Morphology of pain receptors. There are two types of receptors which modulate pain.

Unmyelinated 'C' fibres have a diameter of 0.4 to 1.2 μm, and a speed of conduction of 0.5 to 2 m/s. Their function is to monitor the dull, delayed, diffuse, unpleasant, burning pain.

Small myelinated 'A' delta fibres have a diameter of 2 to 5 μm, and a speed of conduction of 10 to 40 m/s. They monitor the fast pain. When a brief, noxious stimulus is applied, such as a pinprick, you have a double pain: a 'quick' pain, described as sharp and acute, and a second 'slow' pain with a less steep rise and fall of sensation, which lasts longer and is experienced distinctly as dull and less well localised. The difference in character between quick and slow pain can be easily explained. Quick pain with the brief latency, distinct pain and localisation is due to the direct stimulus effect on the receptor.

Slow pain is characterised by the length of time which is taken for
(*a*)   the release of chemical media which activate the receptors;
(*b*)   the chemicals to cover the distance from the stimulated tissue cell to the nearest receptor membrane by means of diffusion;
(*c*)   the transmitting substance to be used up or de-activated
This is only one explanation for fast and slow pain. Probably differences in receptor qualities may influence the character of pain. This is still under investigation.

'A' delta fibres are suppressed by ischaemia, and thus fast pain is abolished before slow pain. Lack of oxygen affects the 'A' fibres and thus cuts out the highly sensitive pressure and contact sensations without changing the pain sensitivity. Local anaesthetics, however, block the pain sensation, while pressure and contact sensitivity remain. There is interrelation between the activity of slow and fast fibres, and when one is blocked there is neural imbalance and diffuse clinical symptoms.

Peripheral mechanisms. As stated earlier, the small, unmyelinated, slow-conducting 'C' fibres mediate pain sensation. The large diameter rapid-conducting myelinated 'A' alpha fibres are responsible for touch and innocuous pressure. Recent experiments indicate that some 'A' delta and 'C' fibres respond primarily to noxious stimuli and others respond to stimuli normally perceived as innocuous. The free pain nerve endings also mediate sensations of touch, pressure and temperature. Thus conduction along different groups of fibres can be slowed or blocked selectively in different ways, and it may explain the way in which some physical agents act on pain.

Chemical stimuli. The most popular accepted theory today is that pain is initiated by the liberation of chemical pain-producing substances. These are plasma kinins such as bradykinin (a nonapeptide) and kallidin (a decapeptide). Brandykinin is produced by the action of a specific enzyme liberated from tissues or leucocytes when these are provoked. It acts on the substrates in the alpha-2 globulin fraction of blood plasma. Bradykinin is readily destroyed by another enzyme present in lymph and circulating cells. Bradykinin and other pain-producing substances produce signs of inflammation such as increased permeability with oedema and vasodilatation. It is not produced in vascular tissues where it is destroyed by a plasma enzyme. It also does not produce pain in the intestinal lumen.

Any physical modality such as short wave diathermy and microwave to the superficial tissues may alter the permeability of cell membranes. Thus diffusion and increased circulation result in the removal of the pain-causing substances.

Muscle receptors. There are non-myelinated 'C' fibres in muscle, but they are not stimulated by stretch. Even a maximal isometric contraction with a force of several kilograms weight cannot excite the fibres. They are excited by deep

Articular nerves

GROUP NUMBER	DIAMETER RANGE μm	STRUCTURE	FUNCTION
I	13 – 17	large myelinated	mechanoreceptor afferent (from ligaments)
II	6 – 12	medium myelinated	mechanoreceptor afferent (from capsule and fat pads)
III	2 – 5	small myelinated	pain afferent
	< 2	unmyelinated	pain afferent vasomotor efferent
IV	2 – 5	small unmyelinated	mechanoreceptors and pain receptors in capsule and adjacent periosteum

(After B. Wyke, 1969)

pressure directly, ischaemia, and a temperature below 20°C or above 45°C. Muscles have three types of stretch receptors and pain receptors. Each functions at its own rate of adaptability and discharge.

Joint receptors. The articular cartilage is without nerves. Pain from a joint is due to irritation or distention of the capsule, tendon sheaths and ligaments, which are rich in myelinated and non-myelinated nerves. Small myelinated fibres and stretch receptors signal small movements. They adapt slowly and discharge readily from the capsule and ligaments, being sensitive to the direction and speed of small movements. Other pacinian structures have large 'A' alpha fibres and are sensitive to rapid movements. They are also present in the capsule. Synovial nerve endings are few and scattered, and are thought to be sympathetic in nature. Their function is not known.

Articular Receptor System

TYPE	MORPHOLOGY	LOCATION	NERVE FIBRES	BEHAVIOR
I	encapsulated globular corpuscles (100 μm × 40 μm)	fibrous capsule (superficial layers)	myelinated (6 μm – 9 μm)	static and dynamic mechanoreceptors; low threshold, slowly adapting
II	encapsulated conical corpuscles (280 μm × 120 μm)	fibrous capsule, deeper layers, fat pads	myelinated (9 μm – 12 μm)	dynamic mechano-receptors; low threshold, rapidly adapting
III	encapsulated fusiform corpuscles (600 μm × 100 μm)	joint ligaments	myelinated (13 μm – 17 μm)	dynamic mechano-receptors; high threshold, very slowly adapting
IV	plexuses and free nerve endings	fibrous capsule, fat pads, ligaments, vessels	myelinated (2 μm – 5 μm) unmyelinated (< 2 μm)	pain receptors; high threshold, non-adapting

(After B. Wyke, 1969)

Bone receptors. Bone responds to pressure, percussion and tension. Subchondral bone is richly supplied with sensory nerves and, if there is a cartilage erosion, pain is stimulated. Areas of bone sclerosis have an increased blood supply which is thought to cause the dull aching pain of advanced joint disease.

NERVE PATHWAYS OF PAIN (by B. Casey)

Somatosensory pathways ascending in the dorsal columns and dorsolateral spinal cord are organised for rapid transmission of spatiotemporal information. The dorsal column fibres, which originate primarily as collaterals of peripheral nerve fibres, synapse in the lower brain stem where the second-order neurons of the dorsal column nucleus send axons to the ventral postero-lateral thalamic nucleus of the opposite side. The dorsal fibres and the lower brain stem neurons to which they project discharge impulses in response to gentle, innocuous stimuli, such as touch or joint movement delivered to relatively small, single and well-defined

The discriminative system

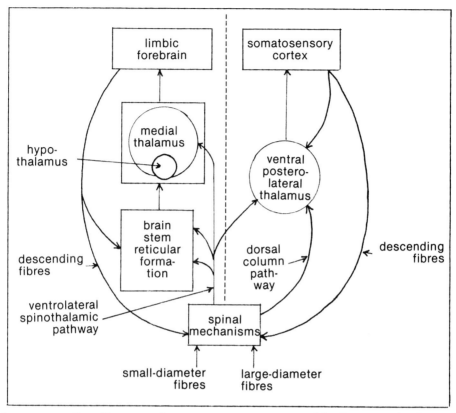

body areas. The fibres and neurons are topographically organised so that elements responding to fore-limb stimulation, for example, are clustered together and are adjacent to neurons receiving input from contiguous body areas.

The ventral postero-lateral thalamic nucleus also receives direct spinothalamic tract input from fibres ascending in the ventrolateral spinal cord, the classic pain pathway. Ventral postero-lateral thalamic neurons, however, do not respond primarily to noxious stimuli. Like the dorsal column system, the ventral postero-lateral thalamus is so organised that each of its neurons responds rapidly to innocuous stimuli delivered to well-localised regions of the body surface.

Pain is projected into the sensory cortex area in the post-central gyrus of the parietal lobe. Perception of pain alone does not require the cerebral cortex. The cortex is apparently concerned with the discriminative exact and meaningful interpretation of pain. Pain is peculiar among the senses as it is associated with a strong emotional component. Information transmitted via the special senses may evoke pleasant or unpleasant sensations, depending upon past experience, but pain alone has a 'built-in' unpleasant affect. This affective response depends on the connections of pain pathways in the thalamus. Interaction of diffuse and direct pathways of the midbrain and hypothalamic levels is probably important for the more complex integrations of pain associated with emotional reactions. The discriminative system operates independently from, but in parallel with, the neural mechanisms subserving the essential motivational-affective dimensions of pain.

The motivational-affective system. Many fibres ascending in the ventrolateral spinal cord do not project directly to the thalamus but instead synapse in the reticular formation of the brain stem, where neurons form a complex network of ascending and descending axons with extensive connections. Other ventrolateral fibres project directly to the medial thalamus. These brain stem reticular and medial thalamic components of the ventrolateral system form a paramedial ascending system which may provide a neural basis for the aversive motivational dimension of pain. The limbic system is now known to play a major role in automatic responses and basic motivational mechanisms underlying aggressive and defensive behavior as well as in responses to rewarding and aversive stimuli. Although these limbic system structures have a role in many other functions, they also provide a neural basis for the aversive drive and affective components of pain.

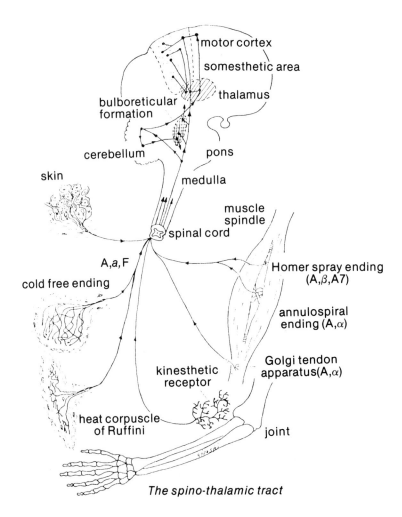

The spino-thalamic tract

NEURAL MECHANISMS UNDERLYING PAIN

The Gate control theory. Melzak and Wall developed a gate control hypothesis in 1965 which has attracted some criticism. Nevertheless it is one of the most widely accepted theories of pain today. The theory postulates a neural mechanism in the dorsal horn of the spinal cord which modulates the somatosensory input before it reaches the central nervous system, that is, before perception occurs.

The cytoarchitecture of the spinal cord consists of a series of six clearly defined laminae. Lamina 1 cells receive information from both the 'A' delta and 'C' fibres when the skin is crushed or burned, and a fraction of them project to higher levels of the spinal cord (Melzack, 1973). Lamina 1 represents, according to Christensen and Perl (1970), a specialised sensory nucleus containing neurons important for nocioception and for detecting thermal changes in the skin.

Lamina 2 and Lamina 3, which together comprise the substantia gelatinosa, play an important role in the pain process as they are thought to have a modulating effect on the input (Melzack). The fibres enter the substantia gelatinosa by way of the dorso-lateral tract. Lamina 4 cells respond to electric stimulation of the 'A' beta myelinated fibres or when gentle pressure is applied to the skin. Lamina 5 is complex and responds to a wide range of pressure stimuli. It receives fine myelinated afferents from viscera, muscle and skin. The afferents have extensive projections to the cerebral cortex mainly through the spino-thalamic tracts and some through the dorsal column systems. Lamina 5 cells respond with increased excitation and facilitation.

Both large and small diameter peripheral nerve fibres enter the dorsal part of the spinal cord. Large diameter cutaneous 'A' alpha fibres inhibit transmission of impulses (close the gate), and the small diameter 'A' delta and 'C' fibres lack this strong inhibitory effect and may facilitate synaptic transmission (open the gate). The difference in the action of the large diameter and small diameter fibres at the spinal level led to the idea of a gate control mechanism.

A negative feedback mechanism activated by the large myelinated 'A' fibres exerts an excitatory effect on the cells of substantia gelatinosa in Lamina 2 and Lamina 3 of the dorsal horn. The substantia gelatinosa, when fired, depolarises the terminals of both large and small fibres on the transmission cells of the dorsal horn via pre-synaptic, and probably the T-cells via post-synaptic inhibition.

Conversely, a large quantity of small fibre activity through an inhibitory effect on substantia gelatinosa results in an increased firing rate of the transmission cells in Lamina 5, a relay station from the dorsal horns to the higher centers. This in turn facilitates subsequent input summation, and prolonged firing and spreading of neurons. The gate is thus kept open and pathways responsible for the perception of pain are activated.

The spinal gating mechanism is influenced by nerve impulses from the brain. Cognitive factors, such as attention and anxiety, exert a powerful influence on the pain process. The brain stem reticular formation exerts a strong inhibitory control over information projected by spinal transmission cells. Reticulospinal influences also cause inhibition of Lamina 5 cells. Fibres from the cortex can influence the spinal activities via the reticulospinal projections and the substantia gelatinosa via the corticospinal fibres. Melzack also refers to a central biasing mechanism which exerts a tonic inhibitory effect (bias) on transmission at all levels of the somatic projection system, including the substantia gelatinosa. Mediating this influence will play an important role in the theory of pain.

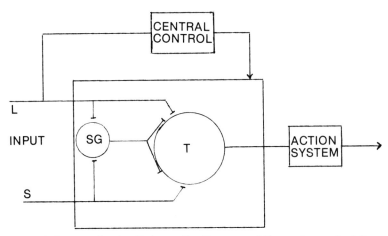

The gate control theory of pain. Schematic diagram of the gate control theory of pain mechanisms: L, the large-diameter fibres; S, the small-diameter fibres. The fibres project to the substantia gelatinosa (SG) and first central transmission (T) cells. The inhibitory effect exerted by SG on the terminals of the afferent fibres is increased by activity in L fibres and decreased by activity in S fibres. The central control trigger is represented by the line running from the large-fibre system to the central control mechanisms; these mechanisms, in turn, project back to the gate control system. The T cells project to the entry cells of the action system.

Today, Melzack and Wall's model is still largely unsubstantiated by physiological evidence. While the presence of large and small fibres on a peripheral level is well established, strong arguments are raised against the central effect of their activity. Despite challenges, Melzack and Wall's model is the most comprehensive in its conceptualisation of the psycho-physical mechanism of pain. It accounts for phenomena such as spreading pain, persistent pain, intermittent pain, referred pain from trigger spots, and allows for the influence of psychological overlay.

Based on the gate control hypothesis, therapeutic intervention of the sensory control of pain can be produced by activating large fibres by low level transcutaneous nerve stimulation (TNS), or by the use of interferential or didynamic currents. The central biasing system can be activated by intense stimulation of the peripheral nerve by acupuncture, sinusoidal currents, interferential and didynamic currents, or any counter-irritation techniques.

REFERRED PAIN

Referred pain is the phenomenon whereby stimuli activating receptors in one area of the body are inaccurately localised so that the patient feels that an entirely different part is being stimulated. Pain is not felt at its true origin. Cyriax calls it an error in critical perception. Generally visceral pain is referred, but superficial pain is not referred. Referred pain may occur in addition to, or in the absence of, deep somatic or visceral pain, for example pain in the arm with angina pectoris.

Pain from a deep somatic region is not referred. Visceral pain often follows a referred pattern. According to Kellergren it is unwise to differentiate between visceral and somatic pain on the basis of referred pain alone. Visceral pain could be diffuse and its distribution may follow the same segmental distribution of soft tissue. Superficial lesions causing pain are not referred.

The segments. In making a diagnosis it is important to understand the segmental distribution of pain. When the foetus is 4 weeks old, the development of segments is started until there is differentiation into dermatomes (skin), myotomes (muscle and other soft tissues), and sclerotomes (bones and fibrous septa). The area of skin supplied by any one spinal nerve through its rami constitutes a dermatome. They vary from person to person.

A myotome is a development of a mesodermal somite which lays the foundation for the development of muscles. Each spinal nerve originally supplies the musculature derived from the myotome of the same segment. Most muscles of the limbs are innervated from more than one segment of the spinal cord. The extent of the relevant dermatome governs the distance that pain arising from any point in the myotome may travel distally.

Since the dermatome often projects further distally than the myotome, pain may be felt to occupy an area more extensive than the myotome from which it arises. For example, the pain arising from supraspinatus tendinitis may reach the radial border of the hand, whereas the fifth cervical myotome does not extend below the elbow. Sometimes the myotome extends further proximally than the dermatome. The C_4 dermatome ends at the shoulder, but the scapula and its muscles form part of C_5 dermatome.

Discrepancies between dermatomes and myotomes. There are eight areas where the skin and the muscle it covers have different dermatomes and myotomes.

Head and face	— Sensation to the face is supplied by the fifth cranial nerve.
	— The muscles of the face are supplied by the seventh cranial nerve.
Scapula and muscles	— The skin overlying these muscles is supplied by the thoracic nerves.
	— The muscles are supplied by the middle and lower cervical segments.
Pectoral region	— The skin is supplied by the thoracic nerves.
	— The muscles are supplied by the cervical nerves.
Hand	— The skin of the radial side is supplied by the C_5 and C_6 segments.
	— The thenar muscles and intcrosseous muscles are supplied by the C_8 and T_1 segments.
Buttock	— The skin of the outer buttock is supplied by L_1 with overlapping from L_2 and L_3.
	— The muscles are supplied by L_4 to S_1.
Thigh	— Patients suffering from $L_{4,5}$ root pressure complain of pain in the buttock, thigh and calf. L_4 and L_5 begin just above the knee.

Exceptions to segmental reference. According to Cyriax the dura mater does not obey the rules of segmental reference. Patients with cervical root pressure symptoms, such as C_7 indicated by muscle weakness, complain of pain running up the neck and through the head ($C_{2 \text{ and } 3}$) and down to the lower scapula region ($T_{3 \text{ to } 6}$). Pain is usually felt in areas derived from a segment other than the affected root. Once the protrusion reaches the nerve root, the pain radiates in the expected way.

Referred tenderness. Trigger spots, which are localised tender spots, have been noted with no cutaneous hyperalgesia. Sometimes these tender spots can be made to shift by mobilisation of the neck. Often when a disc lesion has been resolved, the spots disappear. When pressure is exerted on the dura mater by a bulging disc, a localised tender spot forms within the painful region and when pressed is identified as the root of the trouble by the patient.

Factors affecting the reference of pain. The perception of referred pain depends on four factors:

(a) *Strength of the stimulus* — The stronger the stimulus, the less accurate is the ability of the patient to identify the origin of the pain. In arthritis of the shoulder the patient feels more pain down the arm and nothing in the shoulder. When the pain regresses it is felt more in the shoulder. The increase in intensity of the stimulus leads to a diffusion occurring in the cells of the sensory cerebral cortex, which is interpreted by the patient as an enlargement of the painful area.

(b) *Position of the painful structure* — Pain will be referred a long way if the segment is elongated. This occurs with S_{1-2}, where pain radiates from the buttock to the foot. Generally pain is referred distally and then proximally. Usually diffuse signs occur at the proximal ends if there is a long segment. In structures of the elbow and the knee the pain radiates equally on both sides. The further the lesion from the trunk, the better is the patient able to localise the sensation accurately.

(c) *Depth from the surface* — Lesions occurring in superficial structures are more easily localised. Pain is not referred from the surface. Lesions in deeper structures give rise to diffuse pains and are more difficult to locate.

(d) *Nature of the structure* — In different parts of the nervous system, when subjected to pressure, no symptoms are felt at the point of pressure. Pressure on the spinal cord produces an extra-segmental feeling of pins and needles. Pressure on the dural investment of the nerve roots leads to pain in part of the relevant dermatome. Pressure on a nerve trunk produces distal paraesthesia in the relevant cutaneous distribution of the nerve.

Pain from joint capsules, ligaments and bursae is apt to be diffuse and follows a sclerotome distribution, distal to the point of origin. The pain is described as deep and diffuse with no cutaneous component. If severe, it may produce vaso-vagal responses. Referred pain should always be suspected if a patient complains of a deep burning pain or ache along a limb, or if the patient complains of a deep pain with no boundaries. If the patient complains of numbness, then it is likely to be pressure on a small nerve. Pressure on a nerve trunk generally produces pins and needles distally and no local pain.

Central pain is pain occurring after injury to the pain pathways of the diffuse spino-thalamic system. The injury may result from vascular thrombosis, tumor, aneurysm, demyelinating disease, or incomplete surgical interruption of the pain tracts. The more lateral spino-thalamic tracts allow for rapid access of noxious sensation to the thalamus and thence to the cerebral cortex, whereas the slower diffuse pathways make multiple connections to the regions below the level of the thalamus.

Localisation is the projection of pain to the skin from the site of the lesion. The clarity and extent of the projection can vary. Deep and visceral pain is often described as diffuse and poorly localised.

Projected pathological pain accurately describes the fact that impulses set up anywhere along the pain pathway from nerve to cortex give rise to a sensation projected to the peripheral region served by the end-organ of that pathway. Thus the pain from a ruptured intervertebral disc is not referred but projected, the stimulus is pathological and the projection is normal.

ACUTE AND CHRONIC PAIN

The exact mechanisms that monitor the differences between acute and chronic pain are still being investigated, but the pathophysiology of chronic pain is different to that of acute pain.

In acute pain the sympathetic responses and anxiety predominate. The sensory-discriminative, motivational and cognitive components of the pain phenomenon influence motor mechanisms responsible for the overt responses characteristic of pain. Acute pain produces reactions that include (*a*) local tissue reaction associated with biochemical and metabolic changes, signs of inflammation, local tenderness, and hyperalgesia; (*b*) involuntary (automatic) responses involving segmental and suprasegmental reflex mechanisms which preserve homeostasis and which are manifested by spasm of skeletal or smooth muscle, glandular hyperactivity, vasomotor hyperactivity, cardiovascular and respiratory changes, and alteration of other visceral functions; and (*c*) reactions at the integrative levels involving the cerebral cortex manifested by the complex psychologic and physiologic operant responses, which include verbalisation, moaning, grimacing, and posturing.

The mechanisms of chronic pain states are much more complex. In chronic pain, autonomic changes gradually become habitual and diminish or disappear, and psychological factors play an important role. The aminergic hypothesis of Wall and Sternbach, and Liebeskind and others, suggests that there is depletion of brain serotin and dopamin which accounts for the increase of pain, depression, and other vegetative signs. The frequent use or abuse of drugs, poor physical condition, a pattern of sleep disturbance, loss of appetite, diminished libido, irritability, and hypochondriasis are also associated with chronic pain. The anxiety of acute pain is replaced by depression at times. Treatment of acute pain often proves a failure in the chronic stages.

Persistent reflex responses to trauma or disease are associated with sympathetic hyperactivity, vasoconstriction, local ischaemia, and accumulation of metabolites that form new sources of noxious stimulation and thus initiate and sustain the cycle of pain. This may be the mechanism of causalgia and reflex sympathetic dystrophies. In certain chronic pain states, the inhibitory influence of the central biasing mechanism is impaired or eliminated so that a brief stimulus produces prolonged spontaneous activity at several synaptic levels involving neuron circuits with widespread connections.

Severe emotional stress associated with chronic pain conditions activates psychophysiologic mechanisms that cause skeletal muscle spasm, vasoconstriction and visceral disturbances. This can then lead to local tissue ischaemia and further activation of metabolites that become further sources of noxious stimulation and enhance the cycle of pain.

Operant mechanisms are among the common causes of chronic pain and prolonged disability. The process initiated by noxious stimuli in one part of the body causes a patient to manifest operant or voluntary responses. If these responses produce favorable results, then the patient continues to reinforce the responses and it becomes a part of the chronic pain behavior. Wilbert Fordyce has done considerable work on operant conditioning methods for managing chronic pain. He believes that at times the response or behavior of chronic pain is disproportionate to the underlying condition. A set of actions is termed operants. For example, a patient may describe his pain, walk and move in a guarded way, grimace, ask for medication and decide he will rest by staying in bed. These behavior patterns should not be labelled as 'psychogenic', as they do not respond to psychotherapy.

Principles of diagnosis of chronic pain. Patients with chronic pain do not become accustomed to it, but seem to get more sensitive to pain and suffer more as time passes on.

Protracted pain and long-standing disability produce mental and physical depletions.

General debility, early fatigue, anxiety, malnutrition, and decreased tolerance to pain are some of the clinical features.

The patient shows gradual disinterest in all activities around him. Pain dominates his life.

Iatrongenic complications such as drug addiction, futile surgery, and use of quack medicine are noted.

Factors that cause or aggravate the pain must be ascertained, also those which relieve the pain. Work and home background are important for diagnosis.

The final consideration in understanding chronic pain is how much physical deterioration it is causing, how much mental conflict is manifested as a neurosis and if depression is predominant.

The reverberatory circuits theory. Melzack and Milner explain chronic pain by the so-called *reverberatory circuits of neurons*.

When a neuron is fired, it fires not only its neighbors with which it synapses, but simultaneously a branch of its own axon (a recurrent collateral), which terminates on an inhibitory cell and projects back to the original cell body to inhibit its firing briefly. When this occurs the neuron stops relaying into the collateral and is stopped from inhibiting any further, and resumes spontaneous firing through a rebound excitation without any further additional input. Thus the whole circuit is reactivated, and repetitive bursts of activity occur which spread to adjacent neuron pools.

The mechanism could account for spreading and persistent pain. It could also explain the chronic pain memory-loops with permanent synaptic changes occurring. TCS and interferential therapy could break up the synchronous rhythmic activity in these neural mechanisms. The various pulses of TCS or interferential could come out of phase and break up the neural circuits, which are a closed network of neurons which fire together in sequence and in time establish a pattern of firing independent of input. The activity of the neurons is generally self-exciting and self-sustaining.

MUSCLE SPASM

This is a frequent cause of pain or can be secondary to pathological changes in an underlying bone, joint, tendon or ligament. During muscle spasm the contracting muscle compresses the intra-muscular blood vessels and either reduces or cuts off the blood flow. Muscle contraction increases the rate of metabolism of the muscle. The pain starts as soon as ischaemia sets in and persists after the contraction until after blood flow is re-established. If spasm (tetanic contraction) is maintained, more ischaemia occurs and pain is increased. Pain is thought to be due to the release of a chemical agent, Lewis 'P' factor, which is a normal product of muscle metabolism, in both the resting and active states, and stimulates the pain nerve endings only when it accumulates in large quantities. Cessation of pain requires that the concentration of the 'P' factor be reduced below critical threshold level.

Sustained contractions of skeletal muscle may arise from higher centers or from reflexes of somatic or visceral afferents. Nocioceptive high pressure stimuli on the head give rise to a localised confined pain in the affected area, and tension in the neck muscles associated with a secondary generalised pain (headache).

Explanation of the reflex contraction in the neck muscles is not clear, but it may be due to a change in the inter-neuron pools of the spinal cord. There is no clear experimental evidence of such long-lasting facilitator effects. The muscle contraction may be due to the cycle: deep pain ⟶ sustained muscle contraction ⟶ reflex contraction ⟶ deep pain. The success of procedures such as manipulations, procaine hydrochloride injections, ultrasound, and microwave may depend on their ability to break the cycle.

PSYCHOGENIC PAIN

Emotions not only magnify existing pain, but also cause other types of exaggerated pain. The remarkable feature of psychogenic pain is that it exhibits marked similarity to pain associated with structural lesions or known organic syndromes. Patients generally have associated features such as depression, fear, insomnia, anorexia, loss of libido and potential, lack of energy and interest, and poor ability to concentrate. The main complaint is always pain stemming from the trauma.

PHANTOM PAIN

It is estimated that 95% of all amputees experience phantom sensations of the amputated part some time after surgery. There are three kinds of sensory phenomena in the amputee: (a) mild tingling in the distal part of the limb; (b) strong, momentary pins and needles sensation in the phantom limb, generally triggered by touching neuromas in the stump; (c) occasional intractable severe pain from the amputated leg. This is rare.

Phantom pain generally abates with time. It is believed that the phantom pain is due to integration at the highest levels of the spinal cord or cortex, possibly through the initiation of so-called reverberating circuits, in which a peripheral stimulus sets up a continuous central painful phenomenon. Phantom pain generally involves the distal portion of limbs rather than the proximal ones, because the distal portion of a limb is represented by a larger area of sensory cortex than the proximal.

MYOFASCIAL PAIN SYNDROMES

The myofascial pain syndromes are characterised by the existence of a hyper-sensitive region called the *trigger area*, in a muscle or in the connective tissue, together with a specific painful reaction elicited in some related target area when the trigger area is stimulated. The more common forms of this syndrome have been mapped anatomically. Physiologically they represent a self-sustaining cycle of pain $\longrightarrow$ spasm $\longrightarrow$ pain. It can be broken at several points by attacking either the motor or the sensory part of the mechanism. Consequently local anaesthesia, physical therapy, mobilisation and psychotherapy can all contribute to a cure, and the relief is sometimes dramatic.

The syndrome is characterised by pain, muscle spasm, tenderness, stiffness, limitation of movement, weakness, and occasionally autonomic dysfunction in an area of reference usually at some distance from the trigger point. The disturbances have been previously described as, among other terms, myalgia, myositis, fibrositis, fibromyositis (or myofibrositis), fasciitis, myofasciitis, muscular rheumatism, and muscular strains.

Causes. The most important causes of myofascial pain syndromes are:
(a) Macro-trauma to myofascial structures. After acute injury to muscles, bones and joints, 'trigger areas' are formed in some individuals. These trigger areas may be defined as small, circumscribed, hypersensitive regions in muscles or in connective tissues from which impulses arise and bombard the central nervous system to produce referred pain. The trigger area is so called because its stimulation, like the pulling of the trigger of a gun, produces effects at another place (the target), called the 'reference zone' or 'area of reference'.

(b) Micro-trauma. In addition to severe, acute trauma, made obvious by the prompt onset of symptoms, the trauma of slight injuries may play an equally important part. In the latter case the injury is such that its con-nection with the pain syndrome is not readily traced, and the relationship is overlooked because the symptoms develop gradually. Even less frequently recognised, and yet equally important as a cause of myofascial pain syn-dromes, are the repetitious micro-traumas of daily living and chronic muscular strain, especially in sedentary individuals over the age of 35.

(c) In addition, trigger areas may be initiated by the chilling of fatigued muscles, arthrosis, nerve injuries, and other neuromusculoskeletal disor-ders, and by visceral dysfunction. General fatigue and low metabolic rate, with chemical imbalance, chronic infection, and psychogenic stress may act as predisposing factors in the development of trigger areas.

Symptoms. Stimulation of trigger areas produces pain, tenderness and muscle spasm in a referred area. Pain leads to resistance to any lengthening of muscle, resulting in apparent shortening of affected muscles with limited range of movement and muscle weakness.

High intensity discharges from the trigger areas may be accompanied by autonomic changes such as vasoconstriction and sweating, generally along the reference zone of pain. The pattern of referred pain is usually predictable, and follows a fixed anatomical pathway. The predictable pain pattern makes it possible to locate the myofascial source of pain. It does not follow a dermatomal pattern or a nerve root pattern.

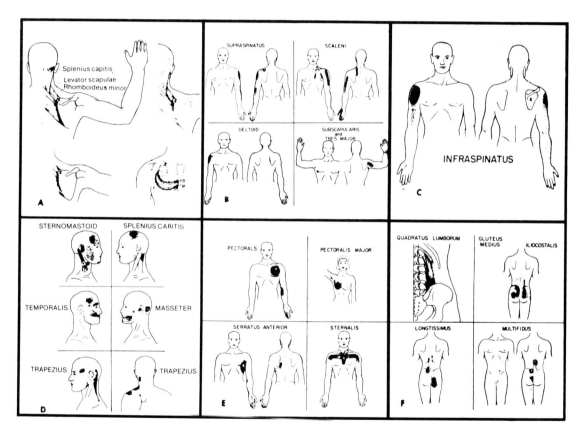

A, diagrammatic representation of scapulocostal syndrome. 'X' represents site of trigger area at superior medial angle of scapula, while stippled areas represent various patterns of pain reference (see text). (After Michele and associates.) B, myofascial pain syndromes of shoulders and arms. Note location of trigger areas (X) and reference of pain in 'essential' (black) and 'spill-over' (stippled) zones of reference. C, infraspinatus syndrome. D, myofascial pain syndromes of the head and neck. E, diagrams showing most important pain patterns (black and stippled) of the chest caused by trigger areas (X) in various muscles. F, various myofascial pain syndromes of the low back. (After Travell and Sola)

Trigger areas in joints or periarticular structures have referred pain close to the areas. A trigger area in muscle is generally referred a considerable distance away. This is not a strict rule. Referred pain is usually dull and aching in character, and its intensity varies from a low tension pain to one of high intensity. It is usually elicited spontaneously as soon as the trigger area is stimulated. The more sensitive the trigger area, the wider is the area of referred pain, including a 'spill over' zone. Tenderness and hyperalgesia persist longer than pain.

Skeletal muscle spasm always accompanies trigger area stimulation. Spasm produced by metabolites can serve as a new harmful stimulus, which excites the internuncial pools, and thus pain will reflexly reinforce abnormal muscle activity, and so a cycle is developed. Unless this cycle is interrupted, the prolonged spasm and pain will lead to organic changes in joints around the area.

Trigger joints act as sympathetic excitants, and as such respond readily to various stress factors, especially those of psychic origin. It has been suggested in the past that some of the cases diagnosed as subacromial bursitis, tendinitis, periarticular rheumatism, and brachial neuralgia were actually myofascial syndromes with trigger areas in the muscles of the back and shoulder girdle and pain referred to the shoulder and arm. Perhaps the two co-exist. A trigger spot sets up joint irritation, which increases the trigger area, causing more joint irritation.

Common trigger areas

TRIGGER AREA	REFERRED PAIN AREA
Lower end of levator scapulae muscle insertion	Pain muscle spasm, tenderness in the posterior part of neck and occipital region of head.
Superior medial angle of scapula	May also overlap into the shoulder and supra-scapular region.
Upper medial angle of scapula and posterior chest wall	Drooping of shoulder girdle, deep-seated pain in shoulder spreading up and down to neck, occiput, and side of head. Later going down to the back of the arm and often to the forearm, wrist, and hand. May go along the course of the fourth and fifth intercostal nerves.
Infraspinatus syndrome, inferior lateral portion of muscle	Anterior lateral aspect of shoulder and region of long head of biceps. Pain may radiate down arm with fatigue of shoulder girdle and weak grip.
Trapezius syndrome, superior margin or inferior infrascapular portion of muscle	Pain is in neck, back of head and sometimes side of head.
Sternomastoid syndrome	Spasm of lateral neck muscles, vasoconstriction of temporal artery.

| Along the length of the sternocleidomastoid muscle | Pain on the forehead, about the hair line, in the ear, in the posterior mastoid process, and in the throat and chin. In addition there is pain of lesser degree through the face. |

Muscles of the sub-occipital region and face — Pain in the upper posterior portion of the neck, the back of the head, and the face.

Insertion of the quadratus lumborum muscle to the transverse process of the upper three lumbar vertebrae and the 12th rib — The pain may be localised to the back but is frequently radiated to the lower abdominal wall and anterior thigh.

Treatment
The trigger areas can be treated with:
(*a*) didynamic current;
(*b*) interferential currents;
(*c*) ultrasound;
(*d*) massage.

Diagnosis
Referred zones can be picked up by the use of didynamic currents.

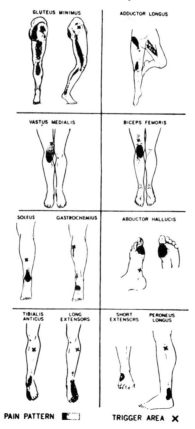

Myofascial pain syndromes of the lower extremities

PAIN PATTERN   TRIGGER AREA X

THE MANAGEMENT OF PAIN

Pain is a multi-dimensional phenomenon which has both psychological and physiological-anatomical correlates, which give it a complexity that must be considered in correct diagnosis as an essential prerequisite for the effective treatment of pain. Pain intensity cannot be measured and pain thresholds vary from individual to individual, or in the same individual from time to time. Our basic understanding of pain is limited, and treatment should embrace the patient as a whole and be carefully selected to relieve the pain in whole or in part without adding in any way to the patient's disability.

Selection of drugs

TYPE OF DRUG	MECHANISM OF INTERFERENCE WITH PAIN
antibiotics anti-inflammatory drugs	Reversal of pathophysiological events such as: Infection Inflammation
anti-pyretic analgesics	Decrease of pain perception. Drugs act at the level of the thalamus. Interference with specific chemical substances involved in pain reception peripherally.
local anaesthetics	Interference with pain pathways.
narcotic analgesics	Interference with central nervous system perception of pain and development of affective responses. When given in the presence of existing pain they generally act only at the cortical level and modify pain interpretation and decrease pain reaction. When given before pain occurs they act at both cortical and thalamic levels and decrease pain perception.
hypnotics	Interference with anxiety, depression, sleeplessness.
tranquillisers ataractic drugs	Act on the cerebral cortex and modify pain interpretation and decrease pain reaction. Ataractic drugs also act at the thalamic and hypothalamic level and may act on efferent nerve endings.
muscle relaxants	Tension of skeletal muscle. Acts on the pain receptors in muscle by blocking the efferent skeletal muscle pathways by action in the spinal cord.
anaesthetics	Interference with consciousness. Produce stupor and coma.
strong hypnotics	Severe pain. Action on the cerebral cortex to decrease pain perception.

Commonly used drugs

ACTION	DRUGS
anti-inflammatory agents	Phenylbutazone (Butazolidin) Oxyphenylbutazone (Tanderil) Brufen Chymoral Indomethacin Corticosteroids
analgesic and anti-pyretics	Acetylsalicylic acid (Aspirin) Codeine Salicylamides Para-aminophenol (Phenacetin acetophenetidin) Aminopyrine Paracetamol
narcotic analgesics	Dihydrocodeine Pentazocine Pethidine Phenazocine Dipipanone Dextromoramide Morphine Heroin Chlorpromazine
drugs for neuralgia	Carbamazepine Diphenyldantoin (Dilantin)
muscle relaxants	Valium Diazepam
hypnotics	Phenobarbiturates Sodium thiopental Amobarbital
tranquillisers	Ataractic drugs Reserpine Chlorodiazepoxide Chlorpromazine Phenothiazines
psychotropic drugs	Amitryptyline
analgesic blocks	Procaine Lidocaine Prilocaine Tetracaine Ethyl acohol Phenol

The problem of acute pain is different to that of chronic pain. Neuralgia, cancer pain, migraine, the pain from reflex sympathetic dystrophy, phantom pain, pain from vascular disorders, psychogenic pain, obstetric pain, visceral pain, and central pain are all pain problems that must be understood from a neurophysiological basis and be carefully evaluated before attempting treatment.

In determining treatment procedures Bonica (1973) suggests that the following must be taken into consideration:

(*a*) cause, site, path, mechanism and probable duration of pain;

(*b*) nature of the causative disease;

(*c*) patient's age, physical and mental status, life expectancy, obligations to family and community;

(*d*) the complications and side effects that may develop from each method of treatment.

Drug therapy

The most common method used by the physician in managing pain today is the systemic administration of analgesics or other drugs. Often the patient referred to physiotherapy departments with the problem of pain is taking drugs of some sort. The side effects and the iatrogenic drug-dependence complications must be considered when evaluating pain management. Physical agents do not have side effects and hence can be a safe and effective tool in the relief of pain.

Neurosurgical relief of pain

Peripheral neurectomy — Decompression of a trapped peripheral nerve.
— Resection of neuromas.
— Resection of peripheral nerves is done in the treatment of malignancies or central nervous system abnormalities.

Sensory rhizotomy — Section of the sensory root of spinal nerves proximal to the spinal ganglion for relief of chronic pain.

Cordotomy — Section of the antero-lateral quadrant of the spinal cord.

Sympathectomy — This is done for causalgia, peripheral vascular disease and malignancy.

TNS implants — Dr. Shealy produced electroanalgesia at the spinal cord by implanting fine wire electrodes above the level of the pain in the spinal cord, which are attached to a coin-sized receiver implanted beneath the skin of the back. A transmitter taped over the receiver sends electric signals into the spine with a flick of a switch. The patient wears a control box at his belt and turns on the stimulator whenever he needs it.

Physiotherapeutic management of pain

Physiotherapeutic techniques can act at several sites in the pain pathway.

INTERVENTION MEASURES

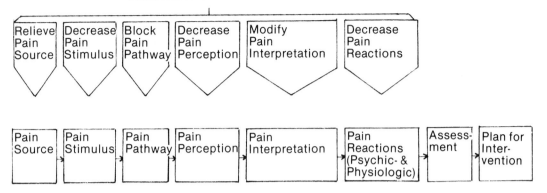

Measures for intervention in the pain pathway

Effect of physical agents on the mechanisms of pain

(a) Cryotherapy

Lowering the temperature of the affected part quickly and with a large drop in temperature the following effects can be obtained. A slow-down of the rate of conduction and a reduction of the size of action potential is seen when the temperature is brought down at least 10°C. Cooling causes a reduction in acetylcholine production and produces an asynchrony of impulses (Clarke, Lind and Helion, 1958). This asynchrony can break the pain pattern and relieve chronic pain. Cold application with an ice cube massage at 0°C will act as an analgesic and a counter-irritant and relieve pain.

Cold can decrease the activity of the fusimotor efferent systems in muscles and thus relieve pain and muscle spasm. The reaction to cold is more long-lasting than the reaction to heat in pain and muscle spasm. This effect is also used for the control of spasticity.

(b) Ultrasound

The conduction velocity of a nerve is reduced if it is insonated with a dosage of 1 to 2 w.cm^{-2} ultrasonic energy. Painful areas which react badly to heat can be treated with pulsed ultrasound, where the micromassage effect will block pain pathways by lowering the nerve conduction velocity. If the cause of the pain is due to adhesions or contractures, then ultrasound is effective in causing depolymerisation of the mucopolysaccharides, mucoproteins, or glycoproteins.

Ultrasound is also able to alter the distribution of ion concentration at the pain receptor sites. It will cause increased diffusion of the algesic plasma peptides and 'H' ion concentrations and thus remove the cause of pain.

(c) Short wave and microwave

Vigorous heating produced by conversive diathermy agents can relieve pain. The physiological process involved is still uncertain. Relief of pain obtained by heat is not long-lasting. If inflammation or chronic swelling is the cause of pain in deeper seated lesions, then the careful use of short wave or microwave targeted on the area can cause absorption of exudate and aid resolution of inflammatory products. A temperature rise to 42°C is essential to get good vasodilatation in muscle.

(d)   Interferential therapy, didynamic currents, sinusoidal currents, through-and-through faradism

Interferential currents and didynamic currents produce a variety of pulses which can be used to relieve pain by two different mechanisms. A suitable current can be used to reduce pain perception by obtaining a counter-irritant effect. Other pulses can block pain pathways by acting on the large 'A' alpha fibres and inhibiting the pain at the spinal level through the presynaptic inhibitory mechanisms.

Sinusoidal currents act as a counter-irritant measure, while through-and-through faradism acts on the large 'A' alpha fibres, 'opening the gate' according to Melzack's 'gate theory'.

Patients suffering from causalgia from partial peripheral nerve lesions or post-herpetic neuralgia are thought to have a loss of conduction of the large 'A' alpha fibres. Pain occurs with the gentlest of stimuli and occurs in paroxysms, characteristic of 'C' fibres. Loss of large 'A' alpha fibres may lead to pathologically increased spinal input via 'A' delta and 'C' fibres. If interferential therapy or didynamic currents are made to activate the large 'A' alpha fibres, then pain can be inhibited at the spinal level.

Pain occurring from reflex sympathetic dystrophy, shoulder-hand syndromes, osteoporosis and vascular disorders can be treated by using interferential currents or didynamic currents on the appropriate sympathetic ganglion, such as the stellate ganglion for the shoulder-hand syndrome.

(e)   Hot packs, paraffin wax, infrared

Hot packs and paraffin wax produce a gentle, slow rise in temperature and are sedative in action as they reduce nerve conduction velocity of the sensory nerves. As their depth of penetration is only to the skin level, it has been found that they reduce the temperature of underlying superficial joints, and in rheumatoid arthritis this reduction of temperature in a joint with inflammation can relieve pain.

Infrared causes a moderate rise in heat which goes to the level of the superficial muscles and also relieves pain.

Use of exercises with physical agents to relieve pain

Pain can be due to lack of movement and function of a part. This is because these factors can cause:

(a)   Aggravation of the biochemical situation at the site of pain, where the local factors causing the nerve fibres to pick up impulses are unresolved.

(b)   Anoxia due to impaired metabolism of muscle circulation. Inactivity increases muscle circulation, but upsets muscle metabolism and the ability of muscle and other soft tissue structures to utilise the nutrition products of circulation.

(c)   Disturbance of the normal transmission of other patterns of afferent stimuli from the local area. These afferent stimuli are coming from stretch receptors in joints and muscles. Others come from the normal thermal, tactile, pressure and vibratory stimuli received on the skin or subcutaneous tissues during activity. The spinal cord receives many messages, but now it has no competition, and the pain stimuli could be facilitated by lack of competition.

Exercise will increase venous and lymphatic return, aid removal of 'P' factors, aid muscle metabolism, and give more stimuli to the spinal cord activity. Thus some of the factors maintaining pain can be eliminated. Of course, at all times the main cause of pain must also be treated.

SUMMARY OF SELECTION OF PHYSICAL AGENTS FOR PAIN MANAGEMENT

A   Acting at the pain source

Adhesions   )   —   ultrasound
Scars   )   —   short wave diathermy
Contractures)   —   microwave
Haematoma   —   ice
             —   ultrasound
             —   short wave diathermy
Inflammation —   short wave diathermy
             —   microwave
             —   ultrasound
             —   hot packs
             —   wax
Infection   —   ultraviolet rays
             —   short wave diathermy
             —   microwave

B   Acting at the level of the pain receptors
By removal of pain metabolites and alteration of cell permeability.
Oedema   )   —   ice
Effusion   )   —   ultrasound
Synovitis)   —   compression unit

C   Acting to block the pain pathway
Interferential currents
Didynamic currents
TNS
Acupuncture
Ice
Ultrasound
Heat
Through-and-through faradism

D   Acting at the level of pain perception and interpretation
A *counter-irritant effect* is produced by:
Interferential currents
Didynamic currents
Acupuncture
Ultraviolet rays
Sinusoidal currents
Renotin ionisation

Pain interpretation is affected by:
Gaining the patient's confidence
Behavior modification

References

Abramson, D J, Chu, L S W, Tuck, S, Lee, S W, Richardson, G, Levin, M, 1966, Effect of tissue temperature and blood flow on motor nerve conduction velocity, *JAMA, 1980,* 1082–1088.

Bishop, B, 1980, Pain: its physiology and rationale for management, *Physical Therapy,* 60, 1, 13–37.

Burton, C, Maurer, D D, 1974, Pain suppression by transcutaneous electronic stimulation, *IEEE, Trans Biomed Eng, BME, 21,* 81–88.

Chambers, R, 1969, Clinical uses of cryotherapy, *Phys Ther, 49, 3,* 245–249.

Clark, W C, Hunt, H F, 1971, Pain in physiological basis of rehabilitation medicine, *W B Saunders Company.*

Currier, D P, Nelson, B S, 1969, Changes in motor conduction velocity induced by exercise and diathermy, *Phys Ther, 49,* 146–152.

Euler, C. Soderberg, U, 1957, The influences of hypothalamic thermoceptive structures on the electroencephalogram and gamma motor activity, *Electroenc Clin Neurophys, 9,* 391–408.

Fields, H L, Adams, J E, Hosobuchl, Y, 1974, Peripheral nerve and cutaneous electrohypalgesia, In J J Bonica, ed, Advances in neurology, *International Symposium on Pain,* 749–754, New York, Raven Press.

Gersten, J W, 1958, Effect of metallic objects on temperature rises produced in tissue by ultrasound, *Amer J Phys Med, 37,* 75–82.

Gersten, J W, 1965, Effect of ultrasound on tendon extensibility, *Amer J Phys Med, 34,* 362–369 (Apr).

Griffin, J E, 1966, Physiological effects of ultrasonic energy as it is used clinically, *Phys Ther, 46,* 18–27.

Griffin, J E, Echternach, J L, Bowmaker, K L, 1970, Results of frequency differences in ultrasonic therapy, *Phys Ther, 50, 4,* 481–485.

Griffin, J E, Echternach, M S, Price, R E, Touchstone, J E, 1967, Patients treated with ultrasonic driven hydrocortisone and with ultrasound alone: A comparative study, *Phys Ther, 47,* 594–601.

Haines, J, 1967, A survey of recent developments in cold therapy, *Physiother, 53,* 222–229.

Handwerker, H O, Iggo, A, Zimmermann, M, 1975, Segmental and supraspinal actions on dorsal horn neurons responding to noxious and non-noxious skin stimuli, *J Pain, 1,* 147–163.

Harris, E D, McCroskery, R A, 1974, The influence of temperature in fibril's stability on degradation of cartilage collagen by rheumatoid synovial collagenase, *New Eng J Med, 290,* 1–6.

Harris, R, 1960, Effect of short wave diathermy on radio-sodium clearance from the knee joint in the normal and in rheumatoid arthritis, *3rd Int Cong Phys Med Rehab,* Washington, 1960, 65–73.

Hartviksen, K, 1962, Ice therapy in spasticity, *Acta Neurol Scand, 38,* (Suppl 3), 79–84.

Horvath, S M, Hollander, J L, 1949, The influence of physical therapy procedures on the intra-articular temperature of normal and arthritic subjects, *Am J Med Sci, 218*, 543-548.

Hovind, H, Nielsen, S L, 1974, Local blood flow after short wave diathermy; Preliminary report, *Arch Phys Med Rehab, 55*, 217-221 (May).

Kane, K, Taub, A, 1975, A history of local electrical analgesia, *J Pain, 1*, 125-136.

King, C A, 1967, The effects of ice or heat: Comparative study on muscle spasm in cases of low back pain, *Phys Can, 19, 4*, 208-211.

Lehmann, J F, Brunner, G D, Stow, R W, 1958, Pain threshold measurements after therapeutic application of ultrasound, microwaves and infrared, *Arch Phys Med, 39*, 560-565.

Lehmann, J F, Johnson, E W, 1958, Some factors influencing the temperature distribution in thighs exposed to ultrasound, *Arch Phys Med, 39*, 347-356.

Lehmann, J F, McMillan, J, Brunner, G D, Blumberg, J B, 1959, Comparative study of the efficiency of short wave, microwave and ultrasonic diathermy in heating the hip joint, *Arch Phys Med Rehab, 40*, 510-519.

Lehmann, J F, Brunner, G D, Martinis, A J, McMillan, J A, 1959, Ultrasonic effects as demonstrated in live pigs with surgical metallic implants, *Arch Phys Med, 40*, 483-488.

Lehmann, J F, Brunner, G D, McMillan, J A, Silverman, D R, Johnston, V C, 1964, Modification of heating patterns produced by microwaves at the frequencies of 2345 and 900 Mc by physiologic factors in the human, *Arch Phys Med Rehab, 45*, 555-563.

Lehmann, J F, Guy, A W, Warren, C G, DeLateur, B J, Stonebridge, J B, 1970, Evaluation of a microwave contact applicator, *Arch Phys Med Rehab, 51*, 143-146.

Lehmann, J F, Masock, A J, Warren, C G, Kobianski, J N, 1970, Effect of therapeutic temperatures on tendon extensibility, *Arch Phys Med Rehab, 51*, 481-487.

Lim, R K S, 1970, Pain, *Ann Rev Physio, 32*, 269-288.

Loeser, J D, Black, R G, Cristman, A, 1975, Relief of pain by transcutaneous stimulation, *J Neurosurg, 42*, 308-314.

Long, D M, 1976, Use of peripheral and spinal cord stimulation in the relief of chronic pain, in J J Bonica, ed, Advances in pain research and therapy, *1*, 395-402, *New York, Raven Press*.

Long, D M, Hagfors, N, 1975, Electrical stimulation in the nervous system: the current status of electrical stimulation of the nervous system for relief of pain, *J Pain, 1*, 109-121.

Melzack, R, Wall, P D, 1965, Pain mechanism: a new theory, *Science, 150*, 971-979.

Melzack, R, 1973, The puzzle of pain, *Penguin, UK*.

Melzack, R, 1974, Psychological concepts and methods for the control of pain, In J J Bonica, ed, Advances in Neurology, *4*, International Symposium on Pain, 275-280.

Melzack, R, 1975, The McGill pain questionnaire: Major properties and scoring methods, *J Pain, 1*, 277-299.

Melzack, R, 1975, Prolonged relief of pain by brief, intense transcutaneous somatic stimulation, *J Pain, 1*, 357-372.

Miglietta, O, 1973, Action of cold on spasticity, *Am J Phys Med, 52*, 198-205.

Nakatani, Y, Sato, T, 1974, Acupuncture for chronic pain in Japan, In J J Bonica, ed, Advances in neurology, *4*, 813-818.

Newton, M J, Lehmkul, D, 1969, Muscle spindle response to body heating and localised muscle cooling: Implications for the relief of spasticity, *Phys Ther, 45*, 91-105.

Ohnhaus, E E, Adler, R, 1975, Methodological problems in the measurement of pain: a comparison between the verbal rating scale and the visual analogue scale, *J Pain, 1*, 379–384.

Olson, J E, Stravino, V D, 1972, A review of cryotherapy, *Phys Ther, 52, 8*, 840–853.

Ruiz, C B, 1958, Ultrasonics in traumatic conditions, *Amer J Phys Med, 37*, 203–205.

Schwann, H P, 1969, Biophysics of diathermy in therapeutic heat, *Connecticut, Elizabeth Licht*.

Shealy, C Norman, 1974, Six years' experience with electrical stimulation for control of pain, In J J Bonica, ed, Adv Neurol, *4*, International Symposium on Pain, 775–782.

Showman, J, Wedlick, L T, 1963, The use of cold instead of heat for relief of muscle spasm, *Med J Aust, 2*, 612–614.

Sternbach, R A, Ignelzi, R J, Deems, L M, Timmermans, G, 1976, Transcutaneous electrical analgesia: a follow-up analysis, *J Pain, 2*, 35–40, March.

Stravino, V D, 1970, The nature of pain, *Arch Phys Med Rehab, 51*, 37–43.

Sweet, W H, Wepsic, J G, 1974, Stimulation of pain suppressor mechanisms: a critique of some current methods, In J J Bonica, ed, Adv Neurol, *4*, 737–747.

Taub, A, Campbell, J N, 1974, Percutaneous local electrical analgesia: peripheral mechanisms, In J J Bonica, ed, Adv Neurol, *4*, 727–733.

Torebjoerk, H E, Hallin, R G, 1974, Excitation failure in thin nerve fibre structures and accompanying hypalgesia during repetitive electric skin stimulation, In J J Bonica, ed, Adv in Neurol, *4*, 733–735.

Valtonen, E J, 1971, Comparative clinical study of the effect of short wave and long wave diathermy on osteoarthritis of the knee and hip, *Scand J Rehab Med, 3*, 109–12.

Wall, P D, Sweet, W H, 1967, Temporary abolition of pain in man, *Science, 155*, 108–109.

Wall, P D, 1975, Editorial, *J Pain, 1*, 1, March.

Wall, P D, 1976, Modulation of pain by non-painful events, In J J Bonica, ed, Adv Pain Res Ther, *1*, 1–15.

Wall, P D, Sternbach, R A, 1976, The need for an animal model of chronic pain, *J Pain, 2*, 2–3, March.

Zottermann, Y, 1939, Touch, pain and tickling: an electrophysiological investigation on cutaneous sensory nerves, *J Physio, 95*, 1–28.

Index